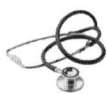

Foreword

One of the tenets of effective public health action is the need for a collaborative approach. The important health protection goal of preventing and controlling infectious diseases in the community, whether they originate from human, animal vector or environmental sources, is an excellent example of this principle.

The generic disease control task can be divided into an afferent arm, whereby the public health authority is made aware of the disease, for example through statutory notification under public health law, and an efferent arm, whereby individuals at risk of the disease (i.e. contacts) are identified, informed of their risk, provided with guidance as to the symptoms to look out for, and where possible offered protective chemoprophylaxis or immunisation. A functional afferent arm will not work without the awareness and acumen of clinical staff who must recognise and report the condition; similarly the efferent arm can only work if the public health tasks of identification and individual management of certain contacts are carried out with the assistance of informed clinical staff. A third partner in the relationship is the pathology laboratory, the support of which is required to carry out the appropriate diagnostic tests. Whilst use of empiric therapy may buy time in clinical management, prompt laboratory confirmation or exclusion of the diagnosis is called for when the public health response to the infectious disease, for example meningococcal infection, measles or tuberculosis, is necessarily complex, labour intensive and liable to engender public concern. Public health physicians and other practitioners devote energy and time to inculcating clinicians with an understanding of the public health law and their public health responsibilities.

The unique and innovative approach taken by the author is to use the case study format to show explicitly the vital roles that clinicians play in the public health response. The reader of these case studies can only conclude that a truly commensal relationship between clinical, laboratory and public health personnel is of great benefit to the infectious diseases patient and to the community from which each patient is drawn.

Professor Mark J Ferson MPH MArtTh MD FRACP FAFPHM FRIPH
Director and Medical Officer of Health
Public Health Unit
South Eastern Sydney and Illawarra Health
Sydney NSW Australia

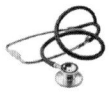

Contents

Foreword	iii
Preface	vi
About the author	vii
Acknowledgments	viii
Introduction	ix–x

Case 1	**Botulism** Peter has an abscess and neurological symptoms …	1
Case 2	**Buruli ulcer** Nelson has a leg ulcer …	15
Case 3	**Cholera** Three adults have diarrhoea …	29
Case 4	**Cryptosporidiosis and Giardiasis** An outbreak investigation …	45
Case 5	**Dengue fever** Otto has a fever …	74
Case 6	**Diphtheria** Boris has a sore throat …	92
Case 7	**Enteric fever** Morgan looks unwell …	105
Case 8	**Hepatitis A** Malini has jaundice …	130
Case 9	**Influenza** Toby's got the flu …	145
Case 10	**Invasive pneumococcal disease** Maurice is very sick …	162

CONTENTS

Case 11	**Legionnaire's disease** Chris is drowsy and has a fever …	177
Case 12	**Listeria** Ted is confused …	197
Case 13	**Measles** Jean-Luc has a rash …	210
Case 14	**Meningococcal disease** Victoria has a sore throat and a rash …	230
Case 15	**Mumps** Kevin has a stiff neck …	252
Case 16	**Pertussis** Hilary has been coughing for weeks …	267
Case 17	**Poliomyelitis** Roger feels weak …	288
Case 18	**Q fever** Ben aches and has a dry cough …	302
Case 19	**Rabies** Desta is acting strangely …	317
Case 20	**Severe Acute Respiratory Syndrome (SARS)** Tommy has a cough and shortness of breath …	334
Case 21	**Tetanus** George has a stiff jaw …	352
Case 22	**Tuberculosis** John has a headache …	364

Index ... 391

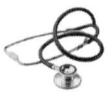

Preface

The premise for this book was to emphasise the importance of the combined roles of clinical and public health teams in managing notifiable infections. I have been fortunate enough to work in both fields (as an Epidemiology Registrar in a public health unit and an Infectious Diseases Consultant in public hospitals); therefore, it is from experience that I can confidently say that both areas represent vital cogs in the fight against infectious diseases. Unfortunately, experience has also taught me that the public health and clinical teams often don't appreciate and even become frustrated with each other while investigating a notifiable infection.

The major purpose of this book, therefore, is to demonstrate how the contribution by both clinicians and public health teams is valuable in controlling notifiable infections. I have chosen a problem-based format to provide a touch of realism to the cases. A scenario is presented with a variety of characters who tackle a notifiable infection. By the end of the chapter, the scenario has covered clinical, diagnostic, therapeutic, prognostic and public health interventions for the infection. I have drawn upon a variety of well-known notifiable infections e.g. vaccine-preventable, communicable, vector-borne, environmental, zoonotic, food-borne or emerging infectious diseases. The only lesser-known infection in this book, Buruli ulcer, was used in order to highlight this disabling and surprisingly widespread infection.

While different countries have varying approaches and resources for preventing and managing notifiable infections, I would hope that the principles presented here are generalisable to any region.

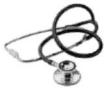

About the author

Dr Sanjaya Senanayake FRACP, MAppEpid, MBBS (Hons), BSc (Med) holds the positions of Infectious Diseases Physician and Director of Hospital in the Home at Canberra Hospital. He is a lecturer at the Australian National University Medical School and conjoint lecturer at the School of Public Health and Community Medicine, University of New South Wales. Dr Senanayake has also written *Common Clinical Cases: A guide to internship*.

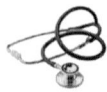

Acknowledgments

To my wife, Dilukshi—it is well known that many wives lose their husbands to golf. It is less well known that a similar phenomenon exists with writing. Thank you for being so patient, supportive and unbelievably efficient during the writing of this book.

To Saesha and Reshmi—when people talk about the joys of having children, they must have been referring to both of you. Please remember this in the future when you make unreasonable demands for mobile phones, laptops and boyfriends.

To our parents—thanks for being there: this simple phrase is economical in words yet full of meaning. Please consider this in the future when we ask you to babysit.

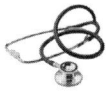

Introduction

> In the criminal justice system, the people are represented by two separate yet equally important groups: the police who investigate crime and the district attorneys who prosecute the offenders. These are their stories.
>
> *Law and Order,* Created/Produced by Dick Wolf

This is the opening line to one of my favourite TV shows, *Law and Order*. The first half of the show is about the police investigation of a crime, which results in an arrest. The second half is about the trial of the defendant and the district attorneys' quest to find him/her guilty. Both police and lawyers work closely together to get a conviction. It has often struck me how similar this is to the management of communicable diseases. With notifiable infections, it is the clinicians (e.g. infectious diseases physicians, general practitioners, microbiologists) who identify and treat the index case or cases. From that point on, their public health counterparts use a combination of outbreak investigation, education and post-exposure prophylaxis to protect the community from further infection.

I have been fortunate enough to work in both systems, namely as an epidemiologist-in-training in a public health unit and as an infectious diseases physician in a large teaching hospital. What has saddened me is that neither group always appreciates the role and expertise that the other has to offer. In fact, given the public health knowledge of some clinicians and the clinical knowledge of some public health practitioners, their combined response to an outbreak should be synergistic. It is not always so. This was one of the main reasons for writing this book.

The book consists of 22 cases and discusses 23 infections in depth. Each case is a complete interactive scenario structured and flagged to identify differential diagnosis **Dx**, investigations **Ix**, treatment **Rx**, prognosis **Px**, isolation measures **M** and public health notification and response **PH**. By the end of each scenario, clinical, laboratory and public health aspects of the infection have been addressed. Hopefully, the reader will then appreciate the teamwork required to control a communicable disease and have a better idea of the roles of clinicians and public health practitioners. Cases are used to provide a touch of realism and a certain degree of 'excitement' for the reader, thereby avoiding the didactic style of a textbook. But, despite this, each case contains thoroughly evidence-based discussions and should be regarded as a review article in itself.

The infections that I have chosen are all notifiable in many countries. They represent a mix of infections: vaccine-preventable, zoonotic, foodborne, waterborne or airborne. The only infection that may be unfamiliar to some readers is Buruli ulcer due to *Mycobacterium ulcerans*. I included this case to highlight an infection the impact (both in terms of morbidity and financial cost) and geographic range of which are grossly underestimated.

The book can be used in two ways, either read from start to finish or used as a reference whenever one of the listed infections is encountered in real-life practice.

I hope that you enjoy it.

Best wishes,
Sanjaya Senanayake

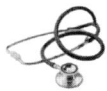

Case 1 Botulism
Peter has an abscess and neurological symptoms ...

Botulism at a glance ...

- **Agents**: family Clostridiaceae; genus *Clostridium;* species *Clostridium botulinum;* toxin is responsible for the disease; there are seven serotypes of toxin (A–G)
- **Geographical distribution**: worldwide
- **Main mode of transmission**: foodborne botulism; infant botulism and its adult equivalent, adult intestinal toxaemia botulism; wound botulism; inhalational botulism
- **Person-to-person transmission**: no (although in theory there is a low risk)
- **Animal-to-person transmission**: no
- **Incubation period**: 18–36 hours (6 hours–10 days)
- **Infectious period**: theoretically, while toxin or spores are present in wounds or faeces; however, no person-to-person transmission has been reported
- **Clinical features**: acute, symmetrical, descending flaccid paralysis
- **Identification**: toxin—mouse bioassay is the best-known test, PCR and ELISA are likely to play important roles in the future; organism—culture of wound and stool
- **Treatment**: supportive therapy, often including mechanical ventilation; human botulinum immunoglobulin (BIG) for infant botulism, if available; equine antitoxin for other forms of botulism; antibiotic therapy (usually penicillin or metronidazole)
- **Prophylaxis**: no
- **Vaccine**: no

CASE 1 BOTULISM

Main characters

Dr Mike Cotic	infectious diseases registrar
Dr Anand Gupta	emergency department resident
Mr Peter Jones	patient with an abscess and neurological symptoms
Shannon	Peter's partner
Dr Rachel Hemly	neurosurgical registrar
Mr Joseph Laber	public health unit officer

Dr Mike Cotic, an infectious diseases registrar in an inner city hospital, gets a page from the emergency department.

'Hi, it's Anand Gupta, one of the residents in emergency. We have a 30-year-old injecting drug user down here. He will be admitted under Neurology because of some blurred vision and upper limb weakness—they are going to see him soon—but an incidental finding is an abscess on his left forearm. He admits to having injected there a few days ago. We would really appreciate some antibiotic advice.'

Mike goes to see the patient. His name is Mr Peter Jones and he is accompanied by his partner, Shannon. He is worried about the abscess but more concerned about his neurological symptoms. Three days ago, he developed blurred vision. Half a day later, he had difficulty talking and yesterday his voice sounded different. Today, his shoulders seem weak.

He injected heroin into his forearm one week ago. The pain and swelling started 48 hours later, two days before the onset of the blurred vision.

On examination, Peter has a fever of 38.5° C. He has a normal heart rate and blood pressure. He is oriented and appropriate in his responses.

Mike elicits the following signs: diplopia with probable left VI and right III cranial nerve palsies, dysarthria secondary to a bulbar palsy, dysphonia and 4/5 weakness of shoulder abduction. The remainder of the cranial nerve and limb examinations are unremarkable.

There is a fluctuant, tender swelling on the left forearm associated with some secondary cellulitis.

Dr Rachel Hemly, the neurology registrar, arrives. Mike tells her, 'I think he may have botulism.'

What is botulism?

Botulism is a disease caused by toxins, usually produced by *Clostridium botulinum*, an anaerobic, spore-forming, Gram positive bacillus. Cases of botulism due to other toxin-producing clostridial species (e.g. *C. butyricum* and *baratii*) have also been reported (Sobel et al., 2004).

The clinical picture is of an afebrile, mentally alert patient with a descending, symmetric, flaccid motor paralysis. The sensory system is unaffected. The cranial nerves are invariably involved first, leading to diplopia, dysphagia, dysphonia, dysarthria (think of the four D's), ptosis and blurred vision. The pupils may be enlarged and sluggishly reactive to light. Descending motor paralysis follows with the risk of respiratory failure (Goonetilleke and Harris, 2004). The clinical picture is similar regardless of the route of exposure to botulinum toxin.

The symptoms are caused by the toxin binding to presynaptic nerve terminals at the neuromuscular junction and at cholinergic autonomic sites. This prevents presynaptic release of acetylcholine, blocking neurotransmission and resulting in the clinical syndrome.

> Rachel says, 'Botulism should not be associated with a fever. How do you explain that?'

Differential diagnoses

Patients with botulism should have no fever. However, this patient also has an abscess on his forearm, which could easily generate a fever, so botulism is still a possibility.

There is a long list of differential diagnoses for botulism (Sobel 2005, Goonetilleke and Harris 2004, Cox and Hinkle 2002), including:

- Guillain-Barré syndrome (GBS)
- Miller-Fisher variant of GBS
- tick paralysis
- diphtheria
- myasthenia gravis
- Eaton-Lambert syndrome
- poliomyelitis
- porphyria
- meningitis/encephalitis
- hypothyroidism
- magnesium toxicity
- organophosphates
- shellfish poisoning
- heavy metals
- carbon monoxide poisoning

> Rachel asks, 'If this is botulism, do you think that the abscess could be involved, or is it an incidental finding?'

C. botulinum is an environmental organism, so wound contamination can occur. Wound botulism is the term for botulism secondary to spores contaminating a wound and was first described in 1951. A recent epidemic of wound botulism occurred in injecting drug users in the US who engaged in 'skin popping' (injecting the drug subcutaneously when the user can't find any veins). Abscess formation in necrotic subcutaneous tissue provides the ideal anaerobic environment for spores to germinate and produce toxin (Werner et al., 2000).

Nevertheless, botulism can have a number of distinct epidemiologies, which should be considered at this point (Sobel, 2005):

Wound botulism discussed above.
Foodborne botulism from ingestion of pre-formed botulinum toxin from contaminated foods.
Infant botulism from infection with *C. botulinum* spores of the intestine of babies under 12 months old. The spores germinate and produce a toxin which is absorbed systemically, leading to botulism.
Adult intestinal toxaemia botulism an adult form of IB. Most adults are resistant to this type of botulism because the adult intestinal flora will not allow colonisation and infection by *C. botulinum* spores. However, it can occur in adults with altered bowel flora (e.g. due to antibiotic use or a functional or anatomical bowel abnormality).
Inhalational botulism from inhalation of the toxin, a possible bioweapon.

The neurological syndrome is similar regardless of the aetiology. However, infant botulism can be difficult to recognise because the history and examination of an infant is not as straightforward as that of an adult. It usually presents as constipation, followed by loss of head control, poor sucking, pooling of secretions or milk in the mouth and lethargy. Infants can also have a neurogenic bladder and be hypotensive early on (Cox and Hinkle, 2002).

Peter confirms that he tried to inject the heroin into a small vein but thinks he failed to do so. Most of the heroin was probably injected subcutaneously.

'Are you sure that this couldn't be foodborne botulism?' says Rachel.

In an adult with botulism, foodborne and wound botulism are the two most likely sources. Inhalational botulism is extremely unlikely outside the setting of a bioterrorist attack or laboratory accident. In the absence of antibiotic use or a bowel abnormality, adult intestinal toxaemia botulism is also unlikely.

Foodborne botulism occurs with the ingestion of preformed toxin in food. The ideal conditions for toxin production and proliferation are an anaerobic environment low in salt, acid and sugar. Fermented and canned foods provide such an environment, and modern industrial canning techniques were developed to address this risk (Sobel, 2005). While this has reduced cases associated with commercial canned foods, home-canned foods are still the major source of foodborne botulism in the US. In the Republic of Georgia, which has one of the highest rates of foodborne botulism in the world, home-preserved vegetables were recently implicated as the major source (Varma et al., 2004). Non-conserved foods (e.g. potato salad, apple pie) and restaurants can also be a source of disease (Sobel et al., 2004).

If Peter does have botulism, Mike should take a thorough history to cover the possible epidemiologies.

On further questioning, Peter reports that four days ago he ate some preserved peaches that his mother had made months ago. Shannon says she ate some too, although much less. Peter denies being on prolonged antibiotic therapy or having a history of bowel problems.

Shannon says, 'I ate the peaches too. Why aren't I sick?'

Although the incubation period of foodborne botulism is usually 18–36 hours, it can range from six hours to 10 days. One factor determining the incubation period is the dose of toxin ingested. Since Shannon ate much less than Peter, it is plausible that her disease may have a longer incubation period, which is why she still is asymptomatic.

Peter asks, 'Shouldn't I have had diarrhoea and vomiting if this was food poisoning?'

Patients with foodborne botulism can experience a gastrointestinal prodrome of diarrhoea or constipation, vomiting and abdominal pain before the onset of the neurological symptoms but this occurs in only 50% of cases (Goonetilleke and Harris, 2004).

Anand asks, 'What tests should I order to confirm botulism and exclude other conditions?'

Investigations

Several investigations are available:

Test serum for the toxin (mouse bioassay)   Serum from the patient is injected intraperitoneally into two groups of mice, one exposed to antitoxin and one not. The test is diagnostic if the unexposed mice develop botulism within 48 hours of inoculation (Goonetilleke and Harris, 2004). This is the most reliable test for isolating toxin. The limiting factor is that very few laboratories are able to perform this test.
Test stool for the toxin and culture it for the organism
Culture the abscess for the organism and examine for toxin
Test the preserved food for the toxin and organism   This should be organised by a public health unit.
Perform electromyography   Botulism can produce a diagnostic triad of EMG changes (originally described by Gutierrez et al., 1994, for infant botulism) consisting of decreased compound muscle action potentials (CMAPs) in at least two muscle groups; tetanic or post-tetanic facilitation (as defined by CMAP amplitudes over 120% of baseline); and prolonged post-tetanic facilitation for >120 seconds without post-tetanic exhaustion. However, these changes may not be present early in the course of the illness, so a negative result does not necessarily exclude the diagnosis but calls for a repeat test in 7–10 days.
Perform a lumbar puncture (LP)   With botulism, the cerebrospinal fluid (CSF) should be normal, unlike many of the conditions that make up the differential diagnoses (e.g. GBS).

Other tests for identifying toxin—such as polymerase chain reaction (PCR) (Akbulut et al., 2005) and enzyme-linked immunosorbent (ELISA) assays—are constantly being improved and likely to play important diagnostic roles in the near future.

Four hours later, Peter has been admitted to the ward and undergone EMG studies and a LP. The EMG shows the triad of changes consistent with botulism; the CSF is normal.

Rachel asks, 'I'm satisfied that this man has botulism. From the infectious diseases viewpoint, should we wait for the toxin and culture results before commencing treatment?'

Treatment

If there is a strong clinical suspicion of botulism, treatment should be commenced promptly. The problem with the toxin and culture assays is that they have a poor sensitivity (33–44%), which decreases with time (Sobel, 2005). In addition, it will take days to get a result, by which time the patient may have progressed to respiratory paralysis and failure.

At this point, Shannon complains that in the last two hours she has been developing blurred vision. On examination, she has ptosis and diplopia—it is likely that she has botulism too.

Rachel asks Mike how to treat the two patients.

The principles of therapy for botulism are:

Admit the patient to an intensive care unit and monitor their vital capacity; deterioration necessitates prompt mechanical ventilation.

Administer botulinum antitoxin As with diphtheria antitoxin, botulinum antitoxin is derived from horse serum, so there is a risk of hypersensitivity. For this reason, skin testing for hypersensitivity should be performed prior to parenteral administration of the antitoxin.

Administer antibiotics, usually penicillin or metronidazole.

For foodborne botulism, consider enemas, gastric lavage and induced emesis if the contaminated food is likely to still be in the gastrointestinal tract.

For wound botulism, debride the abscess This is essential. Nevertheless, botulinum antitoxin should be administered prior to surgery to neutralise any toxin released into the circulation from the operation (Werner et al., 2000).

> Rachel asks, 'Is there any evidence that antibiotics and antitoxin work, or is this all just anecdotal?'

Tacket et al. (1984) report that patients with foodborne botulism who receive antitoxin have a lower fatality rate and a shorter course than those who do not. Those who receive it in the first 24 hours after onset have a shorter course but a similar fatality rate to those who receive antitoxin after 24 hours. It therefore appears that trivalent antitoxin has a beneficial effect on survival and shortens the clinical course of foodborne botulism.

Goonetilleke and Harris (2004) note that the use of antibiotics has not been proven in trials, but the reduction in toxin-producing bacteria probably has some beneficial effect.

> Rachel asks, 'Why bother giving equine antitoxin with its risk of hypersensitivity? I know that a human botulinum immunoglobulin is available. Why not use that?'

A human botulinum immunoglobulin (BIG) has been developed. However, it is not widely available, and the few countries that stock BIG use it for only inhalational botulism—where it has been shown to reduce hospital stay, tube feeding and the need for ventilatory assistance (Cox and Hinkle, 2002)—not foodborne or wound botulism.

> Mike prescribes intravenous penicillin. Rachel asks, 'Will the penicillin be enough to treat the abscess in his arm?'

Abscesses secondary to infected injection sites are likely to be polymicrobial. Mike therefore needs to prescribe an empiric antibiotic regimen with broader cover to address aerobic Gram positive and Gram negative bacteria as well as anaerobes.

Rachel suggests adding ticarcillin/clavulanic acid and gentamicin.

Such a combination will provide the broad antibacterial cover that is required, including *C. botulinum* cover. However, aminoglycosides (gentamicin, tobramycin, amikacin, streptomycin) may potentiate neuromuscular weakness in botulism and should be avoided (Santos et al., 1981). A fluoroquinolone (e.g. ciprofloxacin) could be substituted for gentamicin.

A nurse asks Mike, 'How bad is the outlook?'

Prognosis

The overall mortality for botulism is 10%. It is much lower for inhalational botulism.

The nurse asks, 'Does the patient need any isolation measures?'

Isolation measures

Theoretically, transmission of toxin or spores from faeces or a wound to healthcare workers can occur through broken skin, mucosal surfaces and the eye. However, the risk is low and no cases of person-to-person transmission of botulism have ever been documented (Sobel, 2005). Nevertheless, it would be reasonable to isolate the patient and use standard enteric precautions such as gloving and gowning when entering the room and, of course, good hand washing.

'Does the public health unit need to know about this?' the nurse unit manager wants to know.

Public health notification and response

In most parts of the world, botulism is a notifiable disease because of the public health implications of contaminated food or a bioterrorist attack.

CASE 1 BOTULISM

Mike speaks to Mr Joseph Laber, an officer in the local public health unit. He explains that his two patients may have foodborne botulism. In turn, Joseph speaks to one of his food inspectors to arrange a visit to the patients' home that day to collect food samples. They collect a number of food samples, including the preserved peaches, and send it to their environmental laboratory for *C. botulinum* and toxin testing.

It is now four days since admission. Peter has developed respiratory failure and is now mechanically ventilated. Shannon, who received treatment within 24 hours of the onset of symptoms, is improving rapidly. The reference laboratory confirms that botulinum toxin A was isolated from her serum. Neither toxin or *C. botulinum* was cultured from Peter's wound.

Joseph calls Mike to confirm that toxin A was also identified from the preserved peaches: it is definitely a case of foodborne botulism due to toxin A. 'Is this a common cause of botulism?' Mike asks.

There are seven botulinum toxins, conveniently designated A–G. They are 150 kDa molecules consisting of a light and a heavy chain linked by a disulfide bond. Only four are usually associated with human disease: A, B, E and F. Toxin A causes most cases while F is a rare cause. Toxin A is also the most toxic of the serotypes with a LD_{50} (the amount of toxin that will kill 50% of its victims) of 0.001 μg/kg parenterally and an estimated LD_{50} 0.003–0.07 μg/kg inhalationally (Madsen, 2001). The equine trivalent antitoxin is active against toxins A, B and E.

'I knew that botulinum toxin was dangerous, but I didn't realise it was that strong. How does it compare to toxins like sarin and nerve agent VX?'

Botulinum toxin is the most lethal compound known. It is 15 000 times more toxic than nerve agent VX and 100 000 times more toxic than sarin (Franz et al., 2001).

'Wow. So that's why it has been considered as a bioweapon?'

Although foodborne botulism could be a bioweapon, much of the focus has been on using the aerosolised toxin to cause inhalational botulism. Botulinum toxin is readily aerosolisable (although secondary aerosolisation is insignificant) and it can persist for weeks in non-moving water and in food. Although very dangerous in the aerosolised form (it would take only 8 kg of aerosolised toxin to kill half the exposed people in a 100 km^2 area), it is 20–80 times less toxic compared to the other routes of infection (Franz et al., 2001; Madsen, 2001).

> 'Have there been any cases of inhalational botulism?'

Very few—to our knowledge at least! The best known episode was in three workers in a German laboratory. The neurological syndrome was similar to other routes; however it was preceded by descriptions of a 'mucous plug in the throat', 'the beginning of cold without fever' and later on 'mental numbness'. It is thought that the incubation period of inhalational botulism is 1–5 days (Madsen, 2001).

> A few days later, Joseph receives a call. It is a relative of Shannon's. She has heard about the botulism.
> 'Oh Doctor, this botulism thing sounds so terrible. I was going to eat some preserved sausage but now I'm a bit worried. Can I get botulism from sausages?'

Any improperly canned or preserved food can become contaminated with the toxin, including sausage. In fact, the term botulism is derived from the Latin word for sausage (botulus). This is because the original outbreaks of botulism in Europe were due to contaminated sausage.

> 'How do you kill it, Doctor?'

The toxin can be inactivated by heating to 85°C for at least five minutes; *C. botulinum* spores are destroyed by heating to 121°C under pressure of 15–20 lb/in^2 for at least 20 minutes (Sobel et al., 2004).

> 'Doctor, is botulism like measles in that Shannon and Mike can never get it again?'

Infection is not an immunising process and individuals can develop further episodes (Werner et al., 2000). Currently no vaccine is commercially available, although research is underway (Shukla and Sharma, 2005).

> 'One final thing, Doctor. I have this "friend" who is going to see a cosmetic surgeon to fix some wrinkles. He might give me, I mean my friend, Botox. Is Botox the same thing as this disease?'

Botox™ is botulinum toxin A, the most powerful toxin known. The paralysing effect of the toxin serves a number of medical purposes including the treatment of blepharospasm, dystonias, hypersalivation, sweating, anal fissures and rectal spasms. Its effect on facial wrinkles was an incidental finding during testing for its impact on blepharospasm. The new area of promise for botulinum toxin is in the treatment of pain syndromes; researchers incidentally found that migraine sufferers treated with botulinum toxin for facial wrinkles noted a reduction in the frequency of their headaches (Montecucco and Molgó, 2005).

One problem with toxin use for therapeutic purposes is that it requires several treatments. This can lead to the development of secondary antibodies that neutralise the toxin and render it ineffective (Bakheit et al., 1997).

> 'But Doctor, will my friend get botulism from Botox?'

One reason for the success of botulinum toxin for medical and aesthetic purposes is that its paralysing effect does not spread far from the site of injection. Also, the dose of toxin used for cosmetic effects is generally too small to cause botulism. However, botulism-like symptoms have been reported in people receiving higher doses of toxin for the treatment of muscular disorders (Bakheit et al., 1997; Sobel 2005).

> Two weeks later, Joseph receives another call about botulism. It is the mother of a 10-month-old baby who wants to give the infant some honey but did an internet search and read that it can cause botulism. 'Is this true?' she wants to know.

Chin et al. (1979) examined over 500 food samples to identify vehicles of *C. botulinum* carriage in cases of infant botulism. Honey, soil and one isolate from vacuum cleaner dust were the only sources identified. In the US, 20–35% of cases of infant botulism are from ingesting honey. For this reason, many health authorities recommend that infants under 12 months should not consume honey. It is thought that infants under 12 months are susceptible to colonisation by *C. botulinum* because of their immature bowel flora.

Spika et al. (1989) studied the risk factors for inhalational botulism and identified the following:

- for infants <2 months old: living in a rural area or on a farm
- for infants ≥2 months old: breastfeeding, less than one bowel movement per day for at least two months, or the ingestion of corn syrup

References

Akbulut, D., Grant, K.A., McLauchlin, J. (2005) Improvement in laboratory diagnosis of wound botulism and tetanus among injecting illicit-drug users by use of real-time PCR assays for neurotoxin gene fragments. *Journal of Clinical Microbiology* 43(9), 4342–48.

Bakheit, A.M., Ward, C.D., McLellan, D.L. (1997) Generalized botulism-like syndrome after intramuscular injections of botulinum toxin type A: a report of two cases. *Journal of Neurology, Neurosurgery and Psychiatry* 62(2), 198.

Chin, J., Arnon, S.S., Midura T.F. (1979) Food and environmental aspects of infant botulism in California. *Reviews of Infectious Diseases* 1(4), 693–97.

Cox, N., Hinkle, R. (2002) Infant botulism. *American Family Physician* 65(7), 1388–92.

Dressler, D. (2004) Clinical presentation and management of antibody-induced failure of botulinum toxin therapy. *Movement Disorders* 19(Suppl 8), S92–100.

Franz, D.R., Jahrling, P.B., McClain, D.J. et al. (2001) Clinical recognition and management of patients exposed to biological warfare agents. *Clinics in Laboratory Medicine* 21(3), 435–73.

Goonetilleke, A., Harris, J.B. (2004) Clostridial neurotoxins. *Journal of Neurology, Neurosurgery and Psychiatry* 75(Suppl 3), iii35–39.

Gutierrez, A.R., Bodensteiner, J., Gutmann, L. (1994) Electrodiagnosis of infantile botulism. *Journal of Child Neurology* 9(4), 362–65.

Madsen, J.M. (2001) Toxins as weapons of mass destruction. *Clinics in Laboratory Medicine* 21(3), 593–605.

Montecucco, C., Molgó, J. (2005) Botulinal neurotoxins: revival of an old killer. *Current Opinion in Pharmacology* 5(3), 274–79.

Santos, J.I., Swensen, P., Glasgow, L.A. (1981) Potentiation of *Clostridium botulinum* toxin aminoglycoside antibiotics: clinical and laboratory observations. *Pediatrics* 68(1), 50–54.

Shukla, H.D., Sharma, S.K. (2005) *Clostridium botulinum*: a bug with beauty and weapon. *Critical Reviews in Microbiology* 31(1), 11–18.

Sobel, J. (2005) Botulism. *Clinical Infectious Diseases* 41(8), 1167–73.

Sobel, J., Tucker, N., Sulka, A. et al. (2004) Foodborne botulism in the United States, 1990-2000. *Emerging Infectious Diseases* 10(9), 1606–11.

Spika, J.S., Shaffer, N., Hargrett-Bean, N. et al. (1989) Risk factors for infant botulism in the United States. *American Journal of Diseases of Children* 143(7), 828–32.

Tacket, C.O., Shandera, W.X., Mann, J.M. et al. (1984) Equine antitoxin use and other factors that predict outcome in type A foodborne botulism. *American Journal of Medicine* 76(5), 794–98.

Varma, J.K., Katsitadze, G., Moiscrafishvili, M. et al. (2004) Foodborne botulism in the Republic of Georgia. *Emerging Infectious Diseases* 10(9), 1601–05.

Werner, S.B., Passaro, D., McGee, J. et al. (2000) Wound botulism in California, 1951–1998: recent epidemic in heroin injectors. *Clinical Infectious Diseases* 31(4), 1018–24.

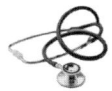

Case 2 Buruli ulcer
Nelson has a leg ulcer …

Buruli ulcer at a glance …

- **Agent**: family Mycobacteriaceae; genus *Mycobacterium*; species *Mycobacterium ulcerans*
- **Geographical distribution**: worldwide
- **Main mode of transmission**: cutaneous
- **Person-to-person transmission**: no
- **Animal-to-person transmission**: theoretically, aquatic insects and mosquitoes could transmit it to humans
- **Incubation period**: 6–12 weeks (1 week to >1 year)
- **Clinical features**: indolent ulcer starting as a painless papule or nodule; a rapidly oedematous form also exists
- **Identification**: organisms in cutaneous lesions through polymerase chain reaction (PCR), culture, direct smear or histology
- **Treatment**: guidelines are evolving; a combination of surgery and adjuvant antibiotic therapy is likely to be best
- **Prophylaxis**: avoid direct skin contact with contaminated water (e.g., by wearing shirts and long trousers in the water)
- **Vaccine**: research continues; there may be some cross-immunity with BCG vaccine

CASE 2 BURULI ULCER

Main characters

Dr Dilukshi Mendez infectious diseases physician
Dr Saesha Wall infectious diseases intern
Mr Nelson Baye young man with a leg ulcer
Dr Gretel Schmidt plastic surgeon
Dr Venura Alba public health physician

Dr Dilukshi Mendez is an infectious diseases physician conducting her weekly outpatient clinic. Dr Saesha Wall, her intern, is sitting in with her. Dilukshi's final patient of the day is a young man, Mr Nelson Baye. The referral from the GP is as follows:

Dear Dr Mendez,
Thank you for seeing 19-year-old Nelson with an ulcer on his right leg. It began as a tiny lump two months ago, three days after pricking his leg at home with glass from a broken jam jar. About four weeks later it began to ulcerate. The ulcer has continued to grow and there is a lot of surrounding erythema. He is an otherwise healthy astronomy student.
A swab of the ulcer last week was reported as showing a light growth of skin commensals.
I commenced him on cephalexin and metronidazole when I first saw him two weeks ago but it hasn't halted the progress. I am grateful for your advice on diagnosis and management.
Yours sincerely,
Dr Reshmi Kuku

Nelson adds that he has never left his home city, apart from a one-week university trip to Malaysia three months prior to the appearance of the nodule. He has no pets, hasn't been sexually active and has not experimented with injecting drugs. Despite the presence of the ulcer, he has felt systemically well. He can't recall any trauma or bites preceding the onset of the papule.

But even an experienced clinician such as Dilukshi is astonished when she sees the ulcer: it is $15 \times 10 \times 1$ cm with a sloughy base; the edge can be undermined easily with a probe; and there is a large area of surrounding erythema and heat. Although it is extensive, the ulcer is barely painful or tender. There is no associated lymphadenopathy. The remainder of the physical examination is normal.

> 'Doctor, what kind of infection could do this?' asks Nelson.
> 'It looks like Buruli ulcer,' Dilukshi says.

What is Buruli ulcer?

The clinical features—a nodule that subsequently ulcerates, undermined edges, minimal pain and no systemic inflammatory response—is consistent with a Buruli ulcer. It is likely that the light growth of skin commensals from the swab represents colonisation or secondary infection, rather than being the primary cause of the ulcer.

Instead of a nodule, Buruli ulcer can also present as a firm plaque or an aggressive oedematous area (usually but not always on a limb) that forms a large ulcer (Wansbrough-Jones and Phillips, 2006).

> 'What's a Buruli?' asks Nelson.

Buruli is the name of a district in Uganda where a number of cases were seen in the 1960s. The disease is also known as the Bairnsdale ulcer or Daintree ulcer, again in recognition of regions (this time in Australia) in which the disease is found.

It is caused by *Mycobacterium ulcerans*, a non-tuberculous mycobacterium. Although the disease was first described in Uganda in 1897, it was only in 1948 in Australia that the organism responsible for the disease was first isolated (Asiedu and Wansbrough-Jones, 2007).

> Saesha listens with interest. 'I have heard of Buruli ulcer but I thought it only occurred in one or two countries and is quite rare. Am I right?'

Buruli ulcer is found in over 30 countries, with African nations having the highest burden of disease. European countries appear to be free of it. It is not rare. For example, the point prevalence in some endemic regions in Ghana is 150.8/100 000 and detection rates in part of Benin are higher than for tuberculosis or leprosy (Johnson et al., 2005a).

> In Nelson's country, Buruli ulcer has been found only sporadically and in a distant region. To Dilukshi's knowledge, Buruli ulcer has

never been detected anywhere near their city. Nelson is also adamant that he hasn't travelled outside of the city, except to go to Malaysia. If this turns out to be Buruli ulcer, he may be the first locally-acquired case.

Saesha is still not happy. 'But I thought that only children developed Buruli ulcer?'

Buruli ulcer is potentially a disease of any age but there are peak ages which vary according to region. In Africa, the majority of cases occur in children aged 5–15 years; in Australia, the disease tends to affect adults, including the elderly (Asiedu and Wansbrough-Jones, 2007).

Saesha is excited at the prospect of possibly seeing the first local case of Buruli ulcer. But she wants to exclude some other possibilities first. 'Could Nelson have contracted this during the Malaysian trip? But that was three months before he noticed the lump on his leg—so that's too long isn't it?'

Differential diagnoses

Malaysia has had cases of Buruli ulcer and the incubation period can be many months (Veitch et al., 1997), so it is a possibility. However, Nelson's activities were limited to travel between the university and his hotel. He did not engage in any outdoor activities, making his risk low.

Chronic ulcers have many causes, infective and non-infective.

The infective differential diagnoses that need to be considered include: tuberculosis (scrofuloderma), non-tuberculous mycobacteria (e.g. *M. abscessus*), cutaneous diphtheria, cancrum oris (although this is usually only found in the face), nocardiosis, fungal infections, tropical phagedaenic ulcer, yaws, cutaneous leishmaniasis and onchocerciasis (Asiedu et al., 2000), so a clinical diagnosis of Buruli ulcer should be confirmed microbiologically.

Saesha asks Dilukshi, 'Shall I get a punch biopsy of the ulcer?'

Investigations

Portaels et al. (2001) do not recommend punch biopsies because they may exacerbate the disease, or lead to secondary infection, and they are often non-diagnostic. Multiple swabs should be taken from the undermined edge of the ulcer and not from the sloughy centre. If the swab is going straight to the laboratory without a long delay, dry swabs are fine. Surgical specimens are also useful and should ideally be full thickness with subcutaneous tissue.

Dilukshi takes a number of dry swabs from the undermined edge of the ulcer.

'What tests should we request on the pathology form, especially for *M. ulcerans*?' Saesha asks.

The microbiological tests for Buruli ulcer and their advantages and disadvantages are outlined in Table 2.1.

Table 2.1 Advantages and disadvantages of tests for *M. ulcerans* from a swab from the ulcer edge

Test	Advantages	Disadvantages
Smear (Ziehl-Neelsen stain)	Quick Good specificity[†]	Poor sensitivity (<50%)
Histology	Good sensitivity	Limited availability in poorly-resourced settings
Polymerase chain reaction (using IS2404 sequence)	Quick Sensitivity and specificity close to 100%	Limited availability in poorly-resourced settings
Culture	Good specificity[†]	Slow (up to six weeks as with tuberculosis) Low sensitivity (60%)

[†]'Good specificity' is used in the context of clinical settings where Buruli ulcer is the likely diagnosis.
SOURCE Johnson et al., 2007; Portaels et al., 1997; Wansbrough-Jones and Phillips, 2006

CASE 2   BURULI ULCER

Osteomyelitis can complicate this infection, either locally or sometimes at distant sites—one study found a rate of osteomyelitis of almost 15% (Noeske et al., 2004)—so a plain X-ray of the affected leg should be ordered.

Also, blood tests, such as C-reactive protein, erythrocyte sedimentation rate (ESR), full blood count, electrolytes, urea, creatinine and liver function tests would provide a useful baseline prior to initiating treatment.

Nelson leaves the clinic, with follow-up planned for one week. Dilukshi has decided to hold off empiric antimicrobial therapy, pending the swab results. The following day, the laboratory reports that no acid-fast bacilli were seen using the Ziehl-Neelsen stain. The blood tests return with the only abnormalities being an elevated C-reactive protein and ESR. The X-ray of the leg is free of osteomyelitis.

However, three days later, Dilukshi receives an email from the mycobacterial reference laboratory: the polymerase chain reaction (PCR) from the swab for *M. ulcerans* is positive. Nelson does have a Buruli ulcer! The laboratory will be able to run further tests to confirm whether it is a Malaysian or a local strain but this may take another few weeks.

Saesha asks, 'Do we need to treat him? I thought that most ulcers would eventually resolve spontaneously.'

Treatment

One study found that one-third of early nodular lesions healed spontaneously. However, this was an incidental finding and not the basis for management recommendations (Revill et al., 1973). Additionally, Nelson's ulcer is large. The optimal management of Buruli ulcer is unclear but probably involves a combination of antibiotics and surgery.

Surgery with wide margins is the mainstay of therapy but access to surgeons is a problem in some countries (Wansbrough-Jones and Phillips, 2006) and the relapse rate is 18–47% (Teelken et al., 2003), possibly due to inadvertent incomplete excision. A PCR study discovered the organism in 3 cm excised margins of seemingly healthy tissue (Rondini et al., 2003). Surgery alone seems most successful in early nodular disease with lesions <5 cm diameter (Wansbrough-Jones and Phillips, 2006).

Recent studies have demonstrated that combinations of antimicrobial therapy, usually in concert with surgery, are an effective means of curing the disease. Successful combinations include rifampicin and amikacin (Marsollier et al., 2003) or rifampicin and streptomycin (Etuaful et al., 2005). However, the former was a study in mice and the latter used human subjects with early non-ulcerated lesions. A prospective study did find that the rifampicin/streptomycin combination healed a number of ulcers after eight weeks of treatment (Chauty, 2005). Clarithromycin and quinolones (e.g. ciprofloxacin) have also been shown to have in vitro activity and may be used with the amikacin/rifampicin or streptomycin/rifampicin combinations (Portaels et al., 1998; Thangaraj et al., 2000). The advantage of using quinolones and macrolides is that they can be administered orally.

Australian guidelines recommend surgery or combined surgery and antibiotics (Johnson et al., 2007) because surgery is readily accessible and the disease tends to affect older patients, for whom parenteral aminoglycosides (amikacin, streptomycin) may be more toxic.

'I've heard that heat therapy can be used too,' Saesha says.

A number of conservative measures have been explored in the treatment of Buruli ulcer; however, they should not be used alone as primary treatment ahead of surgery and/or antibiotic therapy.
They include:

Heat therapy *M. ulcerans* grows optimally at a temperature of 29–33°C, so applying a heating device over the ulcer would inhibit growth. Devices are available commercially.
Hyperbaric oxygen
Topical phenytoin This anticonvulsant has a regenerative effect on surgical wounds and ulcers (this property causes its side effect of gingival hyperplasia) (Bhatia and Prakash, 2004). A recent randomised controlled trial suggested a benefit of topical phenytoin over normal saline dressings, especially for patients <30 years old, lesions where the slough has been debrided, ulcers <30 cm in average circumference and ulcers <1 year old (Klutse et al., 2003).

Dilukshi decides to treat Nelson with the following regimen: IV amikacin (eight weeks) with oral rifampicin and ciprofloxacin

(12 weeks). She also asks the plastic surgical team to review him with a view to debridement and skin grafting in the future.
The plastic surgeon, Dr Gretel Schmidt, looks at the ulcer. 'Are you sure that this is an infection? If you asks me, all the necrosis and underlying erythema reminds me of an envenomation.'

Buruli ulcer does give the appearance of envenomation, such as from a spider bite. Histologically, there are areas of necrosis away from the clumps of mycobacteria and scientists have postulated this is due to a toxin. Subsequently, it was discovered that *M. ulcerans* produces a polyketide toxin, known as mycolactone, which is likely to be an important virulence factor for the organism (George et al., 1999).

The mycolactone expressed by *M. ulcerans* in Australia is different to that found in Africa and this may explain a possible difference in clinical presentation between the two regions, with more Australian cases seemingly presenting with more papules (Asiedu and Wansbrough-Jones, 2007).

Prognosis

Treatment of this infection involves tremendous amounts of patience on the part of both healthcare workers and patients because the condition waxes and wanes. There may need to be a number of surgical debridements before a skin graft is considered; there may be side effects from the antimicrobials; and it will be months before a cure. As well as the psychological impact of the infection, there is also an economic impact. Drummond and Butler (2005) examined the costs of treating Buruli ulcer in Australia. They found that, on average, treatment of a single case cost $AUS14 000 and severe cases cost up to $28 000.

Over the next four months, Nelson undergoes three surgical debridements followed by a skin graft. He develops nausea and lethargy but is able to tolerate the 12 weeks of antibiotics. Two weeks after completing the antibiotic course, the skin graft has taken nicely and his inflammatory markers in the blood are back to normal.

Nelson is delighted and asks, 'Doctor, am I cured?'

Recurrence is well recognised but rates vary in different studies from 6.1% to over 50%. Recurrence usually occurs at the site of the original infection. However, when the primary infection involves bone there is likely to have been spread to multiple sites, so recurrence can occur at a different site. For this reason, it is recommended that all patients with Buruli ulcer be followed up for >1 year (Debacker et al., 2005).

> 'Doctor, did the molecular tests tell you if I got this infection from here or Malaysia?'
> Dilukshi tells Nelson that the molecular testing confirms that Nelson had a local strain of *M. ulcerans*, not a Malaysian strain, the first recorded case.
> 'Well then, how did I get it?'
> Dilukshi tells him that she doesn't know but will attempt to find out. She and Saesha meet with Dr Venura Alba, director of the local public health unit.
> Saesha asks, 'Is it really such a mystery? Nelson told us that he cut his leg with glass while cleaning up a broken jam jar in the kitchen. Three days later, the leg became inflamed. Clearly, the jam was contaminated with *M. ulcerans* which inoculated him when he cut himself with the glass.'

It is hard to ignore the temporal relationship between the glass cut and the onset of infection soon after. Because the epidemiology and mode of transmission of Buruli ulcer are not fully understood, it has been difficult to estimate an accurate incubation period. Nevertheless, both human and animal data suggest that the incubation period is usually between six and 12 weeks, possibly depending on variables such as the infective dose and BCG vaccination status. In animal experiments, differences in these variables led to incubation periods ranging from as little as one week to well over a year (Radford, 1975). Also, glass from a jam jar is an unlikely source of *M. ulcerans*.

Epidemiologic evidence links *M. ulcerans* to marshes, wetlands and stagnant bodies of water. PCR testing of water during an outbreak confirms this (Ross et al., 1997).

> Saesha looks disappointed. 'So do you think that the onset of symptoms soon after the glass cut was purely coincidental?'

There is anecdotal evidence linking trauma to the onset of symptomatic disease. It may be that the individual's skin is already colonised with the organism and trauma allows it to enter subcutaneously and rapidly cause symptomatic disease. Or it may be that the organism is already present subcutaneously in a latent state and that trauma somehow activates the disease process (Debacker et al., 2003): it may well be that Nelson became infected weeks or months ago and that the cut somehow triggered activity.

> Venura calls Nelson to ask about water contact. Nelson lives in a new housing estate where a small lake was built using the run-off from a nearby creek. He had been fly fishing there on and off for six months prior to his illness. This involved his wading in shorts up to his knees in water. Apart from this, he denies any other water contact.
>
> Venura is intrigued and wants to identify more cases. He faxes and emails GPs, surgeons and infectious diseases physicians in the area, informing them that there has been a local case of *M. ulcerans*. The letter educates them about Buruli ulcer and asks them to consider *M. ulcerans* when assessing patients with nodules, plaques or ulcers.
>
> Over the next three months, Venura is contacted about two new cases of *M. ulcerans*. Both individuals also had contact with the lake, swimming there regularly. Venura hypothesises that the lake at the housing estate is the source of infection.
>
> Venura has epidemiologic evidence linking the cases of Buruli ulcer to this lake. Next, he and an environmental health officer collect water samples to send to the mycobacterial reference laboratory. Three days later, they are excited to hear that the *M. ulcerans* was detected through PCR.
>
> 'How can we use this information to prevent more cases?' the officer asks.

Public health notification and response

If the source of this outbreak is the pond, avoiding direct skin contact with the water altogether may prevent a large number of cases. For people going fishing in the pond, studies have shown that wearing long trousers and shirts is protective (Marston et al., 1995; Raghunathan et al., 2005).

Venura updates Dilukshi. She asks, 'So avoiding contact with the pond water will definitely prevent any future cases?'

In Benin, it was shown that Buruli ulcer occurred in people living kilometres away from the water source, although the prevalence of disease was inversely proportional to distance (Johnson et al., 2005b). This may be due to bites from aquatic insects. Marsollier et al. (2002) were able to demonstrate transmission of *M. ulcerans* from aquatic insects to experimental mice. Mosquitoes in Australia have been identified as carrying *M. ulcerans* and therefore might be another potential vector of infection (Fyfe et al., 2007). In fact this outbreak might even be due to an insect vector; therefore collecting and sampling aquatic insects and mosquitoes may be worthwhile. Also, it may be reasonable to advise the use of insect repellants in addition to wearing long-sleeved shirts and long trousers whenever around a pool.

Dilukshi says, 'I guess it's easy to prevent cases here because the pond is the only a recreational source of water, but what about places where farmers need to wade into paddy fields and creeks? Some people would be too poor to buy clothing to cover themselves in the water. Is there a vaccine?'

No vaccine is available (Huygen, 2003). Some data suggest BCG immunisation may be protective (Portaels et al., 2004; Smith et al., 1997) and a study in mice of a DNA vaccine from *M. bovis* produced some encouraging results (Tanghe et al., 2001).

The team recommended avoiding the water and, one year later, no further cases have been reported.

References

Asiedu, K., Wansbrough-Jones, M. (2007) *Mycobacterium ulcerans* infection (Buruli or Bairnsdale ulcer): challenges in developing management strategies. *Medical Journal of Australia* 186(2), 55–56.

Asiedu, K., Scherpbier, R., Raviglione, M (eds) (2000) *Buruli Ulcer Mycobacterium ulcerans Infection.* Available from www.who.int/gtb-buruli/publications/PDF/Buruli_ulcer_monograph.PDF (Accessed 28 August, 2005)

Bhatia, A., Prakash, S. (2004) Topical phenytoin for wound healing. *Dermatology Online Journal* 10(1), 5.

Chauty, A. (2005) Treatment of Buruli ulcer with the combination rifampicin and streptomycin in Bénin. In World Health Organization *Report of the 8th Annual WHO Advisory Group Meeting on Buruli ulcer.* WHO; Geneva, Switzerland. Available from www.who.int/buruli/information/publications/REPORT_2005_FINAL.pdf (Accessed 15 July, 2006)

Debacker, M., Aguiar, J., Steunou, C. et al. (2005) Buruli ulcer recurrence, Benin. *Emerging Infectious Diseases* 11(4), 584–89.

Debacker, M., Zinsou, C., Aguiar, J. et al. (2003) First case of *Mycobacterium ulcerans* disease (Buruli ulcer) following a human bite. *Clinical Infectious Diseases* 36(5), e67–68.

Drummond, C., Butler, J.R.G. (2005) *Mycobacterium ulcerans* treatment costs, Australia. *Emerging Infectious Diseases* 10(6), 1038–43.

Etuaful, S., Carbonnelle, B., Grosset, J. et al. (2005) Efficacy of the combination rifampicin-streptomycin in preventing growth of *Mycobacterium ulcerans* in early lesions of Buruli ulcer in humans. *Antimicrobial Agents and Chemotherapy* 49(8), 3182–86.

Fyfe, J.A., Lavender, C.J., Johnson, P. D. et al. (2007) Development and application of two multiplex real-time PCR assays for the detection of *Mycobacterium ulcerans* in clinical and environmental samples. *Applied and Environmental Microbiology* 73(15), 4733–40.

George, K.M., Chatterjee, D., Gunawardana, G. et al. (1999) Mycolactone: a polyketide toxin from *Mycobacterium ulcerans* required for virulence. *Science* 283(5403), 854–57.

Huygen, K. (2003) Prospects for vaccine development against Buruli disease. *Expert Review of Vaccines* 2(4), 561–69.

Johnson, P.D., Hayman, J.A., Quek, T.Y. et al. (2007) Consensus recommendations for the diagnosis, treatment and control of *Mycobacterium ulcerans* infection (Bairnsdale or Buruli ulcer) in Victoria, Australia. *Medical Journal of Australia* 186(2), 64–68.

Johnson, P.D.R., Stinear, T., Small, P.L.C. et al. (2005a) Buruli ulcer (*M. ulcerans* infection): new insights, new hope for disease control. Available from http://medicine.plosjournals.org/archive/1549-1676/2/4/pdf/10.1371_journal.pmed.0020108-L.pdf (Accessed 12 July, 2005)

Johnson, R.C., Makoutode, M., Sopoh, G.E. et al. (2005b) Buruli ulcer distribution in Benin. *Emerging Infectious Diseases* 11(3), 500–01.

Klutse, E.Y., Adjei, O., Ampadu, E. et al. (2003) Management of Buruli ulcer cases with topical application of phenytoin powder. In WHO *Report of the 6th WHO Advisory Group Meeting on Buruli ulcer.* WHO; Geneva, Switzerland. Available from http://whqlibdoc.who.int/hq/2003/WHO_CDS_CPE_GBUI_2003.8.pdf (Accessed 15 July, 2005)

Marsollier, L., Prevot, G., Honore, D. et al. (2003) Susceptibility of *Mycobacterium ulcerans* to a combination of amikacin and rifampicin. *International Journal of Antimicrobial Agents* 22(6), 562–66.

Marsollier, L., Robert, R., Aubry, J. et al. (2002) Aquatic insects as a vector for *Mycobacterium ulcerans*. *Applied and Environmental Microbiology* 68(9), 4623–28.

Marston, B.J., Diallo, M.O., Horsburgh, C.R. Jr et al. (1995) Emergence of Buruli ulcer disease in the Daloa region of Côte d'Ivoire. *American Journal of Tropical Medicine and Hygiene* 52(3), 219–24.

Noeske, J., Kuaban, C., Rondini, S. et al. (2004) Buruli ulcer in Cameroon rediscovered. *American Journal of Tropical Medicine and Hygiene* 70(5), 520–26.

Portaels, F., Aguiar, J., Debacker, M. (2004) *Mycobacterium bovis* BCG vaccination as prophylaxis against *Mycobacterium ulcerans* osteomyelitis in Buruli ulcer disease. *Infection and Immunity* 72(1), 62–65.

Portaels, F., Johnson, P., Meyers, W.M. (eds.) (2001) *Buruli Ulcer Diagnosis of Mycobacterium ulcerans Disease*. Available from www.who.int/gtb-buruli/publications/PDF/BURULI-diagnosis.pdf (Accessed 28 August, 2005)

Portaels, F., Traore, H., De Ridder, K. et al. (1998) In vitro susceptibility of *Mycobacterium ulcerans* to clarithromycin. *Antimicrobial Agents and Chemotherapy* 42(8), 2070–73.

Portaels, F., Agular, J., Fissette, K. et al. (1997) Direct detection and identification of *Mycobacterium ulcerans* in clinical specimens by PCR and oligonucleotide-specific capture plate hybridization. *Journal of Clinical Microbiology* 35(5), 1097–100.

Radford, A.J. (1975) *Mycobacterium ulcerans* in Australia. *Australian and New Zealand Journal of Medicine* 5(2), 162–69.

Raghunathan, P.L., Whitney, E.A., Asomoa, K. et al. (2005) Risk factors for Buruli ulcer disease (*Mycobacterium ulcerans* infection): results from a case-control study in Ghana. *Clinical Infectious Diseases* 40(10), 1445–53.

Revill, W.D., Morrow, R.H., Pike M.C. et al. (1973) A controlled trial of the treatment of *Mycobacterium ulcerans* infection with clofazimine. *Lancet* 2(7834), 873–77.

Rondini, S., Mensah-Quainoo, E., Troll, H. et al. (2003) Development and application of real-time PCR assay for quantification of *Mycobacterium ulcerans* DNA. *Journal of Clinical Microbiology* 41(9), 4231–37.

Ross, B.C., Johnson, P.D., Oppedisano, F. et al. (1997) Detection of *Mycobacterium ulcerans* in environmental samples during an outbreak of ulcerative disease. *Applied and Environmental Microbiology* 63(10), 4135–38.

Smith, P.G., Revill, W.D., Lukwago, E. et al. (1977) The protective effect of BCG against *Mycobacterium ulcerans* disease: a controlled trial in an endemic area of Uganda. *Transactions of the Royal Society of Tropical Medicine and Hygiene* 70(5-6), 449–57.

Tanghe, A., Content, J. Van Vooren, J.P. et al. (2001) Protective efficacy of a DNA vaccine encoding antigen 85A from *Mycobacterium bovis* BCG against Buruli ulcer. *Infection and Immunity* 69(9), 5403–11.

Teelken, M.A., Stienstra, Y., Ellen, D.E. et al. (2003) Buruli ulcer: differences in treatment outcome between two centres in Ghana. *Acta Tropica* 88(1), 51–56.

Thangaraj, H.S., Adjei, O., Allen, B.W. et al. (2000) In vitro activity of ciprofloxacin, sparfloxacin, ofloxacin, amikacin and rifampicin against Ghanaian isolates of *Mycobacterium ulcerans*. *Journal of Antimicrobial Chemotherapy* 45(2), 231–33.

Veitch, M.G., Johnson, P.D., Flood, P.E. et al. (1997) A large localized outbreak of *Mycobacterium ulcerans* infection on a temperate southern Australian island. *Epidemiology and Infection* 119(3), 313–18.

Wansbrough-Jones, M., Phillips, R. (2006) Buruli ulcer: emerging from obscurity. *Lancet* 367(9525), 1849–58.

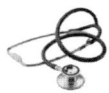

Case 3 Cholera
Three adults have diarrhoea …

Cholera at a glance …

- **Agent:** family Vibrionaceae; genus *Vibrio*; species *Vibrio cholerae*; serogroups O1 and O139 cause epidemic cholera; serogroup O1 has various biotypes (El Tor, classical) and serotypes (Ogawa, Inaba, Hikajima)
- **Geographical distribution:** currently mainly in Africa and Asia
- **Main mode of transmission:** contaminated food or water
- **Person-to-person transmission:** unlikely due to the large infectious dose required
- **Animal-to-person transmission:** no
- **Incubation period:** 2–5 days (as early as 6 hours)
- **Clinical features:** diarrhoea with some vomiting (severity of cases varies)
- **Identification:** cultures of rectal swabs and stool specimens in TCBS medium +/− alkaline peptone water enrichment broth; PCR of stool; dark field microscopy of stool
- **Treatment:** rehydration and maintenance of hydration using oral rehydration solution or intravenous fluids; antibiotics to reduce volume and duration of purging
- **Post-exposure prophylaxis:** probably no role for antibiotics
- **Vaccine:** oral vaccines (killed whole cell vaccine and a live attenuated vaccine); both currently cover only the O1 serogroup

CASE 3 CHOLERA

Main characters

Dr Alain Dupris   infectious diseases physician
Dr Roger Horvath   infectious diseases registrar
Dr Valerie King   director, Centre for Disease Control
Dr Jonah Loewy   naval doctor

Dr Alain Dupris is the on-call infectious diseases physician at a major teaching hospital. He is surprised to receive a call from the department of immigration. A senior official asks him to go to the naval base to assess a boatload of illegal immigrants for gastroenteritis.

Alain takes his registrar, Dr Roger Horvath, to the naval base. On arrival, they meet the director of the Centre for Disease Control (CDC), Dr Valerie King. Alain, Roger and Valerie are met by the naval doctor, Dr Jonah Loewy, who briefs them.

'Six hours ago, a boat with 10 refugees from a South Asian nation was picked up in our waters. They had been sailing for four days. Three of the adults have mild diarrhoea. I am happy to do the usual screening for tuberculosis, HIV and so on, but I wanted your advice regarding the diarrhoea.

'They come from a nation where cholera is endemic. Is cholera a possibility?'

What is cholera?

Cholera is a gastrointestinal infection caused by a toxin-producing Gram negative bacillus, *Vibrio cholerae*. The toxin has two subunits: an active (A) and pentameric binding (B) unit. The B subunit binds the toxin to ganglioside receptors on the surface of epithelial cells. After binding, the A subunit is internalised within the cells, activating the adenylate cyclase enzyme system. This results in active secretion of chloride ions and reduced absorption of sodium ions with resultant loss of electrolytes and water into the gut lumen, leading to dehydration, metabolic acidosis and circulatory collapse (Hill et al., 2006).

The name was created by Pacini, who first identified the Gram negative bacillus in stools from cholera victims in 1854. *Vibrio* means quivering and presumably refers to the chaotic movement of the bacterium under the microscope; *cholera* means flow of bile and refers to a state of anger (Seas and Gotuzzo, 2005).

Cholera has had a dramatic impact on different societies throughout history. For example, the fear of cholera in India was so great that a temple was built specifically to ward off the disease. In the US, cholera led to the creation of the first board of health, with cholera its first reportable disease, and cholera was involved in one of the landmark triumphs of public health medicine and epidemiology when John Snow discovered that water from the Broad Street pump was the vehicle of transmission of cholera during an epidemic in 1854 (Sack et al., 2004).

> Roger looks surprised. 'Isn't cholera almost eradicated?'

In 2005, there were 131 943 reported cases of cholera globally with 2272 deaths (a 1.8% case fatality rate), an increase on the previous year. There is likely to be gross under-reporting both of cases and mortalities, partly due to deliberate attempts to avoid negative impacts on trade and tourism (Sack et al., 2006).

The burden of disease is primarily in developing nations, with Africa and Asia accounting for all but 36 cases of cholera in 2005 (World Health Organization, 2006). Most reported cases from developed nations represent imported disease, although sporadic cases can occur.

> Valerie explains that cholera is certainly a possibility in these refugees. Jonah takes them to the hospital on the naval base where the three refugees with diarrhoea have been placed in isolation. Alain wears a disposable gown and gloves before entering the room and performing an examination. Each patient reported becoming ill a day earlier, with vomiting followed by watery non-bloody diarrhoea with three to six bowel motions per day. They are malnourished but well hydrated.
>
> Alain reports his findings, saying cholera is definitely a possibility. Roger isn't so sure: 'Their only symptoms are vomiting and diarrhoea. Why couldn't it be norovirus infection or something similar?'

After a typical incubation period of 2–5 days—although it can be as short as a few hours—people with cholera suddenly develop profuse watery diarrhoea, sometimes associated with vomiting, which can cause dehydration (Hill et al., 2006). There are few other clinical features, so milder cases can be clinically indistinguishable from other causes of diarrhoeal illnesses, such as norovirus. However, people with cholera can rapidly deteriorate if they are not quickly identified and treated, so Alain is right not to disregard the diagnosis in people with diarrhoea who come from areas where cholera is endemic.

> Roger still isn't satisfied. 'Sorry to be a sceptic, but aren't people with cholera always desperately ill? These three individuals don't sound particularly unwell at all.'

Prognosis

Cholera can be a devastating infection. Severe dehydration occurs in only 5–10% of cases with the remainder being mild-to-moderate or asymptomatic (Hill et al., 2006). Among severe cases, the mortality rate is about 50% if patients are not treated in a timely fashion (Sack et al,. 2004). Given the large numbers of cholera cases globally every year, small percentages such as 5–10% represent large absolute numbers of severe cases. The mortality rate of 50% for untreated severe cases is particularly important in developing nations, which bear the greatest burden of disease, because treatment is not always readily accessible.

In countries where cholera in endemic, it is the extremes of age who are most susceptible to severe illness: there is no immunity in young children and both waning immunity and waning gastric acidity in the elderly (the portal of entry is through the small intestine, so stomach acidity is a defensive barrier: the higher the pH, the lower the infectious dose required). Healthy young adults in endemic countries, on the other hand, are likely to have a degree of immunity and this attenuates the severity of infection (CDC et al., 1999a). Healthy travellers to endemic cholera regions are also more likely to experience asymptomatic or mild disease (Hill et al., 2006).

It is reasonable to assume that the young adult refugees with diarrhoea may have some pre-existing immunity to cholera, which could explain the mildness of their illness.

> All the doctors agree that even the healthy refugees should be carefully observed for the sudden onset of severe diarrhoeal illnesses. In the meantime, Valerie suggests that three stool samples from each refugee with diarrhoea be tested.

Jonah says, 'I presume that I should just order 'microscopy, culture, sensitivities, ova, cysts and parasites (M/C/S, OCP)' for each stool sample. That should pick up *Salmonella, Campylobacter, Shigella*, cryptosporidiosis, giardiasis and *V. cholerae*.'

Investigations

Laboratory scientists asked for M/C/S and OCP will use culture media and tests to detect *Salmonella, Shigella, Campylobacter* and a variety of parasites; however, it is a dangerous assumption that *V. cholerae* will be detected using these measures. *V. cholerae* can potentially be isolated from standard stool culture media but there is no guarantee of this and, even if it grows, it may be in the presence of other colonies that mask it from laboratory staff.

If cholera is being considered, laboratory staff should be alerted either on the request form accompanying the stool specimen or personally, so appropriate tests can be performed. Even if the clinician has not considered cholera as a diagnosis, experienced laboratory staff will often specifically culture for it if the clinical notes in the request form are helpful (e.g. '20-year-old man with diarrhoea after returning from Bangladesh').

Dark field microscopy and rapid immunoassays can be useful in making an early diagnosis of cholera. Dark field microscopy should be performed on a wet mount of liquid stool samples. It typically shows the presence of darting organisms whose motion is halted by the addition of O1 or O139 antiserum (Sack et al., 2004).

Polymerase chain reaction (PCR) for the organism and its enterotoxin is a relatively rapid test which can be highly sensitive and specific. However, it may not be readily available in the developing world (Seas and Gotuzzo, 2005).

The stool samples are examined under dark field microscopy. No motile organisms consistent with *V. cholerae* are seen. Alain doesn't think this excludes the diagnosis. It may simply mean that these partially immune young adults are not excreting large enough numbers of organisms for detection.

> Roger asks whether there is a way to increase the numbers of *V. cholerae* in stool prior to placing it in culture medium.

Faecal suspensions, rectal swabs or liquid stools can be placed in alkaline peptone water (APW) for 6–12 hours. This is an excellent enrichment broth, particularly in situations where there are likely to be low levels of *V. cholerae* present. According to CDC et al. (1999b) these situations include:

- patients in the convalescent phase of illness
- asymptomatic patients
- environmental specimens
- patients likely to have large numbers of other competing organisms

After eight hours of incubating the stool samples in APW, the specimens are plated onto a selective medium for *V. cholerae*, typically thiosulfate citrate bile salts sucrose agar (TCBS). *V. cholerae* colonies are shiny yellow as a result of fermentation of sucrose. Non-sucrose fermenters (e.g. *V. parahaemolyticus*) appear as green or blue-green colonies (CDC et al., 1999b).

> The stool samples are inoculated in TCBS medium. Within 24 hours, shiny yellow colonies consistent with *V. cholerae* appear. Roger looks at the plates with Alain. 'Are any other tests needed to confirm their presence?'

On non-selective agar, an oxidase test should be performed—*V. cholerae* would test positive by turning purple immediately—followed by polyvalent agglutination testing with O1 and O139 antisera for a presumptive diagnosis. The reason that oxidase and agglutination testing of the colonies should be performed on non-selective agar and not TCBS medium is to prevent false-positive and false-negative results (CDC et al., 1999b; Sack et al., 2004). If agglutination with O1 antiserum is positive, the serotype can be confirmed with Inaba and Ogawa antisera.

Oxidase and agglutination testing is performed on the colonies. The results are consistent with cholera. The cultures are also sent to a reference laboratory in the capital city for confirmatory PCR testing. At this stage, the senior lab scientist confidently tells Roger and Alain that the isolate is *V. cholerae* serogroup O1, biotype El Tor, serotype Ogawa.

Roger looks puzzled. 'I understood everything you said up to "*V. cholerae*". What on earth are serogroups, biotypes and serotypes?'

V. cholerae can be classified according to serogroup, biotype and serotype (Sack et al., 2004) see Figure 3.1). Unfortunately, serogroup and serotype can also be referred to as 'serotype' and 'subserotype', respectively (Chen et al., 2006). The serogroup classification is based on the O antigen. More than 200 serotypes of *V. cholerae* have been identified (Sack et al., 2006). Up till 1992, the O1 serogroup was the only *V. cholerae* known to cause epidemic cholera, so serogroups are still commonly divided into O1 and non-O1. In 1992, however, in Bangladesh and India, a new serogroup was found to cause epidemic cholera, serogroup O139. This new serogroup has since spread to 11 other countries and accounts for 15% of laboratory-confirmed cases of cholera in endemic countries in Asia. Nevertheless, serogroup O1 still causes the bulk of epidemic cholera cases (Hill et al., 2006). A more accurate classification of serogroups causing epidemic cholera would be O1, O139 and non-O1/non-O139.

Serogroup O1, but not O139, can be classified into two biotypes, El Tor and classical. Whereas serogroups are determined by the O antigen, biotypes are determined by the biochemical profile of *V. cholerae*. The El Tor biotype was first identified in Indonesian pilgrims passing through the village of El Tor in Egypt.

Both biotypes of serogroup O1 can be further divided into serotypes: Ogawa, Inaba and the rare Hikajima. Further differentiation of the organism can be done through phage typing, clonal typing and electrophoretic typing (Sack et al., 2004).

'Are there any clinical differences between the biotypes?'

CASE 3 CHOLERA

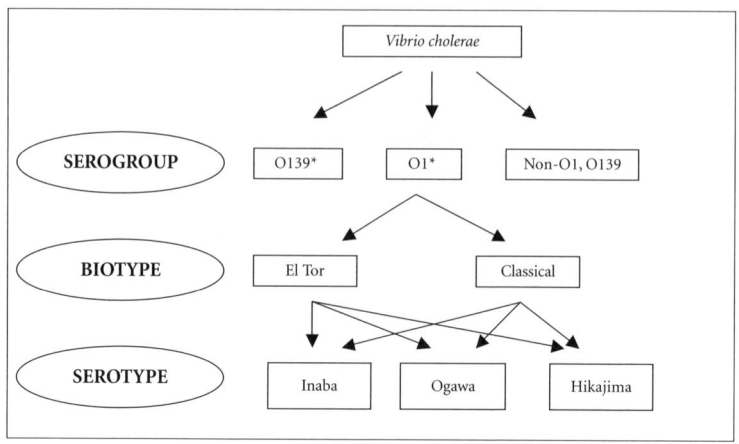

*Serogroups O1 and O139 are the only two serogroups to cause epidemic cholera
FIGURE 3.1 A simple classification for *Vibrio cholerae*

> The classic biotype causes equal numbers of symptomatic and asymptomatic cases. El Tor causes 20–100 more symptomatic than asymptomatic infections (Seas and Gotuzzo, 2005).

'None of the stool specimens contained leucocytes,' Roger comments. 'Is that surprising?'

> *V. cholerae* does not invade the intestinal wall, so it is not surprising to see no or only some leucocytes in stool (Seas and Gotuzzo, 2005).

The isolates are now set up for antibiotic sensitivity testing in the lab. Roger asks Alain, 'Should we prescribe antibiotics now?'

Treatment

> A 1–3 day course of antibiotics reduces the clinical course of cholera by 1–2 days (i.e. from 4–5 days to 2–3 days). This results in a reduced duration and volume of diarrhoea and therefore shortened hospital admissions, a very important factor during cholera epidemics when hospitals in developing nations may be overflowing with cholera patients (Hill et al., 2006; Sack et al., 2004).

'From memory, aren't tetracyclines the drugs of choice?' Roger says.

For adults, a single dose of doxycycline is ideal. Antimicrobials used to treat cholera include tetracyclines, fluoroquinolones, cotrimoxazole and furazolidone (Seas and Gotuzzo, 2005). However, drug resistance is an increasing problem; for example, in Bangladesh nearly all *V. cholerae* strains are resistant to erythromycin, tetracyclines and cotrimoxazole (Sack et al., 2006). For this reason, antibiotic susceptibility testing for all strains of *V. cholerae* is recommended.

'Do we need to notify anyone about the cholera cases?'

Public notification and response

Cholera is a notifiable infection in most parts of the world. The presence of even a single case could potentially herald the onset of a more widespread outbreak with significant morbidity and mortality. Public health units need to be made aware of any cases of cholera in order to identify the source of infection and neutralise it and to identify others exposed to cholera so they can receive prompt treatment. In this case, Valerie from the CDC has been involved from the start of the investigation but she must be told that the diagnosis of cholera has been confirmed so she can launch an outbreak investigation.

Alain informs Valerie and Jonah of these results. Jonah says, 'Actually, I was just about to call you. Our three cholera patients have recovered from their illness. But just about an hour ago, a 10-year-old child from the boat developed watery diarrhoea. Could you please rush over here to assess him?'

Within 20 minutes, Alain, Roger and Valerie are at the naval hospital, assessing the child. Despite the diarrhoea commencing only 90 minutes earlier, he already has signs of moderate dehydration, with reduced skin turgor, restlessness and a dry mouth. His blood pressure is just normal. Unlike the first three cholera patients, he has watery diarrhoea containing mucus.

Roger comments, 'Watery diarrhoea containing mucus—the classical "rice water stool" of cholera, looking like water used to wash rice.'

The poor child is screaming in pain because of leg cramps. 'What causes that?' Roger asks.

In the setting of severe cholera, leg cramps could indicate hypokalaemia caused by diarrhoea. Hypokalaemia would put him at risk of fatal arrhythmias and paralytic ileus. His electrolytes need to be urgently checked and corrected. If his potassium is low, cardiac monitoring would be appropriate, if available.

Jonah says, 'I can't believe how much diarrhoea he has passed in the last 90 minutes.'

Severe cholera can be a terrifying spectacle. Unlike the adult patients, this child probably has no pre-existing immunity and is therefore susceptible to serious disease. Without appropriate treatment, he could be dead within hours from dehydration and its complications.

Alain commences the child on azithromycin and begins rehydrating him. Urgent blood tests confirm that he is hyponatraemic and hypokalaemic with a metabolic acidosis, findings typical of cholera. Cardiac monitoring is commenced.

'What are the principles of rehydrating cholera patients?' Alain asks Jonah.

Rehydration involves six steps.

1. Assess hydration.
2. For dehydrated patients, give an oral rehydration solution (ORS) but use intravenous (IV) fluids instead if they are:
   - severely dehydrated
   - moderately dehydrated but unable to take oral fluids
   - passing >10–20 mL/kg/hr of fluid per rectum.

3. Monitor diarrhoeal output.
4. Replace ongoing fluid losses.
5. Commence an appropriate oral antibiotic as soon as vomiting ceases.
6. Feed the patient as soon as he/she can tolerate it (Sack et al., 2004; Seas and Gotuzzo, 2005).

An ORS is a solution of salts to correct the electrolyte and metabolic derangements caused by the cholera enterotoxin. The WHO recommends a glucose-based solution that contains (in mmol/L) sodium 75, chloride 65, potassium chloride 20, trisodium citrate 10 (instead of bicarbonate) and glucose 75. It has a total osmolality of 245 mmol/L (Department of Child and Adolescent Health and Development and World Health Organization, 2001). A rice-based ORS may have an advantage over the glucose-based WHO ORS in that it reduces the rate of purging. ORS formulations are available in packets, to which water is added, but ORS can be prepared at home by anyone (Sack et al., 2004).

Several types of IV fluids can be used. The most commonly recommended solution is Ringer's lactate, which contains (in mmol/L) sodium 130, chloride 109, potassium 4 and lactate 28. Other IV solutions, such as Dhaka solution, can be used. Normal saline is an option but should be avoided where possible because it does not correct the metabolic acidosis. With initial IV rehydration, the most important point to remember is that it should be given quickly and certainly not for more than four hours (Seas and Gotuzzo, 2005).

> The team agree on WHO ORS for the child. He looks remarkably better two hours later, even though the diarrhoea continues. They use a bedpan to measure the stool volume. Valerie, who worked in cholera-endemic areas in Asia as part of her public health training, says, 'I wish we had a cholera cot.'

A cholera cot is a plastic mattress with a hole around the buttock region under which a bucket can be kept to catch the stool. It allows the patient to rest without moving to empty their bowels and staff to accurately assess the volume of fluid lost.

> The medical staff are all relieved to see that the young boy appears to be over the worst of the diarrhoea. Jonah says to Valerie, 'The incubation period suggests he was infected while on the boat. I presume he caught it from one of the affected adults. Would that be right?'

CASE 3 CHOLERA

Unlike many diarrhoeal infections, person-to-person transmission of cholera through casual contact (e.g. by shaking hands) is extremely uncommon in those with normal gastric acidity because the dose needed to cause infections can be so high (10^8–10^{11} organisms) (Hill et al., 2006).

> Jonah asks, 'If it wasn't person-to-person contact, then how could they have been infected?'

V. cholerae is a remarkable organism. Its natural environment is an aquatic one, where it lives attached to plankton, algae or the shells of crustaceans. When conditions are adverse, it can switch to a dormant state (where it cannot be cultured) but it can thrive and multiply when conditions are optimal, independent of humans (Seas and Gotuzzo, 2005). *V. cholerae* grows best in warm temperatures. This is demonstrated by peaks in cholera activity in Bangladesh in the warm periods before and after the monsoon. In Peru, epidemics of cholera are strictly confined to the warm season (Sack et al., 2004).

Humans come into contact with cholera when the organism contaminates food or water. *V. cholerae* can contaminate rivers, streams, shallow wells, ice or bottled water. Food sources include moist alkaline food in which other organisms have been killed by previous cooking, such as legumes, cooked rice, millet, seafood, lentils and other cooked grains. The organism will survive up to 14 days in food (Seas and Gotuzzo, 2005). Interestingly, the infectious dose is less when cholera is transmitted through food rather than through water. Unsurprisingly, fruits and vegetables grown in sewage and not otherwise decontaminated are a source (CDC et al., 1999a).

> Valerie concludes that a contaminated water or food source on the boat was the most likely vehicle of transmission. She leads an outbreak investigation to identify the source. All three cholera cases drank from the boat's water tank early into the four-day voyage. The 10-year-old boy, who developed cholera after only arriving at the naval base, drank water from the tank only on the last day of the trip when his own water supply had run out.
>
> Valerie's environmental health officers sample the water from the tank. No one is surprised when cultures and PCR confirm that it contains large numbers of *V. cholerae*.
>
> 'Would boiling the water have killed *V. cholerae*?' asks Jonah.

Boiling water or the addition of disinfecting agents, such as chlorine or iodine, will kill *V. cholerae* (World Health Organization, 2007), as will drying and sunlight, but freezing does not (CDC et al., 1999a).

> Jonah also asks, 'With cases of enteric fever, we have to examine stool specimens after recovery to identify chronic carriage. Does the same thing apply to cholera?'

As discussed above, person-to-person transmission of cholera is not important in the spread of disease, so it is not necessary to test the stool of people who have recovered (Sack et al., 2006).

Chronic carriage in the gall bladder/biliary tree has been documented but is uncommon. The most notable case of this was 'Cholera Dolores' who intermittently excreted *V. cholerae* in her stool for years apparently without causing any other cases of cholera (Azurin et al., 1967).

> Jonah wonders whether antibiotic prophylaxis should be given to other crew members.

There is no consensus on this but there is little evidence regarding any benefit of chemoprophylaxis for household contacts of a case (Seas and Gotuzzo, 2005). Also, since it is three days after the refugees left the boat, they would almost be out of the incubation period for cholera.

> Roger says to Valerie, 'I realise the unaffected refugees may already be immune, or have been protected by their gastric acidity, or have had asymptomatic infection. Could something have put the four who did become ill at increased risk?'

Some people have an increased susceptibility to cholera including, for unknown reasons, people with blood group O. One reason for the cholera problems experienced in Peru may be the predominance of blood group O in the population (Hill et al., 2006). Chronic gastritis from *Helicobacter pylori* may also increase susceptibility (CDC et al., 1999a ; Seas and Gotuzzo, 2005).

> A few days later, Jonah updates everyone. There have been no further cases of diarrhoea and the cholera outbreak among the

refugees is over. One refugee is in hospital after cutting her leg on disembarking from the boat and developing an infection. Apparently a Gram negative rod is growing from a leg swab. Jonah jokingly asks if it is cholera.

Non-toxigenic, non-agglutinating strains of *V. cholerae* may rarely cause otitis externa, diarrhoea or wound infections in people who have been in warm and brackish water (Andersson and Ekdahl, 2006).

Alain, whose lab is processing the specimen, confirms that the organism in the cut will probably be an *Aeromonas* species.
Roger says, 'Seeing one sick child with moderately severe cholera was more than enough for me. I hope we never get a cholera pandemic.'

Actually, there currently is a pandemic of cholera, the seventh recorded since 1817. It began in Indonesia in 1961 and reached South America in 1991, three decades later. It is caused by the O1 El Tor biotype.

Roger is worried: 'I'm going to India next year for a conference in New Delhi. Should I get vaccinated against cholera?'

There are two licensed oral vaccines for cholera, a whole cell recombinant B subunit of cholera toxin vaccine (rCTB-WC) and the live attenuated *V. cholerae* O1 strain CVD 103-HgR (Hill et al., 2006).

The whole cell vaccine contains mixtures of El Tor and classical biotypes as well as Inaba and Ogawa serotypes. The presence of the B subunit in the whole cell vaccine reduces the severity of infection in the event that the whole cell component does not prevent disease. (Topps, 2006). The live CVD 103-HgR vaccine has had mixed results in studies, doing well in volunteer trials but performing disappointingly in its only placebo-controlled field trial (Hill et al., 2006).

The optimal use of these new oral vaccines for travellers is unknown. The only certainty is that neither protects against serogroup O139 disease, although trials of other vaccines are continuing.

The risk of disease for travellers is extremely low: 0.001–0.01% per month of stay in a high-risk area (Topps, 2006). Also, travellers often develop milder disease, so it may be reasonable to limit vaccination to travellers assisting in disaster areas or to those visiting cholera-endemic areas with limited medical care (Hill et al., 2006).

For inhabitants in endemic regions, the whole cell vaccine with B subunit potentially could reduce cholera rates. The vaccine provides waning protection over three years, with protective efficacy peaking at 61–86%. This means that booster immunisation would be required every 2–3 years. In addition, the vaccine is not as immunogenic in children under five years old, who would require more frequent boosters (every six months). This immediately raises concerns about the cost–benefit ratio and compliance (Topps, 2006). On the plus side, however, high vaccine coverage leads to indirect herd immunity in neighbouring susceptible contacts (Ali et al., 2005).

During an epidemic (e.g. after a natural disaster), the whole cell vaccine with B subunit is probably even less useful, although an argument could be made for its use. The concern is that it would take three weeks to generate immunity, by which time the disaster would have been controlled. Also, poor immunogenicity in children <5 years means that one of the most vulnerable age groups during a cholera epidemic would not be effectively protected (Topp, 2006).

Interestingly, the cholera enterotoxin is similar in structure to the heat-labile toxin of enterotoxigenic *Escherichia coli* (ETEC), the cause of 15% of travellers' diarrhoea. Immunisation with the whole cell cholera vaccine therefore provides some cross-immunity against ETEC, but there is debate about whether it is worth using the oral cholera vaccine to prevent travellers' diarrhoea (Hill et al., 2006).

Roger asks, 'Didn't there use to be a parenteral vaccine for cholera?'

A cholera parenteral vaccine exists but has been generally criticised for its poor efficacy (50–65% over 3–6 months) and its high rate of adverse effects (50% local reactions, 10–30% systemic features). It has gone out of favour (Hill et al., 2006).

References

Ali, M., Emch, M., von Seidlein, L. et al. (2005) Herd immunity conferred by killed oral cholera vaccines in Bangladesh: a reanalysis. *Lancet* 366(9479), 44–49.

Andersson, Y., Ekdahl, K. (2006) Wound infections due to *Vibrio cholerae* in Sweden after swimming in the Baltic Sea, summer 2006. *Eurosurveillance* 11(8), E060803.2

Azurin, J.C., Kobari,, K. Barua, D. et al. (1967) A long-term carrier of cholera: Cholera Dolores. *Bulletin of the World Health Organization* 37(5), 745–49.

Centers for Disease Control and Prevention, National Center for Infectious Diseases, World Health Organization Regional Office for Africa. (1999a) Chapter 5: Etiology and epidemiology of cholera. In *Laboratory Methods for the Diagnosis of Epidemic Dysentery and Cholera*. Available from www.cdc.gov/ncidod/dbmd/diseaseinfo/cholera/ch5.pdf (Accessed 7 May, 2007)

Centers for Disease Control and Prevention, National Center for Infectious Diseases, World Health Organization Regional Office for Africa. (1999b) Chapter 6: Isolation and identification of *Vibrio cholerae* serogroups O1 and O139. In *Laboratory Methods for the Diagnosis of Epidemic Dysentery and Cholera*. Available from www.cdc.gov/ncidod/dbmd/diseaseinfo/cholera/ch6.pdf (Accessed 7 May, 2007)

Chen, L., Woolley, I.J., Visvanathan, K. et al. (2006) Hypovolemic shock and metabolic acidosis in a refugee secondary to O1 serotype *Vibrio cholerae* enteritis. *Communicable Diseases Intelligence* 30(2), 233–35.

Department of Child and Adolescent Health and Development, World Health Organization (2001) *Reduced Osmolarity Oral Rehydration Salts (ORS) Formulation*. Available from www.who.int/child-adolescent-health/-New_Publications/NEWS/Expert_consultation.htm (Accessed 11 May, 2007)

Hill, D.R., Ford, L., Lalloo, D.G. (2006) Oral cholera vaccines: use in clinical practice. *Lancet Infectious Diseases* 6(6), 361–73.

Sack, D.A., Sack, R.B., Chaignat, C.L. (2006) Getting serious about cholera. *New England Journal of Medicine* 355(7), 649–51.

Sack, D.A., Sack, R.B., Nair, B. et al. (2004) Cholera. *Lancet* 363(9404), 223–33.

Seas, C., Gotuzzo, E. (2005) *Vibrio cholerae*. In Mandell G. L., Bennett, J.E., Dolin, R. (eds) *Principles and Practice of Infectious Diseases*. Churchill Livingstone; Philadelphia.

Topps, M.H. (2006) Oral cholera vaccine—for whom, when and why? *Travel Medicine and Infectious Diseases* 4(1), 38–42.

World Health Organization (2007) *Cholera—Frequently Asked Questions And Information For Travellers*. Available from www.who.int/topics/cholera/faq/en/index.html (Accessed 12 May, 2007)

World Health Organization. (2006) Cholera 2005. *Weekly Epidemiological Record* 81(31), 297–307.

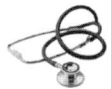

Case 4 Cryptosporidiosis and Giardiasis
An outbreak investigation …

Cryptosporidiosis at a glance …

- **Agent:** Family *Cryptosporidiidae*; genus *Cryptosporidium*; there are at least 15 species; *C. parvum* and *C. hominis* cause the bulk of human disease
- **Geographical distribution:** worldwide
- **Modes of transmission:** waterborne, foodborne, sexual (oral–anal contact)
- **Person-to-person transmission:** yes
- **Animal-to-person transmission:** yes
- **Incubation period:** 7–10 days
- **Infectious period:** infectious oocysts can be excreted from 3–30 days in untreated individuals
- **Clinical features:** acute diarrhoeal illness; extra-intestinal manifestations tend to occur in the immunocompromised
- **Identification:** isolation of the oocysts in stool; need 3 consecutive negative stool samples to exclude infection
- **Treatment:** nitazoxanide for immunocompetent children aged 1–11 years; for HIV patients, antiretroviral therapy to increase the CD4 cell count is vital; a number of anti-parasitic agents can be used in immunocompromised individuals, although data are lacking to make any official recommendations
- **Prophylaxis:** no
- **Vaccine:** no

Giardiasis at a glance ...

- **Agent:** Family Hexamitidae; genus *Giardia;* species *Giardia lamblia* (also known as *G. intestinalis* or *G. duodenalis*); a flagellated protozoan
- **Geographical distribution:** worldwide
- **Modes of transmission:** waterborne, foodborne, sexual (oral–anal contact)
- **Person-to-person transmission:** yes
- **Animal-to-person transmission:** possibly
- **Incubation period:** 1–2 weeks
- **Infectious period:** in the untreated patient, the passage of infectious cysts in the stool can persist for at least 3 months
- **Clinical features:** asymptomatic disease is most common; also, an acute gastrointestinal presentation which can become chronic and be associated with malabsorption, depression and weight loss; extra-intestinal manifestations are rare
- **Identification:** isolation of the cysts or trophozoites in stool, with 3 consecutive negative stool samples needed to exclude infection; invasive diagnosis with duodenal biopsies
- **Treatment:** a number of anti-parasitic agents exist; mainstay of therapy has been the nitroimidazoles (metronidazole and tinidazole); other agents include paromomycin, mebendazole, albendazole, furazolidone, quinacrine, bacitracin zinc and nitazoxanide
- **Prophylaxis:** no
- **Vaccine:** no

Main characters

Dr Mohammed Gebra	general practitioner
Peter Clark	10-year-old boy
Ms Alison Webb	laboratory worker at the local hospital
Mr Socrates Demetriou	infectious diseases nurse at the local public health unit
Dr Emmanuel Gibbs	director, local public health unit
Dr Jane Wylie	general practitioner

> Dr Mohammed Gebra is a rural general practitioner (GP) looking after 10-year-old Peter Clark. He has foul-smelling diarrhoea, crampy abdominal pain and a gurgling tummy. 'I think it might be *Giardia*—I reckon that's going around at the moment,' Mohammed tells Peter's mother.

What is *Giardia*?

In 1681 *Giardia* became the first parasitic protozoan in humans to be seen. This flagellated protozoan is the most common intestinal parasite of humans in developed countries (Fayer, 2004). There are several species (*G. duodenalis, G. psittaci, G. microti, G. ardeae* and *G. muris*) but the one that infects humans is *Giardia duodenalis* (also known as *G. intestinalis* and *G. lamblia*—Vilem Lambl in the late nineteenth century was the first person to provide useful drawings of the protozoan; Cox, 2002). *G. duodenalis* is further divided into assemblages A–F, and only assemblages A and B infect humans (Olson et al., 2004).

Giardia is not an invasive organism and lives in the lumen of the small intestine, typically causing villous atrophy of varying degrees (Fayer, 2004).

Cysts are ingested and excyst in the proximal small intestine, becoming trophozoites. The trophozoites replicate by binary fission. As the trophozoites move towards the colon, they encyst. Both trophozoites and cysts can be found in the stool (Centers for Disease Control, 2004b).

The majority of *Giardia* infections are asymptomatic with cyst excretion (D'Anchino et al., 2002; Pickering et al., 1984). However, well-recognised acute and chronic syndromes occur.

After an incubation period of 1–2 weeks, an acute diarrhoeal illness can occur with malaise, flatulence, abdominal cramping, bloating, weight loss and 'rotten-egg' burps. The diarrhoea is typically malodorous and may vary in consistency from watery to loose to frank steatorrhoea. Fever is an uncommon feature of giardiasis, so its absence should not put one off the diagnosis.

The acute illness can turn into a chronic illness which fluctuates over many months. In chronic giardiasis, steatorrhoea and loose stools are often accompanied by severe weight loss, depression, lactose intolerance and syndromes related to malabsorption of nutrients (Farthing, 1996).

CASE 4 CRYPTOSPORIDIOSIS AND GIARDIASIS

Uncommon or rare manifestations of giardiasis include synovitis/reactive arthritis (Letts et al., 1998), biliary disease (Aronson et al., 2001) and urticaria (McKnight and Tietze, 1992).

> Mohammed orders stool cultures, which Peter's mum duly collects and drops off to the lab at the local hospital.
> The culture results do suggest *Giardia*. Ms Alison Webb, who processed the specimen, notifies the on-call infectious diseases nurse, Mr Socrates Demetriou.
> 'Interesting,' he says. 'Do you know, this is my fourth notification in two days?'
> 'Could it be an outbreak?' Alison asks.

Determining whether there is an outbreak is the first step in a potential outbreak investigation, the steps of which are defined by the Centers for Disease Control and Prevention (2005) as:

- preparing for field work
- establishing the existence of an outbreak
- verifying the diagnosis
- defining and identifying cases
- describing and orienting the data in terms of time, place and person
- developing hypotheses
- evaluating hypotheses
- refining hypotheses and carrying out additional studies
- implementing control and prevention measures
- communicating findings

Establishing the existence of an outbreak is an early step but a vital one before putting the money and resources of an already busy public health unit into an investigation.

An outbreak (also known as an epidemic) refers to a larger number of cases of an infection over a given time period in a certain area; therefore, Socrates needs to know the expected number of cases in his area.

> Socrates quickly pulls up the relevant public health surveillance data: there have been 3–8 cases of giardiasis annually in his area

over the last four years. To get four notifications in two days is certainly above the expected rate and therefore constitutes an outbreak.

Socrates analyses the brief reports from the laboratory. All four patients are children aged 10–12 years. They all are all treated by the same GP: Mohammed.

Socrates calls Mohammed, who has only just received the stool results himself. 'Al, what can you tell me about these *Giardia* cases?'

It turns out that three children (two 10-year old boys and an 11-year-old girl) attend the same school.

Socrates consults his director, Dr Emmanuel Gibbs. Emmanuel has been reviewing recent notifications of a different disease: cryptosporidiosis. This number of these cases is also well above the expected rate and therefore constitutes an outbreak.

What is *Cryptosporidium*?

Cryptosporidiosis is a syndrome due to infection with *Cryptosporidium*, a protozoan. *Cryptosporidium* was first discovered early in the twentieth century by Edward Tyzzer but its impact on humans and its potential for waterborne transmission have been appreciated only since the 1970s (Fayer, 2004). It accounts for 2% of diarrhoea in immunocompetent individuals in developed countries and 6% in developing countries (7 and 12% for children with diarrhoea, respectively). It is present in almost a quarter of patients with both AIDS and diarrhoea (Chen et al., 2002).

There are currently 15 species of *Cryptosporidium*. Most were named according to the host with which they were supposedly associated, for example, *C. felis* for cats, *C. canis* for dogs, *C. hominis* for humans (formerly known as *C. parvum* Type 1). However, it is now clear that most of these species are not specific for their host and are found in many different animals. For example, *C. hominis* (supposedly specific for humans) has been found in creatures as unusual as dugongs (an ocean mammal) (Fayer, 2004). *C. parvum* and *C. hominis* account for nearly all human infections (Leoni et al., 2006).

The thick-walled oocysts enter the body usually through ingestion. Sporozoites are produced when the oocysts excyst; these typically parasitise the cells of the gastrointestinal tract before undergoing asexual and sexual cycles. This ultimately leads to the production of thick-walled oocysts, which are excreted, and thin-walled oocysts, which can cause autoinfection.

CASE 4 CRYPTOSPORIDIOSIS AND GIARDIASIS

Excreted oocysts are immediately infectious (Centers for Disease Control, 2004a). Oocysts retain their infectivity for several months in both salt and fresh water and can remain viable in cool and moist conditions for many months (Sunnotel et al., 2006).
As with giardiasis, acute, persistent or asymptomatic infection can be seen (Chen et al., 2002). The acute illness occurs after an incubation period of 7–10 days and has a median duration of 12 days. The most common manifestation is self-limiting watery diarrhoea with mucus but no blood or white cells. The diarrhoea is often accompanied by nausea, vomiting and abdominal cramping. As with giardiasis, fever is a minor complaint, being present in just over one-third of illnesses. The acute illness can occasionally be quite severe, especially in immunocompromised patients.

A persistent diarrhoeal illness can occur over weeks and may be associated with malnutrition, especially in children in the developing world.

Extra-intestinal manifestations are well recognised and tend to occur in immunocompromised individuals.

> Emmanuel suggests combining the data from the *Cryptosporidium* and *Giardia* notifications. 'How would that help?' Socrates asks.

Both infections have similar modes of transmission (Table 4.1). Therefore, it is possible that the *Giardia* and *Cryptosporidium* outbreaks have a common source.

Table 4.1 Modes of transmission of *Cryptosporidium* and *Giardia* in humans

Mode of transmission	*Cryptosporidium*	*Giardia*
Ingestion of contaminated food	yes	yes
Ingestion of contaminated water	yes	yes
Person-to-person contact[†]	yes	yes
Animal-to-human	yes	maybe
Flies and cockroaches	maybe	maybe

[†]Person-to-person contact refers to faeco-oral transmission through dirty hands or even sexually with oral–anal contact.
SOURCE Graczyk et al., 2005; Mildvan et al., 1977; Sunnotel et al., 2006; Thompson, 2004

Emmanuel and Socrates combine their data and analyse the basic demographic information. All the cases involve children, aged 9–11 years with a mix of boys and girls. They live in different parts of the region. Emmanuel is convinced that the *Giardia* and *Cryptosporidium* cases are linked to a common source; however, he wants to see if he can identify more cases before he launches a full outbreak investigation.

He immediately calls the local division of GPs and expresses his concerns to the CEO. He explains that he wants to send a fax and email to all GPs in the division, asking them to:

- be vigilant for cases of diarrhoea in the next week
- get three stool specimens from all patients with diarrhoea whom they see over the next week
- request that all stool samples be tested for *Cryptosporidium* and *Giardia* in addition to standard tests

'Why the stool testing?' the CEO asks.

Investigations

Not all patients with diarrhoea have stool specimens tested. Diarrhoeal infection can be thought of as a triangle divided into three sections. The lower two sections, making up the bulk of the triangle, represent people with diarrhoea who:
- never seek medical attention and get better
- see their GP but never have their stool tested (When a patient only has a mild diarrhoeal illness, a GP is quite justified in thinking that it is likely to resolve spontaneously without having any public health implications; in addition, the patient may have to pay for the stool to be analysed.)

It is only the tiny area at the top of the triangle (the 'tip of the iceberg') that represents those people with diarrhoea who provide stool specimens and have a microbiological diagnosis confirmed. In other words, Emmanuel is likely to miss the bulk of cases if he does not insist on testing the stool of all patients presenting with diarrhoea to GPs; even then, he will never identify those patients with a very mild illness who never present to their GP at all.

CASE 4 CRYPTOSPORIDIOSIS AND GIARDIASIS

> The CEO is happy for a fax to be sent but wants to clarify a few points. 'Why do we need to send three stool specimens for each patient? Isn't one sample enough?'

One sample is not sensitive enough to detect infection from intermittent excretion of either the cysts or trophozoites. The sensitivity of a single stool specimen for *Cryptosporidium* is 30% and 50–70% for *Giardia* (Blanshard et al., 1992; Hiatt et al., 1995).

> 'Why do we need to specify that the stool be specifically examined for *Giardia* and *Cryptosporidium* in addition to standard microscopy and culture?'

Cryptosporidium can very occasionally be detected through standard microscopy of stool, especially if an iodine solution is used. It cannot be cultured. Generally, special stains or immunoassays need to be performed. Some laboratories may routinely look for *Cryptosporidium* in stool specimens anyway, but if there is uncertainty it is always easier to mention on the request form that you are looking for it.

Giardia, on the other hand, may be detected through routine wet preparation of stool ('wet prep') without making special requests. However, if doctors specifically request an examination for *Giardia* (or 'ova and parasite'), the laboratory will do additional examinations of stool. Such tests include concentration methods, permanent stained smears and immunoassays.

If doctors give sufficient clinical information on the pathology request form, the laboratory will know which tests to perform on the stool sample.

> 'So there are a few ways of detecting these protozoa in stool?'

Giardiasis can be detected through (Centers for Disease Control, 2004b):
- standard stool microscopy
- microscopy of stool prepared for 'ova and parasite' examination
- microscopy of stool using immunofluorescence
- enzyme immunoassay (EIA) examination of stool
- duodenal biopsies/aspirates (an invasive method)

Immunofluorescence and EIA of stool for *Giardia* detect antigen produced by the trophozoites or cysts of the protozoan. They are more sensitive, quicker and economical than the 'ova and parasite' microscopy method (Aziz et al., 2001).

Intestinal cryptosporidiosis can be detected through (Centers for Disease Control, 2004a):
- microscopic examination of stool that has been stained (e.g. using modified acid-fast stains or fluorescent dyes such as auramine)
- microscopy of stool using immunofluorescence
- enzyme immunoassay examination (EIA) of stool
- polymerase chain reaction (PCR) of stool

Immunoassays of stool for *Cryptosporidium* are more sensitive than staining methods, with immunofluorescence being more sensitive and specific than EIAs (Centers for Disease Control, 2004a). PCR for *Cryptosporidium* is not currently used in most clinical laboratories but is likely to become popular in the future. PCR can distinguish between different *Cryptosporidium* species and is more sensitive than stool microscopy (Morgan et al., 1998).

As well as sending the fax to all local GPs, Emmanuel contacts the emergency department, infectious diseases unit, gastroenterology unit and microbiology laboratory at the local hospital to inform them of the possible outbreak.

In the meantime, GP Dr Jane Wylie receives the stool results from three of her patients with diarrhoea: one child has giardiasis and two have cryptosporidiosis.

She calls one of the infectious diseases physicians to ask about treatment. 'Is tinidazole okay for giardiasis?'

Treatment

The antimicrobials used to treat giardiasis are listed in Table 4.2 Although a wide variety of medications are available, the nitroimidazoles (metronidazole and tinidazole) have been the mainstay of therapy for giardiasis. For pregnant women who need treatment for giardiasis, paromomycin (a nonabsorbable aminoglycoside) can be used.

Combination therapy has been used with some success; however, it tends to be used only when monotherapy fails.

Table 4.2 Antimicrobial agents in the treatment of giardiasis

Antibiotic	Duration of treatment (days)	Approximate efficacy (%)
Metronidazole	5–10	80–100 (median 92)
Tinidazole	Single dose	80–100 (median 92)
Nitazoxanide	3	81–85[†]
Furazolidone	7–10	80–96 (median 92)
Albendazole	5–7	94–100
Mebendazole	5	60–90
Quinacrine	5–7	92–95
Paromomycin	5–10	55–88
Bacitracin zinc	10	95

†Although the efficacy of nitazoxanide in the table is lower than that of metronidazole, it actually had superior efficacy to metronidazole (85% versus 80%) in a randomised trial comparing the two agents (Ortiz et al., 2001).
SOURCE Adapted from Gardner and Hill, 2001

> 'What about the two children with cryptosporidiosis? I had an otherwise healthy adult patient with cryptosporidiosis some years ago and one of your colleagues advised me not to treat him. Was he right?'

Treatment for cryptosporidiosis is currently not recommended for immunocompetent adults (Table 4.3) but Jane's two paediatric patients should be treated. The rationale for not treating immunocompetent adults is probably the result of the longstanding absence of effective treatment and a perception that cryptosporidiosis is a self-limiting illness in this group. Nevertheless, studies have already shown that nitazoxanide (a new agent) can be effective in groups other than young children (Rossignol et al., 2006).

Table 4.3 Cryptosporidiosis: when to treat

Group with cryptosporidiosis	Treatment is recommended
Immunocompetent adults	no
Immunocompetent children (1–11 years)	yes
Immunocompromised	yes

Also, it can be argued that cryptosporidiosis is not a rapidly resolving self-limiting illness in immunocompetent adults. One study found that 40% of immunocompetent adults had relapsing gastrointestinal symptoms and were more likely to experience a variety of bothersome symptoms (joint pains, headache, dizziness, eye pains, fatigue) compared to control subjects (Hunter et al., 2004). Therefore, it is possible that the recommendations to treat cryptosporidiosis will change in the near future to include immunocompetent adults.

The recommended antimicrobial treatment for cryptosporidiosis is shown in Table 4.4.

Table 4.4 Cryptosporidiosis treatment recommendations

Group with cryptosporidiosis	Recommended treatment
Immunocompetent children (1–11 years)	nitazoxanide[†]
HIV-infected patients	antiretroviral therapy (ART)[‡]

[†]Nitazoxanide is a synthetic antiparasitic agent approved for use in immunocompetent children with cryptosporidiosis and usually given over 3 days. It is 56–80% effective in resolving symptoms and 52–67% effective in clearing oocysts from stool. It also improves survival in malnourished children with cryptosporidiosis (Demetriou and Saravolatz, 2005). A study of nitazoxanide in immunocompetent older children and adults also showed excellent clinical resolution (96%) and oocyst clearance (93%) compared to control subjects (Rossignol et al., 2006); however, no official recommendations have been made for its use in this age group. [‡]The recommendation for ART is based on the tendency of AIDS patients with CD4 counts less than 100/mm^3 to develop chronic, severe cryptosporidiosis (Chen et al., 2002). The absence of a recommendation to use specific anti-cryptosporidial antimicrobial agents is because of a combination of poor efficacy and limited data (Benson et al., 2005). This does not mean that antimicrobials such as paromomycin and nitazoxanide will not be used, merely that there is currently little evidence supporting their use.

> 'Could you also refresh my memory about prognosis. What should I advise the parents to expect?'

Prognosis

In immunocompetent adults in the developed world, cryptosporidiosis tends to be a self-limiting illness typically of 5–10 days' duration. Nearly 40%, however, can develop recurrent symptoms. In children in the developing world, most cases also resolve quickly but up to 45% of children will have diarrhoea continuing beyond two weeks. Furthermore, cryptosporidiosis in children in the developing world can cause acute malnutrition, which can be further compounded if there was pre-existing malnutrition or if the disease occurred in infancy. In people with HIV, those with CD4 counts <50mm^3 have reduced survival (Blanshard et al., 1992; Clinton White Jr, 2005; Smith and Corcoran, 2004). The more widespread use of antimicrobial agents for cryptosporidiosis in the future, such as nitazoxanide, may further improve the outcome of the disease.

The prognosis for giardiasis is good in countries where antimicrobial therapy is readily available and where rapid re-infection after treatment is unlikely to occur. Even without antimicrobial treatment, the acute diarrhoeal illness often spontaneously resolves after a median duration of twelve days. A proportion of cases go on to develop chronic diarrhoea though; furthermore, in children with a pre-existing poor nutritional status, concomitant giardiasis can impact on both physical and mental development (Chen et al., 2002; Hill, 2005).

> Jane thanks the physician for her advice and prescribes tinidazole for the child with giardiasis and nitazoxanide for the children with cryptosporidiosis.
> 'One final thing,' says Jane. 'Should I restrict the activities of these children for a period of time?'

Untreated cases of cryptosporidium and giardiasis can continue to excrete infectious cysts for 3–30 days (Smith and Corcoran, 2004) and over 3 months (Gilman et al., 1988), respectively. For this reason, restrictions have been suggested (Centers for Disease Control, 2004a; Centers for Disease Control, 2004b; NSW Health, 2006; NSW Health, 2004):

- not swimming in recreational water facilities for two weeks after the diarrhoea has resolved
- food-handlers not handling food till 48 hours after the diarrhoea has resolved
- avoiding jobs involving the care of the elderly, children or sick people till 48 hours after the diarrhoea has resolved
- avoiding faecal contact during sex
- strict handwashing after going to the toilet

Even though Jane's patients are receiving antimicrobials for their infections, treatment is not 100% effective so it may be wise to enforce these measures.

> One week passes and 18 more cases of giardiasis and cryptosporidiosis are notified to the public health unit. This brings the total to 26 cases. Emmanuel's worst fears are confirmed: there is indeed an outbreak.
> He forms an outbreak team consisting of:
> - team leader
> - epidemiologist
> - public health physician
> - environmental health officer
> - three infectious diseases nurses
> - medical microbiologist

A list of all the cases as they arise during an outbreak with pertinent clinical and demographic data is known as a 'line list'. An abridged form of the line list (excluding clinical features) is shown in Table 4.5.

> Socrates asks, 'What does the line list show us?'

CASE 4 CRYPTOSPORIDIOSIS AND GIARDIASIS

Table 4.5 Abridged line list of the cryptosporidial and giardia outbreaks

Number	Initials	Age	Organism	Sex	School	Postcode	Onset of illness
1	PC	10	G	M	UPS	5	13 March
2	FB	11	G	M	UPS	3	13 March
3	SS	10	G	F	UPS	4	13 March
4	IM	10	C	M	UPS	5	13 March
5	MK	11	G	F	UPS	6	14 March
6	MB	10	G	M	UPS	1	14 March
7	CH	11	G	M	UPS	3	14 March
8	MC	10	G	M	UPS	2	15 March
9	BC	10	C	M	UPS	5	16 March
10	BG	10	G	F	UPS	6	16 March
11	SM	10	C	M	UPS	7	16 March
12	CO	11	G	F	UPS	3	17 March
13	PW	11	C	F	UPS	3	17 March
14	IR	10	G	F	MPS	5	17 March
15	TC	11	C	F	MPS	4	17 March
16	KH	11	G	M	MPS	4	18 March
17	BP	10	C	F	MPS	6	19 March
18	AJ	10	G	F	MPS	6	20 March
19	RL	10	C	F	MPS	2	20 March
20	PK	10	G	M	MPS	2	21 March
21	TG	10	C	M	MPS	1	22 March
22	JK	11	C	M	MPS	4	23 March
23	AB	11	C	F	MPS	1	24 March
24	KS	6	G	F	UPS	4	24 March
25	FC	8	G	M	UPS	5	25 March
26	TB	4	G	F	UPS	3	26 March

C = cryptosporidiosis, G = giardiasis, UPS = Utopia Primary School, MPS = Marcellus Primary School

Public health notification and response

The line list shows that:
- There have been 26 cases from the 13 March to 26 March.
- Apart from cases 24–26, all cases are aged between 10–11 years.
- All cases come from two schools (UPS or MPS)
    Apart from cases 24–26, it appears that the cases from UPS occurred first (13–17 March) followed by the cases from MPS (17–24 March)

> 'So why are cases 24–26 in a different age group? And why did their disease start later?'

Cases 24–26 could be secondary cases. They attend UPS, where the earliest cases occurred, so they may have had close contact with the first UPS cases if they are siblings or share a common school activity. But they still could be primary cases.

> 'Are there any other possible scenarios?'

There are a few possibilities:

- Each school has had a class outing to a common site, with UPS going before MPS. During the outing, the children have been exposed to a common source of infection.
- Cases 1–13 from UPS are the primary cases. They then interacted with the children from MPS, infecting them so that they are secondary cases. However, the interval between the onset of illness in the UPS students and MPS students is only four days, which is probably too short for the incubation periods of cryptosporidiosis and giardiasis.
- The UPS and MPS cases have each been exposed to a source of infection within their own school, such as catered food which is prepared externally and supplied to a number of schools or a mobile petting zoo which visited each school. But this would mean that no other classes within the school were exposed, which seems unlikely.
- The infections have nothing to do with school at all and represent some common source in the community; however, it is hard to

explain why the cases come from only two schools and involve mainly 10–11-year-old children.

> It turns out that cases 24–26 are younger siblings of cases 1–3; therefore, they are probably secondary cases.
> 'So, what is the next step?'

At this stage, the outbreak team has completed the first five steps of the CDC guidelines for investigating an outbreak. The next two steps are to develop and evaluate hypotheses.

This is usually done via an observational study, for example, a case-control study or retrospective cohort study. A common misconception is that these studies can only be done for academic or clinical research. In fact, a good observational study is often necessary to solve the mysteries surrounding an outbreak. However, unlike in a research setting, an outbreak team does not have the luxury of time to carefully design the study—they have to be timely and efficient.

> Socrates tells Emmanuel, 'We don't have any good hypotheses at this point to conduct a study on. How can we find some?'

This is a common problem during an outbreak and has led to the development of a 'hypothesis-generating questionnaire'. This involves questioning the cases about every possible exposure to the infection and trying to identify some common exposures between the cases. Once some common exposures have been identified, the outbreak team can determine which exposure is responsible by using an observational study.

The disadvantage is that this can be very time and resource-consuming, for example, questioning *every* case about *every* meal and snack they have consumed during an exposure period which may be many days in duration—and that is only a small part of the whole questionnaire! Often, smaller public health units do not have the resources to use hypothesis-generating questionnaires and enlist the aid of bigger units.

The hypothesis-generating questionnaire will have to be adjusted for different infections (e.g. water-cooling towers need to be considered during a *Legionella* outbreak and bird exposure during a psittacosis outbreak). A hypothesis-generating questionnaire created by OzFoodNet for *Salmonella* outbreaks can be found at mhcs.health.nsw.gov.au/infect/pdf/salmonellosis_questionnaire.pdf. It is a great example of the detail and work required for such a questionnaire.

> Emmanuel 'borrows' some public health officers from the large Centre for Disease Control in a neighbouring city. With their help, they survey the cases using a hypothesis-generating questionnaire. The secondary cases (cases 24–26) are not included in the survey.
>
> A tiring 24 hours later, after all the data have been collected and analysed, two common exposures are apparent (Table 4.6).
>
> It is revealed that the Grade 5 class from UPS attended the camp from 3–4 March. The Grade 5 class from MPS attended the same camp one week later. Exposure and infection at the camp would also fit in with the incubation period of both infections (i.e. the cases from both schools became ill between 1–2 weeks after attending the camp and petting zoo).
>
> Part of the weekend package involved visiting at a petting zoo for half-an-hour on the way to the camp. The hypothesis that can be tested is 'The children were infected at the petting zoo or at Camp Sparta'.
>
> Emmanuel decides to conduct a retrospective cohort study.
>
> Emmanuel liaises with the schools and emphasises the importance of finding the source of the outbreak to prevent further cases.
>
> Another school group is about to visit the camp and petting zoo.
>
> 'Would that be safe?' Socrates asks Emmanuel.

Table 4.6 The common exposures to the cases of giardiasis and cryptosporidiosis

Exposure	Number exposed (%)
Weekend trip to Camp Sparta	22/23 (96)
Petting zoo on way to Camp Sparta	22/23 (96)

Emmanuel cannot be 100% sure that the camp or petting zoo is the source of the outbreak; however, it would be disastrous if another group of children became infected.

CASE 4 CRYPTOSPORIDIOSIS AND GIARDIASIS

> Emmanuel explains the situation to the owners of the petting zoo and camp, who reluctantly agree to close while the investigation continues.
> During this time, the outbreak team visits the petting zoo and camp to gather information and specimens.
> At the petting zoo, the outbreak team learns from the owner that the children stayed for an hour. During this time they had contact with goats, sheep, calves, ponies and rabbits in a small enclosed field. Before leaving the enclosure, they had to wash their hands in running water from a sink in a shed just next to the field. No food or drink is offered to the children during the hour. None of the animals have been unwell.
> 'Wouldn't that be enough to protect them?' the owner asks.

Handwashing, although it is an excellent practice which must be maintained, does not make infection impossible. Children can became infected during their time in the field, before washing their hands. Also, it is hard to be sure if the children washed their hands properly or not.

> 'Are you sure my zoo is the source of the infection?'

Cryptosporidium is likely to be a zoonosis on the basis of strain characterisation and epidemiological studies (Hunter and Thompson, 2005). Humans have been found to be infected with species where the main host is an animal (typically *C. parvum* but occasionally *C. andersoni, C. suis, C. baileyi, C. meleagridis, C. felis. C. muris* and *C. canis*) (Leoni et al., 2006; Fayer, 2004). Sheep and cattle are probably the most important animals in zoonotic transmission of the protozoan (Chen et al., 2002). Furthermore, both outbreaks and sporadic cases of cryptosporidiosis have been linked to animal contact, including visits to farms (Dawson, 2005). The only unknown factor is whether most zoonotic cases of cryptosporidiosis are due to direct animal contact or indirect contact, such as with water that has been contaminated by infected animals (Olson et al., 2004).

For *G. duodenalis*, three of the four subgroups of assemblages A and B have zoonotic potential (Olson et al., 2004). Nevertheless, zoonotic transmission is likely to be a minor source of infection, especially through direct animal contact. There are some communities with poor sanitation where humans and dogs are co-infected with *Giardia*, but it is unclear whether the humans were the primary source of infection rather than the dogs (Hunter and Thompson,

2005; Traub et al., 2004). Consequently, it is worth looking into the animals at the petting zoo as a source of cryptosporidiosis but it is unlikely to reveal the source of giardiasis.

> The outbreak team collected stool specimens from the animals in the petting zoo for analysis at the laboratory.
> 'But if my animals were infected, wouldn't they be sick?'

Both these protozoa cause a diarrhoeal illness in livestock (Olson et al., 2004) but, as with humans, subclinical infection is likely to occur.

> Having finished at the petting zoo, the outbreak team visits Camp Sparta. There are no livestock or pets here. There is a 20 m swimming pool, which the owner chlorinates once a day. He checks the chlorine levels once per week. The drinking and tap water comes from the same source as the rest of the city. Barbecued meat and stir fried vegetables comprise the main meals at the camp with cereal and canned spaghetti used for breakfast. The outbreak team takes samples of:
>
> - 50 L of water from the swimming pool itself and from the filter backwash
> - the food
> - tap water
>
> Further discussion with the owner reveals that the pool is very popular and that it is continuously being hired by primary schools and childcare centres on a daily basis during the week. He reluctantly discloses that there have been a 'few' faecal accidents with toddlers in the pool.
> When a faecal accident occurs, he quickly cleans the affected water without drawing attention to himself; he never evacuates the pool when this happens.
> The samples are sent to the laboratory that afternoon. On the following day, they receive a call: the tap water, food samples and petting zoo samples are negative but the swimming pool water and filter backwash water are positive for both *Giardia* and *Cryptosporidium* (50 and 100 cysts/50 L respectively)!
> 'Is there any point going ahead with the retrospective cohort study now?' Socrates asks.

> The study is conducted and the result for exposure to the swimming pool is the only significant finding (Table 4.7).
>
> Socrates is confused. 'It must be really rare to have *Giardia* and *Cryptosporidium* infections from swimming pools—I thought that it was only from potable water?'

Table 4.7 Two-by-two table for swimming pool exposure and risk of disease

	Disease	No disease
Swimming pool exposure	22	7
No swimming pool exposure	1	30

Relative risk 23.5 (95% CI 3.4, 163.5)

A combination of epidemiological and microbiological evidence always is preferable to one or the other alone.

Contaminated drinking water is certainly an important source of infection but swimming pools are another well recognised source. In fact, the three most common causes of outbreaks in treated recreational water in the US over a 30-year period were *Cryptosporidium* (32%), *Pseudomonas* (31%) and *Giardia* (9%). Both *Giardia* and *Cryptosporidium* were strongly associated with outbreaks where faecal accidents in the pool were seen or suspected (Craun et al., 2005).

As with contaminated drinking water, the swimmer presumably is infected by swallowing the contaminated pool water.

> 'But the chlorine level of the pool was adequate. Why weren't the cysts killed?'

While chlorination of pools is an effective measure against many organisms, *Giardia* and *Cryptosporidium* oocysts are relatively resistant to standard chlorination levels (1–5 mg/L) (Craun et al., 2005). *Cryptosporidium* oocysts are also difficult to filter.

The pool owner will have to superchlorinate the pool (20 mg/L) for at least 12 hours and maintain a pH of 7.2–7.5 in the water for an appropriate period of time before it can be used. He also will need to be educated about how to minimise the risk of and manage faecal accidents in the pool in the future.

Faecal accidents are an all too common occurrence in swimming pools, particularly those frequented by the very young and the very elderly. For this reason, most countries have guidelines on how pool owners should deal with faecal accidents. Most would advise that the pool be evacuated until the faecal organisms have been removed or neutralised. The pool owner of Camp Sparta did not adhere to this, which is probably why the outbreak occurred (Centers for Disease Control, 2001).

The environmental health officer on the outbreak team will also have to talk to him about general maintenance of the swimming pool, including how often he checks the chlorine level and whether the filtration system is adequate. Most guidelines would recommend recording chlorine levels multiple times per day (NSW Health, 1996), but he only checks it once a week!

> 'There were only 50 and 100 cysts in 50 L of the pool water. Is that enough to cause infection?' Socrates asks.

There are two separate questions here:

- What are the infectious doses of *Giardia* and *Cryptosporidium*?
- Can the concentration of cysts in the pool water be used to determine if the infectious dose was reached?

The ID_{50} (median infective dose) for cryptosporidiosis varies between species of the protozoa and between antibody-positive and negative people. Not surprisingly, studies have discovered a range of ID_{50} from as low as nine oocysts to as high as 1880 (Chappell et al., 1999; Okhuysen et al., 1999). The infectious dose for giardiasis is 10–100 cysts (Larocque et al., 2003), which does not seem like a large amount considering that an infected individual can excrete 1×10^8 *Giardia* cysts per gram of faeces (Roxstrom-Lindquist et al., 2006). In other words, humans can be infected with very small doses of the organisms.

It is difficult to say whether the concentration of cysts in the pool water can be used to determine whether the infectious dose was reached. Certainly, the level of cyst contamination in the Camp Sparta pool is consistent with those seen in previous outbreaks (Ichinohe et al., 2005; Lemmon et al., 1996). What cannot be known is how high the levels were at the time the children were infected. Also, some children may have swallowed a volume of water with a particularly high concentration of cysts compared to the rest of the pool.

CASE 4 CRYPTOSPORIDIOSIS AND GIARDIASIS

> A few weeks later, the outbreak is under control. However Jane still has two children who are symptomatic. The first child had giardiasis and got better after a single dose of tinidazole but the diarrhoea returned five days later. She consults the infectious disease physician again for advice.

Before assuming a relapse of giardiasis, the GP must recall that lactose intolerance can complicate acute giardiasis (Farthing, 1996). Jane should get another three stool samples from the child: if giardiasis is present she should treat it but if the stool cultures are negative she should advise a lactose-free diet for a few weeks and monitor the impact. If the child does have giardiasis again, most clinicians would use the same medication for longer and at a higher dose (if possible), use another single agent or use combination therapy.

Examples of combination therapy that have been used for relapsed giardiasis include albendazole-metronidazole, which was 100% effective in 20 refractory patients (Gardner and Hill, 2001), and quinacrine with metronidazole (or tinidazole) (Nash et al., 2001). Experimentally, *Saccharomyces boulardii* and metronidazole may be useful (Besirbellioglu et al., 2006).

> Jane's second patient had cryptosporidiosis. On top of this, she has HIV with a very resistant virus. Her ART for HIV has been ineffective and her CD4 count is only 20 mm^3. Despite taking a course of nitazoxanide for the cryptosporidiosis, her diarrhoea has not resolved although it is better than it was originally; however, over the last few days, she has developed right upper quadrant pain, fevers and her serum alkaline phosphatase (ALP) and gamma glutamyl transferase (GGT) are slightly elevated.
>
> Jane reads up on the management of cryptosporidiosis and HIV.

There is a strong association with HIV and cryptosporidiosis. In fact, the median prevalence of cryptosporidiosis in people with both diarrhoea and HIV is 32% (Hunter and Nichols, 2002). There is also a strong association between CD4 count and outcome of cryptosporidiosis in HIV patients. Patients with CD4 counts over 200 mm^3 tend to have a self-limiting diarrhoeal illness; those with CD4 counts under 100 mm^3 are more prone to chronic and extra-intestinal disease; and cryptosporidiosis in HIV patients with CD4 counts under 50 mm^3 are more likely to have fulminant disease with a median survival of five weeks (Blanshard et al., 1992; Smith and Corcoran, 2004). As this shows, CD4 cells clearly play a role in clearing cryptosporidium from the bowel (Hunter and Nichols, 2002): having a CD4 count over 53 mm^3 is independently associated with survival in HIV patients with cryptosporidiosis (Colford et al., 1996).

Given the impact of CD4 count on the severity of cryptosporidiosis, it is not surprising that the initiation of ART with the subsequent rise in CD4 count is associated with recovery from cryptosporidiosis (Hommer et al., 2003; Hunter and Nichols, 2002). Specifically, protease inhibitors are the class of ART that seem particularly useful against cryptosporidiosis. The impact of protease inhibitors may be through multiple routes, namely a reduction in sporozoite host cell invasion and parasite development in vitro (Hommer et al., 2003), as well as through increased gamma-IFN and IL-2 activity (Maggi et al., 2001).

ART is the only recommended therapy for cryptosporidiosis (apart from symptomatic anti-diarrhoeal drugs) (Benson et al., 2005). Nevertheless, in patients with chronic cryptosporidiosis where immune reconstitution is not possible, specific anti-cryptosporidial can be used although, because data are lacking or the results too disappointing, there are no specific recommendations. According to Kelly (2003) the therapeutic options for HIV patients with cryptosporidiosis where ART is ineffective are:

- nitazoxanide
- paromomycin
- azithromycin and paromomycin
- roxithromycin
- rifaximin

Nitazoxanide is probably the antimicrobial choice for cryptosporidiosis in HIV patients, although more data are needed to determine its true efficacy, dose and duration in the HIV population. Paromomycin has had mixed results in HIV. Azithromycin has had mixed results when used as a single agent (Smith and Corcoran, 2004). One study showed some clinical improvement and a reduction in oocysts excretion with the use of azithromycin/paromomycin combination therapy. The efficacy of roxithromycin and rifaximin is mainly based on cases reports (Kelly, 2003).

The extra-intestinal manifestations of cryptosporidiosis include (Hunter and Nichols, 2002):

- atypical gastrointestinal disease (anything from asymptomatic gastric colonisation to antral narrowing with gastric outlet obstruction)
- cholangitis
- pancreatitis
- respiratory disease (colonisation of the respiratory tract; it is unknown whether symptomatic disease occurs)

With such a low CD4 count, Jane's patient may well have biliary cryptosporidiosis. The cholangitis in this condition can be due to papillary stenosis alone, intrahepatic sclerosing cholangitis alone, papillary stenosis with sclerosing intrahepatic cholangitis or extrahepatic biliary strictures with/without sclerosing cholangitis (Cello, 1989). The diagnosis can be made through endoscopic retrograde cholangiopancreatography (ERCP) with an ampullary biopsy. ERCP also provides an opportunity to treat the cholangitis with a sphincterotomy and stenting if necessary.

Patients with biliary cryptosporidiosis are more likely to die than those without it, but this probably reflects the extent of their immunosuppression rather than the impact of the biliary disease itself (Vakil et al., 1996).

> The parents of the HIV-positive girl with cryptosporidiosis are beside themselves with worry. They want to know how they can prevent this happening again.

To prevent cryptosporidiosis in patients with HIV, US guidelines (Kaplan et al., 2002) recommend educating the patient about modes of transmission of *Cryptosporidium*, strict handwashing after gardening or soil contact and avoiding several key risk factors. They advise:

- avoiding contact with human and animal faeces
- avoiding sexual contact involving oral–anal activity
- avoiding buying dogs and cats aged <6 months of age but if this is unavoidable then having a vet exclude oocyst excretion in the stool
- avoiding contact with calves and lambs, farms and petting zoos
- avoiding drinking untreated water (e.g. from lakes or rivers)
- avoiding swallowing water during recreational water activities, even in a chlorinated swimming pool
- avoiding using bodies of water that may have been contaminated by animal faeces
- boiling potable water during a municipal water-based outbreak of cryptosporidiosis; however, there are insufficient data to recommend routine boiling of drinking water in the non-outbreak setting

(although some countries do recommend routine boiling of water for HIV patients)
- avoiding fruit juices that are unpasteurised
- avoiding eating raw oysters

With regard to medical prophylaxis against cryptosporidiosis, there are no official recommendations; however, rifabutin may reduce rates of infection (Fichtenbaum et al., 2000).

> 'After all our work, we still haven't accounted for one case. Is that common?' Socrates asks.

In a perfect world, every case should have been linked to attending the camp and swimming in the pool but this is not what happens in real life. There are often unexplained cases at the end of the investigation which will never be solved. Similarly, in a food-borne outbreak, there will always be primary cases who became ill despite never eating a dish that was clearly identified epidemiologically and microbiologically as the only source of infection.

> A GP calls Emmanuel: 'One of my patients is the brother of a child with *Giardia* but has been asymptomatic. He underwent screening of his stool and was found to have asymptomatic carriage of *Giardia*. Should I treat it even though he is fine?'

The two common reasons for treating most infections are:
- to cure the symptomatic illness and make the patient feel better
- to prevent transmission of the infection to others

In this case, there is no symptomatic illness to cure, so the issue is whether the sibling needs to be treated to make him non-infectious. The answer depends on how common *Giardia* is locally. For example, in a hyperendemic area in Peru, 44 children with giardiasis were effectively treated with tinidazole. Within six months of treatment, 98% of the children became re-infected with *Giardia* and excreted infectious cysts for a mean of over three months (Gilman et al., 1988). In other words, there is a good argument for not treating asymptomatic carriage of *Giardia* in a hyperendemic region because the risk of rapid re-infection is so high.

However, in countries with low rates of giardiasis, this sibling could be responsible for transmission to many other people, particularly children; therefore, it would be reasonable to treat him.

> The GP says, 'Thanks for that. On a more personal note, I am going camping with my son this weekend. We will be drinking water from rivers and streams. I hate using iodine and chlorine tablets, so I just wanted to know if boiling fresh water is enough to kill the *Giardia* and *Cryptosporidium* cysts?'

Giardia cysts are inactivated by boiling or heating water to a minimum of 70°C for at least 10 minutes (Ongerth et al., 1989). Cryptosporidial oocysts lose their infectivity above 65°C (Sunnotel et al., 2006).

References

Aronson, N.E., Cheney, C., Rholl, V., Burris, D. et al (2001) Biliary giardiasis in a patient with human immunodeficiency virus. *Journal of Clinical Gastroenterology*, 33, 167–70.

Aziz, H., Beck, C. E., Lux, M.F. et al (2001) A comparison study of different methods used in the detection of *Giardia lamblia*. *Clinical Laboratory Science*, 14, 150–54.

Benson, C.A., Kaplan, J.E., Masur, H. et al (2005) Treating opportunistic infections among HIV-infected adults and adolescents: Recommendations from CDC, National Institutes of Health, and the HIV Medicine Association/Infectious Diseases Society of America. *Clinical Infectious Diseases*, 40, S131–235.

Besirbellioglu, B.A., Ulcay, A., Can, M. et al (2006) *Saccharomyces boulardii* and infection due to *Giardia lamblia*. *Scandinavian Journal of Infectious Diseases*, 38, 479–81.

Blanshard, C., Jackson, A.M., Shanson, D.C. et al (1992) Cryptosporidiosis in HIV-seropositive patients. *Quarterly Journal of Medicine*, 85, 813–23.

Cello, J.P. (1989) Acquired immunodeficiency syndrome cholangiopathy: spectrum of disease. *American Journal of Medicine*, 86, 539–46.

Centers for Disease Control and Prevention (2005) *Steps of an Outbreak Investigation*. Centers for Disease Control and Prevention; Atlanta

Centers for Disease Control and Prevention (2004a) *Cryptosporidiosis*. Centers for Disease Control and Prevention; Atlanta

Centers for Disease Control and Prevention (2004b) *Giardiasis*. Centers for Disease Control and Prevention; Atlanta

Centers for Disease Control (2001) Responding to fecal accidents in disinfected swimming venues. MMWR *Morbidity and Mortality Weekly Report*, 50, 416–17.

Chappell, C.L., Okhuysen, P.C., Sterling, C. R. et al (1999) Infectivity of *Cryptosporidium parvum* in healthy adults with pre-existing anti-*C. parvum* serum immunoglobulin G. *American Journal of Tropical Medicine and Hygiene*, 60, 157–64.

Chen, X. M., Keithly, J.S., Paya, C.V. et al (2002) Cryptosporidiosis. *New England Journal of Medicine*, 346, 1723–31.

Clinton White Jr, A. (2005) Cryptosporidiosis. In G.L. Mandell, Bennett, JE., Dolin, R. (eds). *Principles and Practice of Infectious Diseases.* Churchill Livingstone; Philadelphia

Colford, J.M., Jr., Tager, I.B., Hirozawa, A.M. et al (1996) Cryptosporidiosis among patients infected with human immunodeficiency virus. Factors related to symptomatic infection and survival. *American Journal of Epidemiology*, 144, 807-1-6.

Cox, F.E. (2002) History of human parasitology. *Clinical Microbiology Reviews*, 15, 595–612.

Craun, G.F., Calderon, R.L., Craun, M.F. (2005) Outbreaks associated with recreational water in the United States. *International Journal of Environmental Health Research*, 15, 243–62.

D'anchino, M., Orlando, D., De Feudis, L. (2002) *Giardia lamblia* infections become clinically evident by eliciting symptoms of irritable bowel syndrome. *Journal of Infection*, 45, 169–72.

Dawson, D. (2005) Foodborne protozoan parasites. *International Journal of Food Microbiology*, 103, 207–27.

Demetriou, L.M., Saravolatz, L.D. (2005) Nitazoxanide: a new thiazolide antiparasitic agent. *Clinical Infectious Diseases*, 40, 1173–80.

Farthing, M.J. (1996) Giardiasis. *Gastroenterology Clinics of North America*, 25, 493–515.

Fayer, R. (2004) Cryptosporidium: a water-borne zoonotic parasite. *Veterinary Parasitology*, 126, 37–56.

Fichtenbaum, C.J., Zackin, R., Feinberg, J. et al (2000) Rifabutin but not clarithromycin prevents cryptosporidiosis in persons with advanced HIV infection. *AIDS*, 14, 2889–93.

Gardner, T.B., Hill, D R. (2001) Treatment of giardiasis. *Clinical Microbiology Reviews*, 14, 114–28.

Gilman, R.H., Marquis, G.S., Miranda, E. et al (1988) Rapid reinfection by *Giardia lamblia* after treatment in a hyperendemic Third World community. *Lancet*, 1, 343–45.

Graczyk, T.K., Knight, R., Tamang, L. (2005) Mechanical transmission of human protozoan parasites by insects. *Clinical Microbiology Reviews*, 18, 128–32.

Hiatt, R.A., Markell, E.K., Ng, E. (1995) How many stool examinations are necessary to detect pathogenic intestinal protozoa? *American Journal of Tropical Medicine and Hygiene*, 53, 36–39.

Hill, D.R. (2005) *Giardia lamblia*. In Mandell G.L., Bennett, J.E., Dolin, R (eds). *Principles and Practice of Infectious Diseases.* Churchill Livingstone; Philadelphia

Hommer, V., Eichholz, J., Petry, F. (2003) Effect of antiretroviral protease inhibitors alone, and in combination with paromomycin, on the excystation, invasion and in vitro development of *Cryptosporidium parvum*. *Journal of Antimicrobial Chemo*therapy, 52, 359–64.

Hunter, P.R., Thompson, R.C. (2005) The zoonotic transmission of *Giardia* and *Cryptosporidium*. *International Journal of Parasitology*, 35, 1181–90.

Hunter, P.R., Hughes, S., Woodhouse, S. et al (2004) Health sequelae of human cryptosporidiosis in immunocompetent patients. *Clinical Infectious Diseases*, 39, 504–10.

Hunter, P.R., Nichols, G. (2002) Epidemiology and clinical features of *Cryptosporidium* infection in immunocompromised patients. *Clinical Microbiology Reviews*, 15, 145–54.

Ichinohe, S., Fukushima, T., Kishida, K., et al. (2005) Secondary transmission of cryptosporidiosis associated with swimming pool use. *Japanese Journal of Infectious Diseases*, 58, 400–1.

Kaplan, J. E., Masur, H., Holmes, K. K. (2002) Guidelines for preventing opportunistic infections among HIV-infected persons—2002. Recommendations of the U.S. Public Health Service and the Infectious Diseases Society of America. *MMWR Recommendations and Reports*, 51, 1-5-2.

Kelly, M. (2003) Cryptosporidiosis. In Hoy, J., Lewin, S. (eds.) *HIV management in Australasia: a guide for clinical care. 1st ed.* Australasian Society for HIV Medicine.

Larocque, R., Nakagura, K., Lee, P. et al (2003) Oral immunization of BALB/c mice with *Giardia duodenalis* recombinant cyst wall protein inhibits shedding of cysts. *Infection and Immunity*, 71, 5662–69.

Lemmon, J.M., Mcanulty, J.M., Bawden-Smith, J. (1996) Outbreak of cryptosporidiosis linked to an indoor swimming pool. *Medical Journal of Australia*, 165, 613–16.

Leoni, F., Amar, C., Nichols, G. et al (2006) Genetic analysis of *Cryptosporidium* from 2,414 humans with diarrhoea in England between 1985 and 2000. *Journal of Medical Microbiology*, 55, 703–07.

Letts, M., Davidson, D., Lalonde, F. (1998) Synovitis secondary to giardiasis in children. *American Journal of Orthopedics*, 27, 451–54.

Maggi, P., Larocca, A.M., Ladisa, N. et al (2001) Opportunistic parasitic infections of the intestinal tract in the era of highly active antiretroviral therapy: is the CD4(+) count so important? *Clinical Infectious Diseases*, 33, 1609–11.

Mcknight, J.T., Tietze, P.E. (1992) Dermatologic manifestations of giardiasis. *Journal of the American Board of Family Practice*, 5, 425–28.

Mildvan, D., Gelb, A.M., William, D. (1977) Venereal transmission of enteric pathogens in male homosexuals. Two case reports. *Journal of the American Medical Association*, 238, 1387–89.

Morgan, U.M., Pallant, L., Dwyer, B.W. et al (1998) Comparison of PCR and microscopy for detection of *Cryptosporidium parvum* in human fecal specimens: clinical trial. *Journal of Clinical Microbiology*, 36, 995–98.

Nash, T.E., Ohl, C.A., Thomas, E. et al (2001) Treatment of patients with refractory giardiasis. *Clinical Infectious Diseases*, 33, 22–28.

NSW Health (2006) *Cryptosporidiosis: response protocol for NSW public health units.*

NSW Health (2004) *Giardiasis: response protocol for NSW public health units.*

NSW Health (1996) *Public swimming pool and spa pool guidelines.*

Okhuysen, P.C., Chappell, C.L., Crabb, J. H. et al (1999) Virulence of three distinct *Cryptosporidium parvum* isolates for healthy adults. *Journal of Infectious Diseases*, 180, 1275–81.

Olson, M.E., O'Handley, R.M., Ralston, B. J. et al (2004) Update on *Cryptosporidium* and *Giardia* infections in cattle. *Trends in Parasitology*, 20, 185–91.

Ongerth, J. E., Johnson, R.L., Macdonald, S.C. et al (1989) Back-country water treatment to prevent giardiasis. *American Journal of Public Health*, 79, 1633–37.

Ortiz, J.J., Ayoub, A., Gargala, G. et al (2001) Randomized clinical study of nitazoxanide compared to metronidazole in the treatment of symptomatic giardiasis in children from Northern Peru. *Alimentary Pharmacology Therapeutics*, 15, 1409–15.

Pickering, L.K., Woodward, W.E., Dupont, H.L. et al (1984) Occurrence of *Giardia lamblia* in children in day care centers. *Journal of Pediatrics*, 104, 522–26.

Rossignol, J.F., Kabil, S. M., El-Gohary, Y. et al (2006) Effect of nitazoxanide in diarrhea and enteritis caused by *Cryptosporidium* species. *Clinical Gastroenterology and Hepatology*, 4, 320–24.

Roxstrom-Lindquist, K., Palm, D., Reiner, D. et al (2006) *Giardia* immunity—an update. *Trends in Parasitology*, 22, 26–31.

Smith, H.V. Corcoran, G.D. (2004) New drugs and treatment for cryptosporidiosis. *Current Opinion in Infectious Diseases*, 17, 557–64.

Sunnotel, O., Lowery, C.J., Moore, J.E. et al (2006) *Cryptosporidium*. *Letters in Applied Microbiology*, 43, 7–16.

Thompson, R.C. (2004) The zoonotic significance and molecular epidemiology of *Giardia* and giardiasis. *Veterinary Parasitology*, 126, 15–35.

Traub, R.J., Monis, P.T., Robertson, I. et al (2004) Epidemiological and molecular evidence supports the zoonotic transmission of *Giardia* among humans and dogs living in the same community. *Parasitology*, 128, 253–62.

Vakil, N.B., Schwartz, S.M., Buggy, B.P. et al (1996) Biliary cryptosporidiosis in HIV-infected people after the waterborne outbreak of cryptosporidiosis in Milwaukee. *New England Journal of Medicine*, 334, 19–23.

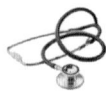

Case 5 Dengue fever
Otto has a fever …

Dengue fever at a glance …

- **Agent:** family Flaviviridae; genus *Flavivirus*; species dengue virus
- **Geographical distribution:** endemic to Asia, Africa, Central and South America and the South Pacific; autochthonous transmission can occur in non-endemic regions where the mosquito vector is present
- **Mode of transmission:** mosquito-borne infection; principal vector is the *Aedes aegypti* mosquito; *A. albopictus* and other Aedes mosquitoes can transmit the disease
- **Person-to-person transmission:** nosocomial transmission is rare but documented
- **Incubation period:** 4–7 days (3–14 days)
- **Clinical features:** most infections are minimally symptomatic or completely asymptomatic, especially in children <15 years; classic dengue consists of fever, severe myalgias, arthralgias, rash, retro-orbital pain and headache; severe infections manifest as dengue haemorrhagic fever or dengue shock syndrome
- **Identification:** most commonly, detecting a positive dengue virus IgM in primary infection after 4–5 days but serology in secondary infections can be more difficult to interpret; detection of the dengue virus through culture, antigen detection, nucleic acid hybridisation and reverse transcriptase polymerase chain reaction (RT-PCR), if available
- **Treatment:** supportive only
- **Post-exposure prophylaxis:** nil
- **Vaccine:** still at the research stage

OTTO HAS A FEVER ...

Main characters

Dr Barbra Wall	infectious diseases registrar
Mr Otto Trump	man who may have dengue fever
Dr Branson Hughes	public health physician
Mr Richard Parker	medical student doing an infectious diseases rotation
Mrs Leanne Trump	Otto's wife
Dr Annabel Marks	public health physician

Dr Barbra Wall, the infectious diseases registrar, is called to review a febrile patient in the emergency department.

There is a letter from the GP:

Dear Dr,

Thank you reviewing Mr Otto Trump, a 41-year-old man, who might have dengue fever. He had been holidaying in Samoa for three weeks and returned home two days ago. He developed fevers yesterday and came to see me. I ordered an urgent dengue IgM. Fortunately, the dengue reference lab (your hospital lab) is close to my practice and they were able to process the specimen quickly. I received the result today: he is IgM positive for dengue (IgG pending).

Interestingly, he had a dengue-like illness three months ago while in Sri Lanka but no blood tests were ever performed. He has recently been diagnosed with rheumatoid arthritis and is currently on a non-steroidal anti-inflammatory drug (NSAID) but he is otherwise well.

Thank you for your advice about diagnosis and management.

'Can you jog my memory—what's dengue fever?' asks her medical student, Mr Richard Parker.

What is dengue fever?

Dengue fever is a clinical syndrome caused by a flavivirus transmitted by mosquitoes. The word dengue is Spanish and refers to the mannerisms presumably related to the patient's stiff gait and fear of motion; however, the term is likely to have originated from the Swahili phrase 'ki denga pepo' (a kind of sudden cramp-like seizure from an evil spirit or plague) (Rigau-Pérez, 1998).

'That's right. I remember lectures on it last year. But isn't it an arbovirus, not a flavivirus?'

The term arbovirus is a shortened form of arthropod-borne virus, that is, a viral infection transmitted by invertebrates, usually blood-sucking insects. Since dengue fever is transmitted by mosquitoes, it certainly is an arbovirus but it also belongs to the family Flaviviridae: therefore, dengue virus is both an arbovirus and a flavivirus.

Classic dengue fever has an incubation period of 4–7 days (3–14 days) and is characterised by the following (Wilder-Smith and Schwartz, 2005):

- fever (can be biphasic)
- retro-orbital pain
- headache
- severe myalgias and arthralgias (hence the name 'break-bone fever')
- rash

Accompanying these classic symptoms can be lymphadenopathy, flushed face, conjunctival injection, sore throat with injected pharynx, and gastrointestinal and respiratory symptoms. Rarely, rhabdomyolysis, neurological syndromes and myocarditis can occur.

However, dengue infections can have a wide variety of presentations and the majority of cases are minimally symptomatic or completely asymptomatic, especially in children <15 years (Rigau-Pérez et al., 1998).

Otto indeed confirms that he became unwell two days ago, one day after returning from Samoa, with fevers, shoulder and lower back myalgias and a retro-orbital headache. He hasn't had a rash and his physical examination is remarkable only for a fever of 39.5°C and a heart rate of 78/minute.

'I'm surprised he's not tachycardic (heart rate >100/minute) with such a high fever,' says Richard. 'Why is that?'

Differential diagnoses

In most infections, patients with a fever as high as 39.5°C should be tachycardic. However, some infections can cause a relative bradycardia, which can be helpful in pointing to a diagnosis. These infections include typhoid fever, Q fever, Legionnaire's disease, pneumonia due to

Chlamydia spp., dengue fever and sandfly fever (Ostergaard et al., 1996; Wittesjo et al., 1999). Formulae have been described that assess for relative bradycardia (Cunha, 2000).

But before attributing a relative bradycardia to infection, make sure that the patient does not have a cardiac pacemaker and is not on medications that can cause bradycardia, such as beta-blockers, calcium channel blockers or digoxin.

Wilder-Smith and Schwartz (2005) list some of the differential diagnoses for fever, headache and myalgia:

- typhoid fever (irrespective of vaccination status for typhoid)
- malaria (irrespective of the use of anti-malarial prophylaxis)
- leptospirosis
- Epstein-Barr virus (EBV)
- cytomegalovirus (CMV)
- HIV seroconversion illness
- Chikungunya (a mosquito-borne alphavirus infection)
- West Nile virus
- measles
- rubella

There are features that would make dengue fever more likely. A Thai study demonstrated that the combination of a positive tourniquet test and leukopenia of <5000/mm^3 had a sensitivity of only 74% but a specificity of 85% and positive predictive value of 83% (Kalayanarooj et al., 1999). The tourniquet test reflects capillary fragility (Cao et al., 2002). To perform a tourniquet test, place a sphygmomanometer cuff around the arm, inflate the cuff to between the systolic and diastolic blood pressures for five minutes and observe a 2.5 × 2.5 cm area on the volar aspect of the forearm just distal to the antecubital fossa. If ≥20 petechiae appear within that area, the test is positive.

Barbra performs the tourniquet test on Otto and it is positive. She orders a number of blood tests, including thick and thin films for malaria, a Monospot, two sets of blood cultures and baseline serology for HIV, CMV, EBV and leptospirosis. Results of a full blood count, electrolytes and liver function tests taken earlier are now available (Table 5.1). Richard asks whether these are consistent with dengue.

CASE 5 DENGUE FEVER

Table 5.1 Otto's full blood count, electrolytes and liver function tests (normal ranges in brackets)

White cell count: 2.2×10^9/L ($4-11 \times 10^9$/L)
Platelets: 130×10^9/L ($150-400 \times 10^9$/L)
ALT: 100 IU (<45 IU)
AST: 115 IU (<45 IU)
Sodium: 131 mM (135–145 mM)
Blood film comment: atypical lymphocytes seen

Investigations

Although leukopenia is not exclusive to dengue fever, the combination of leukopenia and a positive tourniquet test means there is a >80% chance of the diagnosis being correct.

Thrombocytopenia is commonly seen in a number of infections in travellers, including dengue fever, where it may appear in the first few days of illness. The presence of atypical lymphocytes on the blood film favours a viral aetiology. Doctors, especially those in non-endemic regions for dengue, would most commonly associate atypical lymphocytes with infectious mononucleosis due to EBV or CMV but dengue fever is a recognised cause.

Mild or occasionally large rises in liver transaminases are non-specific for dengue fever but are seen in up to two-thirds of patients (Souza et al., 2004). Hyponatraemia is another non-specific sign.

In conclusion, these results, along with Otto's history, support dengue fever but are not diagnostic.

Richard shakes his head and says to Barbra, 'Why are you hesitant to call this dengue fever? Remember that the GP checked his dengue IgM yesterday and it was positive. You can't deny that.'

The IgM enzyme-linked immunosorbent assay (ELISA) can be a useful diagnostic tool for acute dengue fever and is one of the most commonly used tests to confirm a diagnosis of dengue. However, as Wilder-Smith and Schwartz (2005) point out, it has its limitations:

- it is usually positive only after 4–5 days of illness
- false-positives can occur due to cross-reactivity with other flaviviruses (e.g. Japanese encephalitis)
- false-positives can occur in patients with rheumatoid factor
- IgM may remain elevated for 3–6 months after an acute episode

Barbra therefore has three reasons for questioning the relevance of the positive IgM:

- Otto has rheumatoid arthritis and therefore is rheumatoid factor-positive
- his dengue-like episode three months ago could explain the positive result
- one day's illness is too early for a dengue IgM ELISA to become positive

Interpretation of dengue serology requires understanding the primary and secondary antibody responses (Teles et al., 2005). A primary antibody response occurs in a primary dengue infection. After a few days of infection, IgM is produced in large amounts, peaking at about two weeks but persisting for many months. Unfortunately, the antibodies cannot be detected until Day 4–5 of illness. Low levels of IgG are produced just after the IgM.

In the early stages of primary infection, the infecting serotype of dengue can be determined because the IgM is serotype-specific. However, it can be difficult to determine the serotype in the convalescent stage. This is because individuals who have encountered flaviviruses previously, either through immunisation (e.g. with Japanese encephalitis or yellow fever vaccine) or through previous infection (including infection with another dengue serotype) can produce cross-reactive antibodies. This is called a secondary antibody response.

In these people, there is something of a role reversal: a large IgG response occurs and peaks at about two weeks, decreasing over 3–6 months. However, the IgM response is much lower, sometimes not even detectable, and of shorter duration compared to the IgG response. The only diagnosis that can be made is of acute flavivirus infection.

However, there are other serologic techniques used in dengue fever, including enzyme immunoassay (EIA or ELISA), haemagglutination inhibition (HI), complement fixation test (CFT), dot-blot immunoassay and neutralisation tests (Teles et al., 2005). EIA is a sensitive assay that can determine whether dengue virus is responsible or not and differentiate primary from secondary infections, using the IgM/IgG ratio. HI is a very sensitive test but has problems with cross-reactivity and often requires paired baseline and convalescent sera for a diagnosis. CFT can only detect antibody 7–14 days after the onset of illness.

Neutralisation tests use live virus and so require biosafety level 3 precautions. In a primary dengue infection, neutralisation will detect moderately specific antibodies in the convalescent stages. In secondary infection, cross-reactivity can occur, with neutralising antibodies from the first dengue infection often higher than those responsible for the current one. Neutralisation is prone to inhibition by serum factors other than the dengue antibody and usually requires paired sera. Hybrid chimeric viruses have been used in neutralisation tests to differentiate between flaviviruses.

Dot-blot immunoassay can be very sensitive and specific, although interpretation may require experienced scientists in a large laboratory. Dengue virus can also be diagnosed through culture, antigen detection and genome detection (using nucleic acid hybridisation and reverse transcriptase polymerase chain reaction [RT-PCR]). There are several issues with culture. It takes days to weeks to produce a result, the dengue virus is heat labile (and so may not survive transportation), it takes time and money to equip a laboratory, and there is a lower yield in secondary infection because of the high antibody titres. Dengue viral antigen has the advantage of being detectable for longer than viral RNA.

RT-PCR is more sensitive and faster than viral culture techniques and can be used as an epidemiologic tool to rapidly detect infecting serotypes. It is ≥90% sensitive in detecting the dengue virus in serum early in the disease; however, after one week, the sensitivity plummets to only around 10%, presumably due to clearing of the viraemia (Teles et al., 2005).

Otto's serum is also tested for dengue virus RT-PCR. The hospital's lab is the national reference laboratory for dengue virus and is doing a dengue RT-PCR run tomorrow, so Barbra will have the luxury of a prompt result.

'Will any radiological tests help?' Richard asks.

Radiological investigations have traditionally played little, if any, role in the diagnosis of dengue fever. A recent study examined the role of abdominal ultrasound (Venkata Sai et al., 2005), concluding that the sensitivity of

- gall bladder wall thickening (at Days 2–3 or 5–7 after the onset of fever) was 100%
- ascites (at Days 5–7 after the onset of fever) was 96%
- right pleural effusions (at Days 5–7 after the onset of fever) was 87.5%

However, specificity could not be determined because of the absence of a control group.

> Barbra is called to assess Otto the following day because of a rash. He is on no medications apart from paracetamol (acetaminophen) for pain. Barbra suspects a dengue fever rash.

The dengue fever rash, which can be itchy and uncomfortable, may not appear until a few days into the illness. Rigau-Perez et al. (1998) list three types of rash:

- petechial rash
- confluent erythematous rash intermingled with patches of normal skin
- maculopapular rash

> Otto has a confluent itchy erythematous rash consistent with dengue fever. He is still febrile but, overall, feels better. He also tells Barbra and Richard that he had a nosebleed this morning, but it resolved pretty quickly.
>
> Richard looks alarmed. 'Epistaxis—he must be developing dengue haemorrhagic fever!'

The term dengue *haemorrhagic* fever (DHF) has led to a misconception that any haemorrhage in a patient with dengue fever heralds the onset of DHF. However, patients with classic dengue fever can have haemorrhagic manifestations, such as epistaxis and gum bleeding, and occasionally serious bleeding episodes can occur.

> 'So, how do we know if Otto has DHF?'

CASE 5 DENGUE FEVER

The WHO's case definition for DHF requires four manifestations and is outlined below (World Health Organization, 2005)

- current or recent fever AND
- platelet count ≤100 000/mm^3 AND
- haemorrhagic manifestations AND
- objective evidence of plasma leakage caused by increased vascular permeability, manifested by at least one of the following:
    - elevated haematocrit (≥20% over baseline or a similar drop after intravenous fluid replacement)
    - pleural or other effusion (e.g. ascites)
    - low protein

However, this definition has two limitations. First, hospitals with limited laboratory facilities, such as many in the developing world, would not be able to check haematocrits and platelet counts. Second, dengue patients with plasma leakage may initially not have the specified degree of thrombocytopenia.

One suggestion has been to stop using the term DHF and just use the terms 'dengue fever' and 'severe dengue fever', where severe dengue fever refers to dengue infection with increased vascular permeability (World Health Organization, 2005).

> So, Otto does not have DHF at the moment. However, Richard has more questions. 'Is DHF the same as dengue shock syndrome (DSS)? I often hear of the two terms being used together.'

DSS is a severe form of DHF. It is common to see the terms being used together (i.e. DHF/DSS). The WHO's (2005) case definition is:

- dengue haemorrhagic fever AND
- rapid and weak pulse AND
- narrow pulse pressure (<20 mm Hg) OR systolic hypotension (<80 mm Hg if age <5 years; <90 mm Hg if age ≥5 years) AND
- cold clammy skin and restlessness

Clinical signals of impending DSS include severe abdominal pain, restlessness, sweating, prostration, tender hepatomegaly and a change from fever to hypothermia (Rigau-Pérez et al., 1998).

Otto's wife, Leanne, is naturally concerned about his condition and asks, 'Doctor, what drugs can you give him to treat the dengue fever?'

Treatment

There is no in vivo evidence to support the use of antiviral agents, corticosteroids or drugs such as carbazochrome that reduce vascular permeability in the management of uncomplicated dengue fever. (Wilder-Smith and Schwartz, 2005). Analgesics are used for pain and antipyretics for fever. The management of DHF and DSS is purely supportive, but supportive measures—such as whether to use a colloid or crystalloid IV fluid—have been extensively researched and documented (World Health Organization, 1997a).

It is important to check haematocrits and blood counts daily to monitor for impending DHF or DSS.

'Is my husband going to die, Doctor?'

Prognosis

Although people with dengue fever feel awful, it is usually a self-limiting illness that resolves without complication. Death is a rare event. Even DHF can have a mortality rate <1% in well-resourced units with medical staff experienced in its management (in other settings, however, the mortality can be as high as 10–20%). DSS can have a mortality rate around 40% (Wilder-Smith and Schwartz, 2005).

Barbra tells Leanne that they will watch him closely, but he should be fine if he just has dengue fever.

'But how do you know he won't develop the haemorrhagic fever, Doctor?'

The risk factors for DHF are not fully understood but include (Halstead, 2005; Kalayanarooj and Nimmannitya, 2005; Stephens et al., 2002; Stephenson, 2005):

Age Young children are the most susceptible, with a slight increased risk in older patients. Ninety-five percent of cases of DHF/DSS occur in children <15 years. Older teenagers and young adults have the lowest risk. Plasma leakage plays an important role in DHF, so the physiological changes in microvascular permeability seen with age may explain the susceptibility of young children.

Repeat dengue infections Pre-existing antibodies from an earlier dengue infection prevent re-infection with that same serotype. However, they are not capable of neutralising infection with a different serotype. These pre-existing antibodies can still generate an immune response, which can be deleterious to the host. According to the antibody enhancement hypothesis, the presence of Fcγ receptors on cells is critical for increasing both the number of infecting cells and the level of viraemia, through the creation of a co-receptor on the permissive cell.

Viral genotypes with increased pathogenicity The Asian strain (genotype) of DENV-2 is supposedly more virulent than its American DENV-2 counterpart, causing more cases of DHF. In dengue patients from Peru, serum antibodies to DENV-1 infection were able to neutralise American DENV-2 viruses more effectively than Asian DENV-2 viruses (Kochel et al, 2002). However, the evidence for genotypes with increased pathogenicity is tenuous. For example, the supposedly less virulent American strain of DENV-2 has caused DHF in Venezuela and the Pacific Islands. Also, the American DENV-2 genotype has been associated with high transmission rates of almost 90%, a characteristic typically associated with more virulent strains.

Genetic factors Studies on South-East Asian populations show that HLA class I alleles influence the outcome of subsequent dengue infections in individuals previously infected with another serotype. Also, people of African descent living in the Americas are less susceptible because of the presence of a resistance gene.

Nutritional status Probably as a result of their reduced cellular immunity, malnourished children are less likely to develop dengue fever or DHF. Conversely, obese children are more prone. However, if malnourished children do develop DHF, they are more likely to experience a severe form (i.e. DSS).

Otto continues to improve over the next three days. However, after a ward round a worried-looking nurse comes over. 'Doctor, I took the patient's blood earlier and accidentally stuck myself. Could I get dengue fever from the needlestick injury (NSI)?'

Nosocomial transmission of dengue fever through NSI has been documented (Wagner et al., 2004). However, it is now Day 6 of Otto's illness: his level of viraemia is probably quite low, making the risk of transmission very small.

Since the risk is low and there is no post-exposure prophylaxis for dengue fever, Barbra can only educate the nurse about the symptoms of dengue fever and ask her to seek help if she becomes ill. As with any occupational exposure, both nurse and patient need to be assessed for the risk of hepatitis B and C and HIV transmission.

> On the following day, Otto's platelet count is almost normal and he has been afebrile for 48 hours. He is discharged home, grateful for the medical care but annoyed at himself for getting dengue.
>
> 'I bet you I got it at night. I used to sleep without covering myself with sheets and I didn't use mosquito nets because I'm claustrophobic. I barely got bitten during the day.'
>
> Is Otto right about being infected at night?

The *Aedes* genus of mosquitoes is the vector for dengue virus, with *A. aegypti* the main vector. Only the female mosquito can transmit infection to humans, and they are daytime feeders. Therefore Otto is incorrect in believing that he was infected at night.

> 'I love travelling to tropical countries, and I will continue to go despite this attack of dengue. What precautions should I take in the future?'

Wilder-Smith and Schwartz (2005) recommend that travellers to dengue-endemic regions should use measures to avoid mosquito bites such as:

- permethrin-impregnated clothing, with as little skin exposure as possible
- DEET (N,N-diethyl-methylbenzamide) repellents
- insecticides

Returned travellers who have recovered from a primary dengue infection often voice concerns about the risk of developing DHF with subsequent travel. Infection with one dengue serotype provides lifelong immunity against that serotype. Therefore, if travellers are returning to a region where only that one serotype exists (a hypoendemic region), there is little or no risk of DHF.

Even if they are travelling to a region with different serotypes to their primary infection, the overall risk of developing DHF is likely to be low. Using the figures of 100 million cases of dengue fever per year and 250 000 cases of DHF per year, the overall risk of DHF is 1:400 (0.0025) (Gibbons and Vaughn, 2002). However, this total number of 100 million cases per year is likely to be an underestimate, given the number of asymptomatic or minimally symptomatic cases, so the risk of developing DHF is probably even lower. If the traveller is an adult rather than a young child, this further reduces the risk of DHF.

While anti-mosquito measures do not prevent mosquito-borne infections, they do reduce the risk and travellers are more likely to be compliant with anti-mosquito measures for the short duration of their trip than longstanding inhabitants are.

> 'Will I be completely safe if I spend as much time indoors as possible?'

Being indoors does not make people completely safe because *A. aegypti* mosquitoes spend resting time indoors (for example, under furniture and in closets) so they are not just found in the outdoor environment (World Health Organization, 1997b).

> 'What about a vaccine?' Otto asks.

Unlike with the other flaviviruses (Japanese encephalitis and yellow fever), there is no vaccine for dengue virus. However, research is ongoing. Live attenuated vaccines have been tested in human subjects with encouraging results but, until their safety and efficacy is fully understood, such vaccines will not be commercially available (Stephenson, 2005).

> 'Do we need to let the public health unit know about him?' asks Richard.

Public health notification and response

Dengue fever is notifiable in most regions of the world, whether the infection is endemic or not. This reflects the growing global problem of dengue, with the vector and virus becoming more widespread, more epidemics occurring, DHF appearing in new regions, and more than one serotype appearing in the same region (Wilder-Smith and Schwartz, 2005).

> Barbra informs the local public health physician, Dr Branson Hughes. A few weeks later, Branson is attending a routine teleconference with other public health figures from around the country to discuss weekly disease surveillance. Out of interest, Richard attends. One representative, Dr Annabel Marks, informs everyone that her district has had autochthonous transmission of dengue.
> 'What does that mean?' Richard asks.

Autochthonous transmission is the introduction of dengue fever to regions where the virus is not endemic but the vector is present. It usually occurs when an infected traveller returns to the region and is bitten by a mosquito. The infected mosquito can now transmit the virus to other people. Autochthonous transmission is not exclusive to dengue and is often described with another mosquito-borne infection: malaria.

> Branson asks Annabel, 'But you don't have *A. aegypti* mosquitoes in your area, do you?'

Although *A. aegypti* is the principal vector for dengue, other mosquitoes from the *Aedes* genus (e.g. *A. albopictus* and *A. polynesiensis*) have been implicated in disease transmission (Lopez Antunano and Mota, 2000).

> It appears that a number of military personnel returning from assignment in Thailand developed dengue fever soon after arriving in Annabel's district. Unfortunately, there is a dense population of *A. albopictus* mosquitoes there. Within two weeks of the onset of sickness in the military personnel, household contacts and neighbours developed illnesses that have now been confirmed as dengue. This second generation of cases had not travelled overseas to an endemic region within the specified incubation period of dengue, so the endemic *A. albopictus* mosquitoes must have started a chain of local transmission.

CASE 5 DENGUE FEVER

> The group discusses the issue and decides that vector eradication measures should be undertaken to minimise further transmission, followed by long-term vector surveillance.
>
> Richard asks how vector surveillance and control could be accomplished.

The WHO (1997b) outlines the following options for vector surveillance and control:

Vector surveillance

- Monitor larvae or pupae population size using different indices (e.g. house index, Breteau index or container index).
- Monitor the population size of adult mosquitoes (e.g. landing rate).
- Given that vectors can be imported from endemic regions, have ongoing surveillance of airports, seaports, cemeteries and even tyre-retreading facilities. In fact, tyres shipped from infested areas have introduced the vector to previously vector-naive areas (Laird et al., 1994). Some regions are so concerned about the problem of *Aedes* mosquitoes being introduced to naive regions through tyres that legislation has been created to address the issue, such as the Illinois *Waste Tire Act* (Novak, 1995).

Vector control   (broadly divided into environmental management and chemical control)

- Environmental management
  - Improve the domestic water supply.
  - Reduce water storage in containers that provide a habitat for the vector. Have a 'dry day' once a week where water containers are emptied, killing larvae.
  - Cover water storage containers or render them mosquito proof to reduce the chances of infestation.
  - Reduce, reuse, recycle or effectively dispose of containers that can serve as a habitat for mosquitoes (e.g. plastic containers and used tyres).
  - Modify the artificial habitats to prevent mosquito infestation (e.g. place buckets upside down or store containers inside).
- Chemical control
  - Perform focal (or larvicidal) treatment of containers with drinking

water. Larvicides include 1% temephos sand granules, methoprene briquettes and BTI (*Bacillus thuringiensis* H-14). The water is still safe to drink after application.
- Perform perifocal treatment with hand or power sprayers to kill both larvae and adult mosquitoes. This can be used in containers with or without non-potable water. The insecticides include malathion, fenitrothion and some pyrethroids.
- Arrange space spraying (spraying insecticide into the air to kill adult mosquitoes). This is used during an outbreak of dengue fever to reduce the number of new cases. The two common forms of space spraying are thermal fog and ultra-low-volume aerosols/mists. The dispersal of aerosols or mists can be achieved with portable machines, generators mounted on vehicles or aerial spraying with helicopters or planes. Organophosphates (e.g. malathion, fenitrothion, naled, pirimiphos-methyl) and pyrethroids (e.g. deltamethrin, resmethrin, bioresmethrin, permethrin) can be used.

Another method of vector control for dengue is to use sterile insect techniques in which mass populations of male mosquitoes are artificially rendered sterile and released in large numbers into the environment to mate with females. However, this is still a theoretical approach for dengue (Esteva and Yang, 2005).

> Annabel decides to launch a space spraying operation to reduce the number of mosquitoes. Branson still has one concern. 'How do we know if the mosquitoes are resistant to the insecticides?'

Due to many decades of chemical control of *Aedes* mosquitoes, resistance to many insecticides has emerged. The WHO has kits to test the vector's susceptibility to different insecticides and they advise obtaining sensitivity testing prior to using insecticides and at regular intervals afterwards (World Health Organization, 1997b).

> The space spraying operation is a success and the dengue epidemic ends. Afterwards, the affected district institutes a strict vector surveillance program.

References

Cao, X.T., Ngo, T.N., Wills, B. et al. (2002) Evaluation of the World Health Organization standard tourniquet test and a modified tourniquet test in the diagnosis of dengue infection in Viet Nam. *Tropical Medicine & International Health* 7(2), 125–32.

Cunha, B.A. (2000) The diagnostic significance of relative bradycardia. *Clinical Microbiology and Infection* 6(12), 633–34.

Esteva, L., Yang, H.M. (2005) Mathematical model to assess the control of *Aedes aegypti* mosquitoes by the sterile insect technique. *Mathematical Biosciences* 198(2), 132–47.

Gibbons, R.V., Vaughn, D.W. (2002) Dengue: an escalating problem. *British Medical Journal* 324(7353), 1563–66.

Halstead, S.B. (2005) More dengue, more questions. *Emerging Infectious Diseases* 11(5), 740–41.

Kalayanarooj, S., Nimmannitya, S. (2005) Is dengue severity related to nutritional status? *Southeast Asian Journal of Tropical Medicine and Public Health* 36(2), 378–84.

Kalayanarooj, S., Nimmannitya, S., Suntayakorn, S. et al. (1999) Can doctors make an accurate diagnosis of dengue infections at an early stage? *Dengue Bulletin* 23, 1–9.

Kochel, T.J., Watts, D.M., Halstead, S.B. et al. (2002) Effect of dengue-1 antibodies on American-2 viral infection and dengue haemorrhagic fever. *Lancet* 360(9329), 310–12.

Laird, M., Calder, L., Thornton, R.C. et al. (1994) Japanese *Aedes albopictus* among four mosquito species reaching New Zealand in used tires. *Journal of the American Mosquito Control Association* 10(1), 14–23.

Lopez Antunano, F.J., Mota, J. (2000) Development of immunizing agents against dengue. *Pan American Journal of Public Health* 7(5), 285–92.

Novak, R.J. (1995) A North American model to contain the spread of *Aedes albopictus* through tire legislation. *Parassitologia* 37(2-3), 129–39.

Ostergaard, L., Huniche, B., Andersen, P.L. (1996) Relative bradycardia in infectious diseases. *Journal of Infection* 33(3), 185–91.

Rigau-Pérez, J.G. (1998) The early use of break-bone fever (Quebranta huesos, 1771) and dengue (1801) in Spanish. *American Journal of Tropical Medicine and Hygiene* 59(2), 272–74.

Rigau-Pérez, J.G., Clark, G.C., Gubler, D.J. et al. (1998) Dengue and dengue haemorrhagic fever. *Lancet* 352(9132), 971–77.

Souza, L.J., Alves, J.G., Nogueira, R.M. et al. (2004) Aminotransferase changes and acute hepatitis in patients with dengue fever: analysis of 1,585 cases. *Brazilian Journal of Infectious Diseases* 8(2), 156–63.

Stephens, H.A., Klaythong, R., Sirikong, M. et al. (2002) HLA-A and -B allele associations with secondary dengue virus infections correlate with disease severity and the infecting viral serotype in ethnic Thais. *Tissue Antigens* 60(4), 309–18.

Stephenson, J.R. (2005) Understanding dengue pathogenesis: implications for vaccine design. *Bulletin of the World Health Organization* 83(4), 308–14.

Teles, F.R., Prazeres, D.M., Lima-Filho, J.L. (2005) Trends in dengue diagnosis. *Reviews in Medical Virology* 15(5), 287–302.

Venkata Sai, P.M., Dev, B., Krishnan, R. (2005) Role of ultrasound in dengue fever. *British Journal of Radiology* 78(929), 416–18.

Wagner D., de With K., Huzly, D. et al. (2004) Nosocomial acquisition of dengue. *Emerging Infectious Diseases* 10(10),1872–73.

Wilder-Smith A., Schwartz, E. (2005) Dengue in travelers. *New England Journal of Medicine* 353(9), 924–32.

Wittesjo, B., Bjornham, A., Eitrem, R. (1999). Relative bradycardia in infectious diseases. *Journal of Infection* 39(3), 246–47.

World Health Organization (1997a) Chapter 3 Treatment. In *Dengue Haemorrhagic Fever: Diagnosis, Treatment, Prevention And Control. 2nd Edition.* World Health Organization; Geneva. Available from www.who.int/csr/resources/publications/dengue/024-33.pdf (Accessed 9 March, 2006)

World Health Organization (1997b) Chapter 5 Vector surveillance and control. In *Dengue Haemorrhagic Fever: Diagnosis, Treatment, Prevention And Control. 2nd Edition.* World Health Organization; Geneva. Available from www.who.int/csr/resources/publications/dengue/048-59.pdf (Accessed 9 March, 2006)

World Health Organization (2005) *Dengue, Dengue Haemorrhagic Fever And Dengue Shock Syndrome In The Context Of The Integrated Management Of Childhood Illness.* World Health Organization; Geneva. Available from www.who.int/child-adolescent-health/New_Publications/ CHILD_HEALTH/DP/WHO_FCH_CAH_05.13.pdf (Accessed 7 March, 2006)

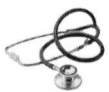

Case 6 Diphtheria
Boris has a sore throat …

Diphtheria at a glance …

- **Agent**: family Corynebacteriaceae; genus *Corynebacterium*; species *Corynebacterium diphtheriae*
- **Geographical distribution**: respiratory diphtheria—worldwide but the burden of disease is mainly in the developing world; cutaneous diphtheria—worldwide but in the developed world tends to occur in underprivileged groups
- **Main modes of transmission**: droplet transmission; physical contact with cutaneous lesions or soiled articles; milk
- **Person-to-person transmission**: yes
- **Animal-to-person transmission**: no
- **Incubation period**: 2–5 days
- **Infectious period**: 2–4 weeks; uncommonly, up to six months
- **Clinical features**: respiratory tract inflammation associated with a pseudomembrane (can be anatomically divided into anterior nasal, faucial, laryngeal and tracheobronchial); cutaneous ulcers; invasive disease from non-toxigenic strains
- **Identification**: culture of the organism; toxin identification (Elek test, polymerase chain reaction, enzyme immunoassay)
- **Treatment**: antibiotics (usually penicillin or macrolides) and antitoxin
- **Post-exposure prophylaxis**: antibiotics (usually penicillin or macrolides)
- **Vaccine**: toxoid vaccine available, usually in combination with other vaccines

Main characters

Dr Ann Chong	infectious diseases registrar
Mr Boris Uranov	man with fever and a sore throat
Dr Laurence May	infectious diseases consultant
Dr Trinity DeSouza	microbiologist
Dr Michael Burn, PhD	public health officer

Dr Ann Chong is the infectious diseases registrar in a busy hospital. She is called to the emergency department to see a patient with pharyngitis. Mr Boris Uranov is a normally healthy 50-year-old man who looks unwell.

It appears that Boris was well up till three days ago. Then he developed a sore throat, which has become progressively worse. It is difficult for him to swallow because of pain. He has had low-grade fevers around 38°C. His GP examined him today but referred him to hospital because the throat looked very inflamed and she thought he might benefit from intravenous antibiotics and fluids.

On examination, Boris looks tired and is tachycardic. He has bilateral cervical lymphadenopathy. The tonsils and posterior pharynx are coated with a greyish covering. The remainder of the examination is normal, apart from a systolic ejection murmur. Scraping the greyish material for culture results in bleeding.

Ann reviews the blood results. Apart from a mild neutrophilia and raised C-reactive protein, the blood profile is unremarkable. She speaks to her consultant, Dr Laurence May. After hearing about the throat findings Laurence asks, 'Do you think it could be diphtheria?'

What is diphtheria?

A greyish pseudomembrane in the pharynx that bleeds after scraping is typical of diphtheria. Diphtheria is caused by a non-spore-producing, Gram positive bacillus, *Corynebacterium diphtheriae*. It is further divided into three biotypes: intermedius, mitis and gravis.

A pseudomembrane is a collection of inflammatory cells, organisms, fibrin and epithelial cells. The word diphtheria is Greek for leather, describing the leathery appearance of the pseudomembrane.

CASE 6 DIPHTHERIA

> Ann looks puzzled and says, 'Diphtheria? Really? But we never get diphtheria in developed nations—and haven't vaccination programs eradicated it in the developing world?'

Diphtheria is still a major problem in many parts of the globe, with the burden of disease mainly in the developing world. Mattos-Guaraldi et al. (2003) give some examples of endemic areas: Africa, India, Bangladesh, Vietnam, the tropics, parts of South America and the Newly Independent States (NIS) of the former Soviet Union.

Developed nations rarely see cases of diphtheria. For example, Australia has only had one notification since and the US only 0–4 cases annually up till 2003 (National Notifiable Diseases Surveillance System, 2005a). Note that neither US nor Australian data include cutaneous disease (National Notifiable Diseases Surveillance System, 2005b). Most doctors in developed nations, including most infectious diseases specialists and microbiologists, never see a case. Nevertheless, diphtheria can occur in travellers returning from an endemic region.

> Ann is still puzzled. 'Even so, I think of diphtheria as a childhood disease. This patient is 50 years old—isn't he too old?'

In the early twentieth century, when diphtheria was a global problem, 70% of cases occurred in children <15 years. More recently, the situation has reversed. In a massive outbreak of diphtheria in the NIS in the early 1990s, 70% of cases occurred in people >15 (Galazka and Tomaszunas-Blaszczyk, 1997). Explanations include (Galazka and Tomaszunas-Blaszczyk, 1997; Gidding et al., 2000):

- less overcrowding and better living conditions, resulting in preschool children who are less likely to encounter circulating strains
- childhood immunisation, resulting in a further reduction in circulating toxigenic strains and thereby reducing opportunities for adults to boost falling immunity years after immunisation

The problem of waning immunity in adults has been addressed by many countries, including the US, UK, Australia and Canada, with the addition of booster doses of diphtheria vaccine. In addition to the three vaccinations in the first year of life, it is recommended that boosters be given around the age of five years and during the teenage years. Even then, immunity can wane later in adult life, so some countries recommend a booster at the age of 50 years (National Health and Medical Research Council, 2003).

> 'Oh well. Maybe it is diphtheria then. His wife and daughter recently returned from a trip to India but neither of them have a respiratory illness. Just the usual mosquito bites et cetera.'
> Laurence says, 'Does he have cats or drink unpasteurised milk?'
> Ann is surprised. 'Why do you ask?'

C. ulcerans is another toxin-producing *Corynebacterium*, which can cause a similar illness to *C. diphtheriae*. However, *C. ulcerans* is a zoonosis usually associated with drinking unpasteurised milk and contact with dairy animals and sometimes with cats (Hatanaka et al., 2003). Unlike *C. ulcerans*, humans are the only carriers of *C. diphtheriae*.

> 'I have just collected a sample of that greyish membrane over the tonsils. Will the microbiology lab need to use special media to identify diphtheria or is it just normal blood agar?' asks Ann.
> Laurence isn't sure ('I've never seen a case before either,' he admits) and tells Ann to speak to the microbiologist, Dr Trinity DeSouza.
> Trinity thanks Ann for telling her about the throat swab because the lab will indeed need to set up special culture media to isolate the organism. She recommends tellurite-containing media such as Tinsdale medium
> She outlines the laboratory clues to a diagnosis of *C. diphtheriae* (Efstratiou et al., 2000):
>
> - 'Chinese character' appearance of Gram positive rods
> - black colonies with a grey-brown halo on Tinsdale medium
> - metachromatic granules with Loeffler's stain
> - distinctive enzyme pattern after further culture on an agar plate (pCUP: positive catalase and cytinase, urease and pyrazinamidase negative)

Investigations

Ann's discussion highlights the importance of communicating with the microbiologist, especially about uncommon conditions. If Ann had not spoken to Trinity or written on the pathology request form that she was concerned about diphtheria, the specimen would not have been cultured on the correct media.

> Trinity also tells Ann that the best samples are the pseudomembrane itself ('I've already got that') and a swab of the tissue from under the pseudomembrane.
> 'Can you test for the toxin too?' Ann asks.

Because of the public health implications of finding a toxigenic strain, it is routine to demonstrate toxin production.

Toxigenic strains of *C. diphtheriae* carry the tox gene in a lysogenic corynebacteriophage. The expressed toxin consists of two chains, A and B (Hadfield et al., 2000). Diagnostic tests are identified in Table 6.1.

Many countries will only have a single reference laboratory to test for diphtheria toxin.

> 'One more thing, Trinity. I know that we isolate non-diphtheria *Corynebacteria* species from standard culture media all the time, from blood cultures and wound swabs and so on, so why can't we isolate *C. diphtheriae* by inoculating a throat swab into normal culture media?'

Actually, *C. diphtheriae* will grow on standard blood agar media. The problem is that all the other throat flora will grow on the same media too, making it difficult to pick out the *Corynebacterium* from the other bacterial colonies.

Table 6.1 Tests for *C. diphtheriae* toxin

Test	Comment
Elek test	Filter paper containing antitoxin is placed over a culture plate of the organism.
Polymerase chain reaction (PCR)	This detects the toxin structural gene. It is useful in excluding diphtheria if negative but a positive result can be difficult to interpret.
Enzyme immunoassay	One study showed 100% correlation with the Elek test.

SOURCE Efstratiou et al., 2000

Ann thanks Trinity for her assistance. She returns to the patient and informs him about the possibility of diphtheria. The patient looks surprised. 'Is there anything else that this could be?'

Differential diagnoses

The differential diagnoses of severe pharyngitis includes:

- viral pharyngitis
- streptococcal pharyngitis
- infectious mononucleosis (IM)
- Vincent's angina
- acute epiglottitis

MacGregor (2005) notes that streptococcal pharyngitis is associated with higher fevers, more severe dysphagia and more intense pharyngitis than diphtheria. Infectious mononucleosis (IM) is associated with a membrane but this tends to be localised to the tonsils, be white rather than grey, and not to bleed after scraping. Acute epiglottitis presents very acutely and is not associated with a membrane. Vincent's angina has gingival involvement with Gram stain demonstrating spirochaetes and fusobacteria.

However, early in the course of respiratory diphtheria there may only be a red pharynx and no pseudomembrane, which can make it very difficult to distinguish it from other conditions; even when the pseudomembrane first appears, it can be white rather than grey, which can lead to confusion with IM. Some cases of respiratory diphtheria are not even associated with a pseudomembrane. Consequently, diphtheria of the pharynx is not always an easy diagnosis to make.

Because of the possibility of these other diagnoses, in addition to standard blood tests and swabs Ann should ask for a Monospot test (for IM) and serology for Epstein-Barr virus, cytomegalovirus and Group A streptococcus (baseline now and convalescent serology in 10–14 days).

The nurse looking after Boris approaches Ann and says, 'My father had diphtheria when he was a boy in Pakistan. I remember him saying it only affected his nose—he didn't have pharyngitis. Could that have been diphtheria?'

Respiratory diphtheria can be limited to the following areas (Hadfield et al., 2000):

Anterior nasal disease This is usually mild, presenting with seropurulent or serosanguineous nasal discharge, although deep ulceration can occur.
Faucial disease (tonsils and proximal pharynx) This is the most common site.
Laryngeal and tracheobronchial disease This is uncommon but very dangerous because suffocation can result from airway swelling or aspiration of the pseudomembrane.

The nurse now asks, 'Does he need to be isolated?' Ann says that she thinks so, but isn't confident of the duration and degree of isolation. She calls Dr Michael Burn, PhD, an officer from the local public health unit, who confirms her suspicion.

Isolation measures

Diphtheria is a communicable disease. If Boris has diphtheria (and Ann has to assume so till cultures prove otherwise), then he should be placed in a single room and staff and visitors should observe droplet precautions by donning masks, gowns and gloves on entering the room.

These precautions should continue till two cultures of the nose and throat, each at least 24 hours apart and at least 24 hours after stopping antimicrobial therapy, are negative for diphtheria (Bonnet and Begg, 1999).

Ann asks Michael, 'Do you need to start contact tracing at this stage?'
'Yes. We don't wait for the diagnosis to be confirmed, because contacts can themselves develop diphtheria or else be carriers, possibly transmitting the bacteria to others.'

Public health notification and response

A person with untreated disease is infectious for up to four weeks, but carriers may be infectious for longer (National Health and Medical

Research Council, 2003). Public health units begin making a contact lists as soon as possible, namely:

- household members
- sexual partners
- healthcare workers involved in airway management of the index case, such as mouth-to-mouth resuscitation or intubation (Bonnet and Begg, 1999)

Contacts at childcare centres, schools and work may be contacts, depending on the length and proximity of contact with the individual. According to Bonnet and Begg (1999), a reasonable approach to managing contacts is to:

- Take pharyngeal swabs for diphtheria culture.
- Provide antibiotic prophylaxis, irrespective of the results of pharyngeal cultures. Antibiotic prophylaxis can be a single dose of intramuscular benzylpenicillin or a seven-day course of oral erythromycin. Pharyngeal swabs should be repeated at the end of treatment from those contacts whose original swabs were positive for *C. diphtheriae*. If cultures are still positive after the initial course of antibiotics, a further 10 days of erythromycin is warranted. Other macrolides may be used in place of erythromycin, such as clarithromycin or azithromycin.
- Assess clinical status daily for seven days since the last contact with the index case OR ask contacts to call the public health unit if they develop symptoms suggestive of diphtheria within seven days of their last contact of the index case. The incubation period of respiratory diphtheria is generally 2–5 days. If contacts have not developed symptomatic infection by a week since their last contact with the index case, they are unlikely to develop clinical disease.

Ann thanks Michael for his input. The nurse organises a single room for Boris. 'Now what antibiotics are you going to treat him with?'

Treatment

Antibiotics are recommended for treatment of respiratory diphtheria. This makes sense because killing the organisms will reduce the spread of pharyngeal disease and also reduce toxin production (by reducing the number of bacteria that can produce toxin).

MacGregor (2005) notes that only penicillin and erythromycin have been studied in controlled trials against diphtheria, although it is sensitive to a number of agents in vitro—other macrolides (azithromycin, clindamycin), fluoroquinolones, tetracyclines and rifampicin—so penicillin or erythromycin should be given for 14 days. Erythromycin is slightly better in clearing carriage of diphtheria but has the disadvantage of more adverse effects (gastrointestinal side effects with oral treatment, phlebitis with intravenous [IV] medications).

The other advantage of these antibiotics is that they are usually effective against streptococcal pharyngitis, if Boris does not turn out to have diphtheria.

He should receive diphtheria antitoxin (DAT). Although it would be ideal to wait to see if the strain is producing toxin before giving DAT, this may take a few days, by which time the patient could be extremely sick or even dead. The dose and route of administration (IV or intramuscular) depends on the site, severity and duration of illness (Bonnet and Begg, 1999).

Because DAT is derived from horse serum, it can be associated with severe hypersensitivity reactions. The risk is considered so serious that all patients should receive a test dose (e.g. an intradermal dose followed by a small parenteral dose). Nevertheless, DAT is so important in treating diphtheria that hypersensitivity may not completely preclude its use. In hypersensitive patients, treating physicians may consider concurrent administration of steroids, antihistamines or adrenaline (epinephrine) (National Health and Medical Research Council, 2003).

The nurse asks Ann, 'Will he need any type of monitoring?'

Prognosis

Boris needs close monitoring for toxin-related cardiac complications, which usually occur in the second week of illness. Diphtheria toxin is regarded as a very potent toxin; in fact, scientists have tried to incorporate the diphtheria toxin into plague bacteria as a biological weapon (Miller et al., 2002).

Almost 30% of patients with diphtheria will develop ECG abnormalities and, clinically, diphtheric myocarditis is associated with conduction disturbances and dilated cardiomyopathy. Up to 60% of diphtheria patients with myocarditis will die and death from cardiac damage accounts for one-third of all deaths from diphtheria (Dung et al., 2002; Lumio et al., 2004).

Boris therefore requires daily 12-lead ECGs. If they become abnormal, he will need continuous ECG monitoring, if such facilities are available, and possibly interventions such as temporary pacing and antiarrhythmic agents.

His respiratory status will also have to be monitored closely. The slightest deterioration in respiratory function may be an indication for intubation or a tracheostomy.

The other major complication mediated by toxin is neurological disease. The risk of neurological disease is proportional to the severity of the presenting diphtheria infection, with up to 75% of patients with severe primary infection developing neurological complications (MacGregor, 2005). Unlike cardiac disease, neurological disease often begins in the first few days of infection. The soft palate and pharyngeal wall tend to be the first sites of paralysis, followed by other cranial nerve palsies and then a peripheral neuropathy. However, the neuropathy tends to resolve with time.

> The nurse makes a note to inform the ward nurses that Boris needs daily 12-lead ECGs. She now asks, 'Didn't you say that he had a heart murmur? Do you think that he already has endocarditis?'

> Ann suspects a flow murmur related to Boris' serious infection and tachycardia. However, diphtheria can be associated with invasive disease outside the respiratory tract, for example, endocarditis, bacteraemia, splenic abscesses or septic arthritis. Interestingly, these invasive manifestations tend to be associated with non-toxigenic strains of *C. diphtheriae* rather than toxin-producing ones (Holthouse et al., 1998).

> Boris is admitted to the ward. He improves on IV penicillin and DAT; the ECGs remain normal. On Day 3 of admission, Trinity calls Ann to let her know that the cultures of the throat swab have isolated a toxigenic *C. diphtheriae*.
>
> Ann immediately calls the public health unit with the news. 'It's good to know that our contact tracing wasn't in vain,' Michael says.

> 'But I still can't work out how he was infected.'
> 'I think I know—Boris's daughter, who was recently in India, is the source.'
> Ann is puzzled. 'But she hasn't had a respiratory illness, just some infected mosquito bites.'
> 'Exactly!' says Michael.

Michael is suggesting that the daughter's 'mosquito bites' are, in fact, cutaneous diphtheria.

> 'What's cutaneous diphtheria?' asks Ann.

Cutaneous diphtheria is the most common extra-respiratory manifestation of the disease. It can occur as chronic non-healing ulcers with no clear cause or be a complication of insect bites (de Benoist et al., 2004). Cultures of the ulcers are often polymicrobial, growing *Staphylococcus aureus* and Group A streptococcus (*Streptococcus pyogenes*) as well as *C. diphtheriae*.

Cutaneous diphtheria is important because it can serve as a reservoir for transmitting toxigenic strains to contacts, resulting in respiratory diphtheria.

Cases can be imported following travel to developing nations with endemic diphtheria or can occur in developed countries in socially disadvantaged groups (MacGregor, 2005).

> But Ann is still not convinced. 'Boris told me his children's immunisations are completely up to date. He even had his wife double check their records. That daughter is fully immunised against diphtheria. So how could she have the disease?'

As with most vaccine-preventable diseases, immunisation is not a guarantee of protection. There are case reports of fully immunised individuals developing cutaneous diphtheria (de Benoist et al., 2004) and immunised people can also develop respiratory disease, although the infection tends to be less severe.

Neither immunisation nor the immunity induced by infection prevent carriage of the organism.

> Michael arranges for the daughter to be reviewed by Laurence. He takes a swab of her ulcer, which isolates *S. aureus* and *C. diphtheriae*—she is the source of Boris's infection. Laurence commences her on a combination of antibiotics and DAT.
> Both Boris and his daughter complete treatment for diphtheria without incident. All other contacts complete prophylaxis without *C. diphtheriae* being isolated from the pharyngeal swabs prior to commencing antibiotics.
> Laurence calls Michael to clarify some issues: 'Do Boris and his daughter need to vaccinated or would the disease itself have induced sufficient natural immunity?'

Respiratory diphtheria does not always induce adequate immunity, so Boris will need a booster or another immunisation course, depending on his immunisation history. The only exception to this is if Boris received a booster within the last twelve months (Bonnet and Begg, 1999).

Cutaneous diphtheria, however, is more likely to induce natural immunity. Nevertheless, many centres would still immunise people with cutaneous diphtheria in the convalescent stage of treatment.

> 'His wife works at a café three times per week. Boris said that the public health unit had told her to stay away from work initially. Is this true?' Laurence asks.

Diphtheria transmission can occur through food handlers, especially those handling milk. Boris's wife should have been excluded from work and stay away until tests confirm she is no longer a carrier. Others who should be excluded are people working with potentially unimmunised children, such as healthcare workers and childcare centre staff (Bonnet and Begg, 1999).

References

Bonnet, J.M., Begg, N.T. (1999) Control of diphtheria: guidance for consultants in communicable disease control. World Health Organization. *Communicable Disease and Public Health* 2(4), 242–49.
de Benoist, A.C., White, J.M., Efstratiou, A. et al. (2004) Imported cutaneous diphtheria, United Kingdom. *Emerging Infectious Diseases* 10(3), 511–13.

Dung NM, Kneen R, Kiem N. et al. (2002) Treatment of severe diphtheric myocarditis by temporary insertion of a cardiac pacemaker. *Clinical Infectious Diseases* 35(11), 1425–29.

Efstratiou, A., Engler, K.H., Mazurova, I.K. et al. (2000) Current approaches to the laboratory diagnosis of diphtheria. *Journal of Infectious Diseases* 181(Suppl 1), S138–45.

Galazka, A., Tomaszunas-Blaszczyk, J. (1997) Why do adults contract diphtheria? *Eurosurveillance* 2(8), 60–63.

Gidding, H.F., Burgess, M.A., Gilbert, G.L. (2000) Diphtheria in Australia, recent trends and future prevention strategies. *Communicable Diseases Intelligence* 24(6), 165–67.

Hadfield, T.L., McEvoy, P., Polotsky, Y. et al. (2000) The pathology of diphtheria. *Journal of Infectious Diseases* 181(Suppl 1), S116–20.

Hatanaka, A., Tsunoda, A., Okamoto, M. et al. (2003) *Corynebacterium ulcerans* diphtheria in Japan. *Emerging Infectious Diseases* 9(6), 752–53.

Holthouse, D.J., Power, B., Kermode, A. et al. (1998) Non-toxigenic *Corynebacterium diphtheriae*: two cases and review of the literature. *Journal of Infection* 37(1), 62–66.

Lumio, J.T., Groundstroem, K.W., Melnick, O.B. et al. (2004) Electrocardiographic abnormalities in patients with diphtheria: a prospective study. *American Journal of Medicine* 116(2), 78–83.

MacGregor, R.R. (2005) *Corynebacterium diphtheriae*. In Mandell, G.E., Bennett, J.E., Dolin, R. (eds) *Principles and Practice of Infectious Diseases*. Churchill Livingstone; Philadelphia.

Mattos-Guaraldi A.L., Moreira L.O., Damasco P.V. et al. (2003) Diphtheria remains a threat in the developing world—an overview. *Memorias do Instituto Oswaldo Cruz* 98(8), 987–93.

Miller J., Broad W., Engelberg S. (2002) *Germs: biological weapons and America's secret war*. Simon & Schuster Adult Publishing Group.

National Health and Medical Research Council (2003) *Australian Immunisation Handbook. 8th Edition*. National Health and Medical Research Council; Canberra. Available from www9.health.gov.au/immhandbook/ (Accessed 2 November, 2005)

National Notifiable Diseases Surveillance System (2005a) *Number of notifications of diphtheria, Australia, in the period of 1991 to 2004 and year-to-date notifications for 2005*. Available from www9.health.gov.au/cda/Source/Rpt_3.cfm (Accessed 2 November, 2005)

National Notifiable Diseases Surveillance System (2005b) *Summary of Notifiable Diseases*. Available from www.cdc.gov/epo/dphsi/annsum/2003/03graphs.htm (Accessed 2 November, 2005)

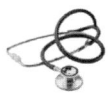

Case 7 Enteric fever
Morgan looks unwell …

Enteric fever at a glance …

- **Agents:** family Enterobacteriaceae; genus *Salmonella*; species *Salmonella enterica* serotypes Typhi and Paratyphi
- **Geographical distribution:** most commonly in Asia (especially South-Central Asia and South-East Asia), the Caribbean, Latin America, Africa, Oceania (excluding Australia and New Zealand); sporadic cases can occur almost anywhere
- **Main mode of transmission:** faeco-oral
- **Person-to-person transmission:** always (food, drink or sex may be the vehicle)
- **Animal-to-person transmission:** no
- **Incubation period:** 7–14 days (3 days–2 months)
- **Infectious period:** from the first week of illness till clearance of bacteria from stool
- **Clinical features:** uncomplicated disease—stepladder fever, transient truncal rash in light-skinned people, myalgias, dry cough, headache, abdominal symptoms, relative bradycardia, splenomegaly; complicated disease—most commonly, gastrointestinal haemorrhage, viscus perforation and encephalopathy
- **Identification:** most commonly through isolation of bacteria from blood, stool, bone marrow or urine cultures; serological tests are available but not as reliable as cultures; nested polymerase chain reaction (PCR) may be a promising test for the future
- **Treatment:** rehydration and antibiotic therapy (antibiotic choice is complex); dexamethasone for severe typhoid fever
- **Post-exposure prophylaxis:** nil
- **Vaccine:** oral live attenuated vaccine; intramuscular capsular polysaccharide vaccine; a promising conjugated typhoid vaccine is available; typhoid vaccines do not protect against *S.* Paratyphi A

CASE 7 ENTERIC FEVER

Main characters

Dr Dustin Mann	infectious diseases physician
Dr Renée Silver	infectious diseases registrar
Mr Morgan Sutherland	patient with enteric fever
Dr Marian Motaba	medical microbiologist
Dr Richard Manetta	public health unit director
Mr Kevin Goodman	food inspector
Marion	food-handler

> Dr Dustin Mann is the infectious disease physician on-call at a large hospital. His mobile rings—it's his registrar, Dr Renée Silver.
> 'Hello, Dustin. I'm down in the emergency department with a patient who was called back with positive blood cultures.'

Large numbers of patients are seen in busy emergency departments every day. Most are not admitted to hospital and are sent home to be followed up by their local doctor. Sometimes patients have a febrile illness and, although blood cultures are taken, they are deemed too well to be admitted to hospital and are discharged. Occasionally these blood cultures become positive and patients have to be re-called.

> Dustin walks down to the department and reviews the patient. Mr Morgan Sutherland is a 45-year-old man who looks moderately unwell.
> Nine days ago, he became ill. He felt lethargic with generalised myalgias and feeling hot with slight chills. His temperature was about 37.7–37.8°C. Over the next few days, he developed a frontal headache and dry cough. The shivers and fevers seem to have worsened in the past few days and he now is measuring temperatures of 38.7–39°C. He presented yesterday to hospital when his wife noticed a fine rash over his chest and abdomen. His blood tests that day demonstrated a mild leukopenia and mildly elevated liver function tests.
> He was reviewed by an intern who assessed him as having 'a viral illness' and suggested resting at home. The intern thought

the rash was a viral exanthem; however, it had disappeared by the time Morgan returned home.

He specifically denies shortness of breath, urinary symptoms and diarrhoea; in fact, he has been constipated for the last few days. Morgan is usually healthy apart from taking a proton pump inhibitor for reflux oesophagitis. He dislikes taking medicine and has not used antibiotics at this stage.

On examination, he looks tired. He has a fever of 39°C and a regular pulse of 85/minute. The only other positive findings are a white-coated tongue and mild splenomegaly. He has no neck stiffness.

Dustin asks Renée, 'Am I right in saying that the blood culture bottles contain Gram negative bacilli?'

Renée looks surprised. 'Yes, that's right. The lab won't be able to give us more information about the organism till tomorrow. How did you know though? This doesn't look like Gram negative sepsis to me.'

Dustin replies, 'This man has enteric fever.'

What is enteric fever?

Enteric fever is an infection caused by *Salmonella enterica* serotype Typhi (*S.* Typhi) or *S. enterica* serotype Paratyphi (*S.* Paratyphi); the former produces typhoid fever, the latter paratyphoid fever (Basnyat et al., 2005). It is a big public health problem, with over 200 million cases in 2000 alone (Crump et al., 2004). *S.* Typhi make up 90% of cases of enteric fever and *S.* Paratyphi 10%, although the proportion of cases due to *S.* Paratyphi may be increasing in some areas (Bhutta, 2006).

> Renée is still astonished. 'We live in an industrialised country. Morgan hasn't travelled to an endemic region for enteric fever for years. How could he have contracted it here?'

The burden of enteric fever is in the developing world (Table 7.1) and residents of developed nations usually contract enteric fever in the context of recent overseas travel to an endemic region. Travellers to developing nations have an incidence of typhoid fever ranging from 3–30/100 000 (Basnyat et al., 2005); however, sporadic cases of enteric

Table 7.1 Regions with medium and high rates of endemic typhoid fever

High endemicity (>100/10⁵ cases/year)	South-Central Asia, South-East Asia
Medium endemicity (10–100/10⁵ cases/year)	Caribbean, Latin America, Africa, rest of Asia, Oceania†

†Oceania, for the purposes of this table, excludes Australia and New Zealand.
SOURCE Adapted from Crump et al., 2004

fever can occur in developed nations, even in the absence of recent overseas travel.

> Dustin asks his registrar, 'What features in the history, examination and blood results support a diagnosis of enteric fever?'

Several features of Morgan's illness suggest enteric fever:

Fever pattern Morgan's fever has been gradually increasing over the last nine days from the high 37s to the high 38s. This is known as a stepladder pattern of fever and is typical of typhoid. Classically, the fever increases in this stepladder fashion during the first week before plateauing in the second week and decreasing over the third and fourth weeks (Bal and Czarnowski, 2004).

Coated tongue By itself, this is not a particularly sensitive or specific sign. However, in combination with bradycardia, loose bowel motions and a stepladder rise in fever, a coated tongue has a specificity of 94% (Haq et al., 1997).

Transient truncal rash This may have been rose spots, which are red-pink spots 2–4 mm in diameter usually found on the chest and abdomen in enteric fever. Its usefulness as a diagnostic sign is limited by its transient appearance and the difficulty of finding them on people with darker skin. For these reasons, it is recognised in less than 30% of cases of enteric fever (Klotz et al., 1984; Parry et al., 2002; Thisyakorn et al., 1987).

Constipation Because of the association of various *Salmonella* spp with acute diarrhoeal illnesses, many healthcare workers assume patients with enteric fever will also have loose bowel motions. However, many patients with enteric fever become constipated (30% in a study by Tran et al., 1995), although diarrhoea can occur and is more common in young children and in HIV-positive individuals (Parry et al., 2002).

Myalgias, dry cough and headache These non-specific symptoms are common in enteric fever (Basnyat et al., 2005). One study found they occurred in around 20%, 33% and 70% in patients with enteric fever, respectively (Tran et al., 1995).
Relative bradycardia This is common in enteric fever (Basnyat et al., 2005). See Case 5 for more information.
Splenomegaly This is common but alone is a non-specific sign.
Leukopenia and abnormal liver function tests These are common laboratory features of typhoid fever. The full blood count tends to be normal or reduced (anaemia, leukopenia, thrombocytopenia) and hepatic enzymes are elevated usually no more than 2–3 times baseline levels (Parry et al., 2002). In children, though, leucocytosis is not uncommon (Bhutta, 2006).

> 'Now can you tell clinically whether Morgan's enteric fever is due to typhoid or paratyphoid fever?'

It is difficult to distinguish clinically between the two causes of enteric fever (Vollaard et al., 2005).

> Morgan listens to this conversation with some alarm. 'I could have typhoid? Are you sure it couldn't be anything else?'

Differential diagnoses

There is a broad differential diagnosis for enteric fever, including: (adapted from Basnyat et al., 2005; Parry et al., 2002)

- malaria
- dengue fever
- leptospirosis
- amoebic liver abscess
- infectious mononucleosis
- HIV seroconversion illness
- brucellosis
- tuberculosis
- rickettsial disease
- Q fever
- influenza

However, in this case, Dustin has the luxury of knowing that the blood cultures are positive for Gram negative bacilli, ruling out many of these other conditions. In the absence of a positive blood culture, the diagnosis would have been much more difficult to make.

In some countries with endemic malaria and enteric fever, even experienced clinicians empirically treat patients for both infections because they cannot distinguish clinically between the two (Nsutebu et al., 2003).

Dustin asks Renée about empiric treatment. She recommends gentamicin for now.

Treatment

Despite in vitro studies showing that S. Typhi and S. Paratyphi can be sensitive to gentamicin, as well as first and second-generation cephalosporins, these antibiotics are ineffective in vivo (Basnyat et al., 2005).

Antibiotic choice is difficult because resistance patterns change continually. Traditional agents, such as ampicillin, cotrimoxazole and chloramphenicol, have not been used as empiric therapy recently because of resistance. Multidrug-resistant strains (i.e. those resistant to ampicillin, chloramphenicol and cotrimoxazole) have become endemic in some parts of the world (Parry, 2004). The risk of having an adverse outcome is greater in cases of enteric fever with a multidrug-resistant organism (Bhutta, 2006).

Fluoroquinolones (e.g. ofloxacin, ciprofloxacin) have become the antibiotic group of choice in recent times but fluoroquinolone failure has become an increasing problem in Asia. This has been driven by increased use associated with over-the-counter access and cheap prices in developing nations (Parry, 2004; Walia et al., 2005). To complicate matters further, while fluoroquinolone resistance is increasing, some isolates are becoming more and more sensitive to traditional agents such as chloramphenicol, to which they had been previously resistant (Lakshmi et al., 2006).

Both azithromycin and the parenteral third-generation cephalosporins (cefotaxime, ceftriaxone) are effective alternatives to the fluoroquinolones in treating enteric fever (Table 7.2). A Cochrane review detected no difference between fluoroquinolones and azithromycin in treating enteric fever. The same review found no difference in microbiological failure or relapse between fluoroquinolones and ceftriaxone, although the fluoroquinolones had a relatively reduced clinical failure (Thaver et al., 2005). Cefixime, an

Table 7.2 Efficacy of fluoroquinolones, ceftriaxone and azithromycin in enteric fever

	Time to defervescence (days)	Primary clinical treatment failure (%)	Relapse rate (%)	Chronic stool carriage (%)
Fluoroquinolones	<4	<4	<2	<2
Ceftriaxone	7	5–10	3–6	<3
Azithromycin	4–6	3–4	<3	<3

SOURCE Adapted from Basnyat et al., 2005; Parry et al., 2002

> oral third-generation cephalosporin, is used despite questions about its efficacy (Basnyat et al., 2005).
>
> A reasonable empirical approach would be to use a parenteral third-generation cephalosporin or oral azithromycin while awaiting sensitivities.

Renée decides to prescribe oral azithromycin 500 mg/day.

'Dustin, if the organism turns out to be sensitive to fluoroquinolones, then can I stop the azithromycin and switch him to oral ciprofloxacin?'

> Fluoroquinolones are still the drug of choice for enteric fever isolates that are sensitive to fluoroquinolones (Bhutta, 2006). Treatment duration depends on disease severity and antibiotic choice (Table 7.3).

Table 7.3 Duration of treatment

	Drug	Duration
For uncomplicated typhoid fever	Fluoroquinolones	5–7 days (3 days in an epidemic setting)
	Azithromycin	7 days
	Ceftriaxone	10–14 days
For severe or complicated typhoid fever	Use all the above agents (Bhutta, 2006)	10–14 days

'I presume he will need to be isolated?'

Isolation measures

Morgan has been infectious to the public, staff and other patients from the first week of his illness and will be so till his stools are cleared of the infection (Skull and Tallis, 2001). He should be placed in a single room with his own shower and toilet. Staff and visitors should enter the room wearing gloves and gowns and wash their hands before and after entering the room.

Dustin asks Renée to inform the microbiology lab that Morgan may have enteric fever.
'They've found Gram negative bacilli in the blood cultures, so how will it help them further if we say we're thinking of enteric fever?'

Investigations

It is always important to give the microbiology staff as much information as possible. Giving a possible clinical diagnosis may allow them to use tests that they would not have otherwise chosen and therefore identify the organism more quickly. Also, they would be interested to know the clinical history behind the positive cultures. Finally, it is simply a matter of courtesy!

Renée calls Dr Marian Motaba, the microbiologist, and passes on their suspicions.
'Thanks for telling me, Renée. Normally, we just put our positive blood cultures on horse blood agar, chocolate agar and MacConkey agar. Since we know that you are thinking of enteric fever, we will also set up an XLD plate and do some agglutination studies tomorrow on the new colonies.'
Renée is a bit puzzled. 'Marian, I haven't done my laboratory training as yet, so I hope you don't mind if I ask some questions. Firstly, if it is a *Salmonella* species, will it grow on MacConkey agar?'

MacConkey agar is a culture medium specifically devised to grow Gram negative bacteria. This culture medium further categorises Gram negative bacteria on the basis of whether they ferment lactose or not: the fermenters produce red colonies and the non-fermenters white-transparent colonies. Virtually all *Salmonella* spp are non-lactose fermenters producing white-transparent colonies; however, 1% of *Salmonella* spp are lactose fermenters, which can be confusing if other methods to identify *Salmonella* are not used (Pegues et al., 2005).

'But I assume that *Salmonella* species aren't the only non-lactose fermenters, meaning that you need more information to distinguish it from other bacteria. Is that right?'

XLD (xylose-lysine-deoxycholate) agar will identify *Salmonella* spp as red colonies. Furthermore, *Salmonella* spp that produce hydrogen disulfide (H_2S) grow red colonies with black centres (Isenberg et al., 1985). Nearly all *S*. Typhi strains produce H_2S while only 10% of *S*. Paratyphi A do (Kelly et al., 1985).

'What are the agglutination studies for?'

Salmonella can be divided into serogroups based on three major antigens:

- O antigen (somatic)
- H antigen (flagellar)
- Vi antigen (capsular)

Peripheral laboratories may only use basic kits that classify *Salmonella* spp into serogroups (A–E) on the basis of their O antigen alone (Pegues et al., 2005). This can still be useful in enteric fever, where *S*. Typhi is serogroup D (*S*. Paratyphi strains can occur in different serogroups).

'Marian, using all these special culture media and agglutination tests is interesting, but why don't you just whack the isolate into the Vitek® to get an answer?'

Vitek® is an automated machine. The scientist puts a card with the colonies from the culture plate into the machine and it provides a name and drug susceptibilities. It is a very useful tool in any microbiology laboratory but, like any machine, it is not always correct. Therefore, it is important to have other corroborative evidence, especially in unusual cases.

Morgan may have enteric fever despite the absence of a travel history to an endemic region. Isolating *S.* Typhi or *S.* Paratyphi would be unusual, so it is important to support the finding from the Vitek® machine with the XLD plates and agglutination studies.

> 'If his blood cultures had been negative, could we have isolated the organism from elsewhere?'

S. Typhi or *S.* Paratyphi can be isolated from blood, bone marrow and stool. Bone marrow culture is the most sensitive site for culturing these organisms but the test is more invasive and difficult to arrange than a blood culture. Even urine cultures can be positive, especially if there are structural abnormalities in the urinary tract or schistosomiasis. According to Basnyat et al. (2005) and Parry et al. (2002), the sensitivity of cultures at the usual sites are:

- bone marrow: 80–95% (even if antibiotics have been used)
- blood: 60–80% (sensitivity reduced by antibiotics)
- stool: 25% in adults, 60% in children (usually positive only after the first week of illness)

> 'What about serology?'

The gold standard for diagnosing enteric fever is culture of the organism. However, in developing countries with high rates of enteric fever and limited resources, a rapid antibody test that is both sensitive and specific for the condition would be preferable.

For over a hundred years, the serological test used for diagnosis of typhoid fever (enteric fever due to *S.* Typhi) has been the Widal test, invented by F. Widal in 1896. This agglutination test uses killed *S.* Typhi as the antigen (Olopoenia and King, 2000). Problems both with sensitivity and specificity limit its use but some endemic regions find it a useful test if the cut-off point for a positive diagnosis is adjusted locally (Parry et al., 2002). According to Olopoenia and King (2000), the causes of false-positive results are:

- previous immunisation against typhoid fever
- infection with other *Salmonella* spp that share the O antigens used in the test
- other infections (e.g. miliary TB, brucellosis, chronic liver disease, dengue fever, malaria and other Enterobacteriaceae)
- variability in the use of the commercial antigen for the test.

The cause of false-negative results are:

- an amount of infecting antigen too small to elicit a positive response
- variability in the use of the commercial antigen for the test
- individuals who are carriers
- inaccurate reading of the result by technicians.

New commercial antibody kits have been developed which use subunit antigens rather than whole killed organisms but the results have been variable (Dutta et al., 2006; Kawano et al., 2007). These tests do not target *S.* Paratyphi, an important cause of enteric fever, so serology has not displaced culture as the gold standard for diagnosis.

Molecular tests, such as polymerase chain reaction (PCR), have been developed but are not available for identification of *S.* Typhi or *S.* Paratyphi in most hospital laboratories. However, nested PCR of blood for *S.* Typhi appears to have a very high sensitivity and specificity and may one day become the gold standard for diagnosis (Bhutta, 2006).

On the following day, Morgan still feels unwell and has high fevers; however, he isn't worse than the previous day.

Marian calls from the lab to confirm that the organism is a non-lactose fermenter, is growing black-red colonies on XLD agar and is serogroup D on agglutination tests. She is now waiting for the Vitek® machine to confirm that this is *S.* Typhi. By tomorrow, they should have sensitivities. The specimen will have to be sent interstate to the national reference laboratory for further typing of the isolate. It is Day 10 of his illness.

On the following day, Marian calls again: 'That fellow with the typhoid fever has a multidrug-resistant organism, so ampicillin, chloramphenicol and cotrimoxazole are useless. It has a ciprofloxacin-sensitive isolate but it has reduced susceptibility with a minimum inhibitory concentration (MIC) of 0.25 mg/L.'

Renée is confused. 'Can I use ciprofloxacin?'

The isolate is sensitive to ciprofloxacin in vitro since the MIC is ≤1 mg/L but this does not necessarily mean there will be clinical efficacy. The MIC to ciprofloxacin means nothing without knowing the isolate's sensitivity to nalidixic acid. This antibiotic is a quinolone rarely used in clinical practice today. It has been shown that *Salmonella* spp that are sensitive in vitro to fluoroquinolones but resistant to nalidixic acid are unlikely to be successfully treated with fluoroquinolones such as ciprofloxacin (Clinical and Laboratory Standards Institute, 2006).

'The isolate is resistant to nalidixic acid, so I wouldn't advise ciprofloxacin. The azithromycin he's on should be fine.'

Renée asks whether Marian has alerted the public health unit.

Public health notification and response

Marian should have alerted the local public health unit. In many parts of the world, enteric fever is a laboratory-notifiable disease, that is, there is a legal requirement for the laboratory to tell the health department whenever *S.* Typhi or *S.* Paratyphi is isolated in cultures. This allows public health officials to identify close contacts at risk of infection from the index case. They may also identify the source of the index case's infection, thereby preventing further spread.

After five days of treatment, Morgan still has high fevers although he hasn't deteriorated. On Day 6 of his admission, he begins to complain of generalised abdominal pain.

On examination, he doesn't look well. He is drowsy and confused and has a new tachycardia, a blood pressure lower than previously and signs of peritonitis.

'What's happening?' the nurse looking after him asks.

Prognosis

Overall, the mortality rate is low (<1%) and probably even less in travellers with enteric fever (Basnyat et al., 2005). However, about 10–15% of patients with enteric fever develop complications. These can be wide-ranging, including:
- intestinal perforation
- gastrointestinal bleeding (usually not life threatening)

- hepatitis
- encephalopathy
- nephritic syndrome
- osteomyelitis (usually in patients with haemoglobinopathies)
- endocarditis
- myocarditis
- pneumonia
- disseminated intravascular coagulation (Carlson and Dobozi, 1994; Katafuchi, 2005; Parry et al., 2002; Wani et al., 2004)

The most important complications are gastrointestinal haemorrhage (due to necrosis in Peyer's patches into a blood vessel), intestinal perforation and encephalopathy. Complications tend to occur in those who have been sick for over two weeks (Parry et al., 2002).

An erect chest X-ray demonstrates subdiaphragmatic air, confirming a perforated viscus. Morgan is resuscitated with intravenous (IV) fluids and surgeons are urgently consulted. Renée asks Dustin, 'Should we give him corticosteroids?'

Although the data are limited, it appears that 48 hours of six-hourly dexamethasone (1mg/kg) following a bolus dose (3mg/kg) reduces mortality in those with severe typhoid fever. Features of severe typhoid fever include delirium, obtundation, shock, coma or stupor (Pegues et al., 2005).

Morgan is in shock, has an altered mental state and is delirious; therefore, he has features of severe typhoid fever and should receive 48 hours of IV dexamethasone, advises Dustin.

He is rushed to the operating theatre. The surgeons examine the bowel carefully and find only a single perforation in the ileum. A small segment of bowel is resected and Morgan is sent to the intensive care unit, still on azithromycin. Over the next few days, he continues to improve and soon is afebrile.

He has been traumatised by the severity of this illness and, worried, asks, 'This won't come back again, will it?'

Unfortunately, relapses occur in 5–10% of cases, usually within 2–3 weeks of the fever resolving (Parry et al., 2002). As Table 7.2 demonstrates, antibiotic choice also contributes to the relapse rate.

CASE 7   ENTERIC FEVER

> Morgan shakes his head in wonderment. 'I can't believe I became so ill. Up till today, I had been completely healthy apart from a bit of reflux oesophagitis.'
>
> 'Actually', says Dustin, 'the medication for your reflux may have made you more susceptible.'

The portal of entry for *S.* Typhi or *S.* Paratyphi into the body is through the small intestine, so stomach acidity is a defensive barrier: the higher the pH, the lower the infectious dose required. Morgan has reflux oesophagitis and takes omeprazole, a proton pump inhibitor that increases the gastric pH (making the stomach less acidic), thereby reducing the infective dose of *S.* Typhi or *S.* Paratyphi needed to cause an infection (Parry et al., 2002). The infectious dose for enteric fever varies between 1000 and 1 000 000 organisms (Hornick et al., 1970).

> Morgan recalls that a public health doctor spoke to him by phone early in his admission. He can't remember the conversation very well because he was so sick at the time but thinks there was something about testing his family for typhoid. Dustin promises he will follow this up with the public health unit director, Dr Richard Manetta. He contacts him later that day.
>
> 'Richard, our typhoid patient was keen to know how your contact tracing investigation was going. My understanding of contact tracing protocols was that they vary from place to place.'

The public health approach to enteric fever is controversial. Skull and Tallis (2001) examined the guidelines for managing cases of typhoid and their contacts in Australia, the US and England and found that those from the Australian state of Victorian were the only ones to define typhoid carriers and discuss their management. Furthermore, there was little conformity between guidelines especially with regard to:

- the follow-up of cases (timing and number of stool specimens)
- exclusion from food-handling/work/school
- determining who contacts are
- determining how contacts are followed up (timing and number of stool specimens)

Given the low yield of positive stool cultures from secondary contacts of the index case, researchers have questioned whether it is worth screening contacts at all (Thomas et al., 2006).

> Richard goes through the local guidelines for identifying and following up contacts:
> - Contacts are household contacts, carers and those exposed to the same source of the infection (if this is known).
> - To clear a case of infection, three consecutive stool specimens taken more than 24 hours apart are required. These should only be submitted ≥1 month after the onset of the illness and ≥48 hours after ceasing antibiotics.
> - To clear a contact of infection, two consecutive stool specimens ≥24 hours apart are required.
> - Positive stool samples mean three more consecutive stool samples must be collected every month until all three are negative.
> - All contacts should be educated about the symptoms of enteric fever and be urged to seek medical attention if these develop.
> - For both cases and contacts, good hygienic practices must be emphasised to minimise the risk of faeco-oral transmission.
>
> Dustin asks, 'Do you usually request urine specimens from the index case?'

Follow-up urine specimens are usually required if the urine cultures during the acute illness were positive or if there is a history of urinary tract infection or schistosomiasis (NSW Health, 2004).

> 'This patient did not travel overseas, so he must have acquired this locally. Have you had any other cases of locally-acquired S. Typhi recently?' Dustin asks.
> It turns out that there have been six typhoid notifications from this part of the country in the last four weeks, all in people with no history of recent travel.
> 'So does this mean that you have an outbreak on your hands?'

CASE 7   ENTERIC FEVER

An outbreak (also known as an epidemic) refers to a larger than usual number of cases of an infection over a given time period in a certain area. Certainly, six cases of locally-acquired typhoid in four weeks would constitute an outbreak in a developed nation.

> 'But is it the same strain of *S*. Typhi?' asks Dustin.
> 'Yes,' replies Richard. 'All six cases have the same phage type.'

S. Typhi can be differentiated into further strains. If a single strain of *S*. Typhi is identified as being responsible for a cluster of cases of typhoid fever, this is further evidence that there is an outbreak, probably from a single source. Bacteriophage typing (phage typing) is a commonly used method of identifying strains of *Salmonella* spp.

In simple terms, a bacteriophage is a virus that infects and can kill bacteria. The diagnostic role of bacteriophages is based on the principle that certain phages infect certain species of bacteria. Phage typing is usually performed in a reference laboratory for *Salmonella* spp. It generally takes only one day to get a result after the test has been set up in the laboratory.

Other methods used to identify strains of *S*. Typhi include pulsed field gel electrophoresis (PFGE) and identifying variable-number tandem repeats (Liu et al., 2003).

Since the phage can infect and kill bacteria, it is logical to wonder about a role as an antibacterial agent. In Georgia (in the former Soviet Union), phage therapy is used as an alternative to antibiotics to treat bacterial infections (Parfitt, 2005). Recently, the US Food and Drug Administration approved the use of a bacteriophage in meat and poultry products to combat *Listeria monocytogenes* contamination (Lang, 2006).

> 'Given that you have an outbreak on your hands, how are you going proceed?' Dustin asks.

Richard should initiate the outbreak investigation steps outlined in Case 4.

> Over the next three days, Richard and his outbreak team investigate the typhoid cluster. None of the six cases know each

other and a brief history reveals no obvious connection. A hypothesis-generating questionnaire is then used, identifying that within the incubation period:

- 6/6 (100%) had eaten cheesecake (bought however from six different bakeries)
- 6/6 (100%) had drunk milk
- 5/6 (83%) had eaten apples
- 5/6 (83%) had eaten bread
- 4/6 (67%) had drunk orange juice

The team initiates a case-control study using 18 controls randomly chosen from the electoral roll and the six typhoid cases to examine these variables.

The epidemiologist on the outbreak team completes the statistical analysis. The odds ratio for each variable are given in Table 7.4.

There is unlikely to be an association between the typhoid cases and the apple, bread or orange juice because the lower limits of the 95% confidence intervals are below 1.0. The reason that the cheesecake and milk both have odds ratios of infinity is because there were no cases of typhoid who did not have these items. Therefore, it is important to look at a two-by-two tables for these food items to see which are more likely to be involved in the outbreak (Table 7.5).

Of the 18 controls who did not have typhoid, only one ate cheesecake. This is in contrast to 17 controls who drank milk. In other words, there

Table 7.4 Odds ratio of food groups associated with the outbreak of typhoid fever

Item	Odds ratio (95% confidence intervals)
Cheesecake	infinity
Milk	infinity
Apples	5 (0.5–51.8)
Bread	1.4 (0.1–16)
Orange juice	1.0 (0.1–78.1)

Table 7.5 Two-by-two tables of number of cases and controls who did and did not consume the milk or cheesecake

	Typhoid	No typhoid
Cheesecake yes	6	1
Cheesecake no	0	17
Milk yes	6	17
Milk no	0	1

were more people exposed to milk than cheesecake who did not develop the disease, so the cheesecake is more likely to be the source of infection. This is circumstantial evidence, but often that is all that an outbreak team has to go on.

> The epidemiologist tells Richard, 'I saw a case of *Salmonella* infection associated with contaminated eggs in a cheesecake. Do you think that the eggs in the cheesecake are the culprit?'

There are species of *Salmonella* that can be transmitted through eggs or animals but the *S.* Typhi and *S.* Paratyphi that cause enteric fever are purely human pathogens—they are not transmitted through animals or animal products (Parry et al., 2002). Despite the cheesecake being the culprit in this typhoid outbreak, any contamination of the food item has come from an infected human, probably during preparation of the cheesecake.

Given the faeco-oral transmission of enteric fever from person to person, it is not surprising that sexual activity between men has been documented as a means of transmission of typhoid fever (Reller et al., 2003). Presumably heterosexual activity involving ano-oral contact is also a risk factor.

> The food inspector on the outbreak team, Mr Kevin Goodman, talks to the stores that sold cheesecake to each of the typhoid patients. It turns out that they all use the same cheesecake manufacturer, 'Say Cheese'. None of the typhoid cases have any

cheesecake left so the inspector takes a cheesecake from each of the stores for analysis at an environmental laboratory.

Kevin also investigates the manufactor and finds that some hygienic practices are inadequate. There are 15 employees involved in handling the food. Kevin gets all their names and asks them to provide stool samples for typhoid. One or two are reluctant to do so but he reminds them that he can detain them under a public health order if they fail to comply with his instruction.

Two days later, samples from two of the cheesecakes taken from the six stores grow Gram negative bacilli consistent with a *Salmonella* sp. Richard immediately uses his public health powers to close the cheesecake manufacturer, issue a recall of all cheesecakes distributed to other stores, and advise members of the public not to consume cheesecake bought from any of the distribution stores.

Three days later, the first stool specimen of one of the food-handlers at 'Say Cheese' is found to contain a *Salmonella* sp, which later is found to be the outbreak strain. The source, Marion, was one of the food-handlers who initially refused to supply stool specimens. He appears shocked because, even though he has travelled to countries where typhoid fever is endemic, he can't recall an enteric fever-like illness.

'Is he lying?' his boss asks.

This man is likely to be a chronic typhoid carrier and it is recognised that up to 25% of typhoid carriers have no recollection of a typhoid-like illness (Parry et al., 2002).

Unfortunately for Marion, the public health unit is able to tap into a national database of typhoid cases. They find that Marion did, in fact, have typhoid fever in another state 18 months earlier. After speaking to the local public health unit there, they learn that he was a waiter at that time. His initial stool specimens post-treatment were still positive and he was advised to seek medical attention for antibiotics to eradicate carriage. He was also advised not to be a food-handler until he had been cleared of typhoid carriage in the stool. Unfortunately, Marion disappeared soon after this and

> was unable to be contacted. It now appears that he has continued working as a food-handler despite being instructed not to do so.

Marion's case is not unlike another asymptomatic typhoid carrier. Mary Mallon (the infamous 'Typhoid Mary') was an asymptomatic typhoid carrier who continued to handle food despite being instructed not to by the New York health department in the early twentieth century (Chan and Reidpath, 2003).

> Over the next few weeks, Marion again disappears, despite being told that he needs close medical follow-up. A public health order for detention is issued and he is soon found by the authorities. Detention orders are a last resort for public health officials but are deemed necessary if the community at large is at risk from an individual. He is admitted to hospital where he is given four weeks of antibiotics. Three follow-up stool cultures show successful clearance of the infection and he is released.
>
> Morgan's attempt to clear the infection is not as successful. His initial stool cultures post-treatment grew *S. Typhi*. Despite a course of antibiotics for some weeks, his stool cultures continue to be positive more than three months later. Dustin tells him that he is a chronic carrier.
>
> 'What do you mean by chronic carrier?' Morgan asks.

Chronic excretion of enteric fever organisms can occur in the stool or, less commonly, in the urine (especially those with pre-existing urinary tract abnormalities or schistosomiasis). Up to 10% of patients will excrete the organisms for up to three months and up to 3% will do so for more than a year (Parry et al., 2002).

> 'Is there any way to fix this, Doctor?'
> Dustin nods and says that cholecystectomy (removal of the gall bladder) might be the solution.
> 'How does that work?'

After the bacteria that cause enteric fever are ingested, they travel to the small intestine where they enter the underlying lymphoid tissue. The bacteria are then drained into the mesenteric lymph nodes, liver and spleen, where they multiply within mononuclear phagocytic cells during the incubation period of the infection. Then bacteraemia occurs, during which the bacteria spread to many sites, especially the bone marrow, liver, spleen and Peyer's patches of the terminal ileum.

The gall bladder can also be invaded, either directly as a result of the bacteraemia or indirectly from the liver and biliary tree. Once the gall bladder is infiltrated, organisms will be excreted in the stool or re-infect the small intestine. This is why cholecystectomy is an option for chronic carriers who do not respond to antibiotics. Not surprisingly, chronic colonisation of the gall bladder with *S.* Typhi or *S.* Paratyphi is more likely in those with cholelithiasis (gallstones); also, chronic carriage is more common in the elderly and in women (Parry et al., 2002).

> Morgan then asks, 'My 20-year-old daughter is going to India in a few months. She saw how sick I was with the enteric fever and doesn't want to get it. Is there a vaccine that she can take before going overseas?'

There are two types of commonly available typhoid vaccines, an oral vaccine (live attenuated strain) and an intramuscular capsular (Vi) polysaccharide vaccine. These vaccines provide up to 50–80% protection against *S.* Typhi but this is only temporary (Basnyat et al., 2005). Boosters need to be given every three years if individuals are likely to be re-exposed to typhoid, such as during further overseas travel (National Health and Medical Research Council, 2003). Boosters for the oral vaccine need only be given every five years if a four-dose course rather than a three-dose course is taken. A study found that nearly all travellers returning to the US with typhoid fever had not been vaccinated (Steinberg et al., 2004), so it is worth taking.

Another reason for vaccinating Morgan's daughter, irrespective of her upcoming holiday, is that she is the household contact of a chronic carrier of typhoid (National Health and Medical Research Council, 2003).

The vaccines are highly safe, with few adverse reactions. Since the oral vaccine is live, it cannot be taken by immunocompromised individuals. Both vaccines have age limits and are contraindicated in those <6 years for the oral live vaccine and <2 years for the capsular polysaccharide vaccine (National Health and Medical Research Council, 2003).

> 'Only 50–80% protection? That's not very good,' Morgan says. 'Isn't there anything better?'

A typhoid vaccine conjugated to a non-toxic *Pseudomonas aeruginosa* has been developed and has protective efficacy rates >90% in young children (Canh et al., 2004). It appears promising and may be an option in the future.

> 'Will it protect her against the other cause of enteric fever, the paratyphi bug?'

The available vaccines do not appear to induce immunity against *S.* Paratyphi A (Basnyat et al., 2005). The <100% efficacy of the vaccines against *S.* Typhi and their lack of protection against *S.* Paratyphi A mean good hygienic and dietary practices while overseas remain important, irrespective of vaccination status.

> 'Now, my daughter is only going to India for two weeks. Is it really necessary for her to have the immunisation for such a short trip?'

An American study found that about 16% of travel-associated cases of typhoid fever occurred in people who were overseas for two weeks or less (Steinberg et al., 2004), so even short trips are potentially risky.

> Renée listens to this conversation with interest. She asks Dustin, 'Do all travellers need to have the typhoid vaccine if they are travelling to endemic areas?'

It is probably reasonable to offer it to all travellers to typhoid-endemic regions. According to Ryan and Kain (2000), people at risk of complicated typhoid fever should be particularly encouraged to be immunised, including those with:

- severe atherosclerosis
- internal prostheses

- cholelithiasis
- immunocompromise

> Renée has one final question: 'Where did the name typhoid come from?'

It derives from the word tuphos, which refers to a stuporous state (Saab and Doshi, 2006).

References

Bal, S.K., Czarnowski, C. (2004) A man with fever, cough, diarrhea and a coated tongue. *Canadian Medical Association Journal* 170(7), 1095.

Basnyat, B., Maskey, A.P., Zimmerman, M.D. et al. (2005) Enteric (typhoid) fever in travelers. *Clinical Infectious Diseases* 41(10), 1467–72.

Bhutta, Z.A. (2006) Current concepts in the diagnosis and treatment of typhoid fever. *British Medical Journal* 333(7558), 78–82.

Canh, D.G., Lin, F.Y., Thiem, V.D. et al. (2004) Effect of dosage on immunogenicity of a Vi conjugate vaccine injected twice into 2- to 5-year-old Vietnamese children. *Infection and Immunity* 72(11), 6586–88.

Carlson, D.A., Dobozi, W.R. (1994) Hematogenous *Salmonella typhi* osteomyelitis of the radius. A case report. *Clinical Orthopaedics and Related Research* (308), 187–91.

Chan, K.Y., Reidpath, D.D. (2003) 'Typhoid Mary' and 'HIV Jane': responsibility, agency and disease prevention. *Reproductive Health Matters* 11(22), 40–50.

Clinical and Laboratory Standards Institute (2006) *Performance standards for antimicrobial susceptibility testing: sixteenth informational supplement.* Clinical and Laboratory Standards Institute; Wayne, Pennsylvania

Crump, J.A., Luby, S.P., Mintz, E.D. (2004) The global burden of typhoid fever. *Bulletin of the World Health Organization* 82(5), 346–53.

Dutta, S., Sur, D., Manna, B. et al. (2006) Evaluation of new-generation serologic tests for the diagnosis of typhoid fever: data from a community-based surveillance in Calcutta, India. *Diagnostic Microbiology and Infectious Disease* 56(4), 359–65.

Haq, S.A., Alam, M.N., Hossain, S.M. et al. (1997) Value of clinical features in the diagnosis of enteric fever. *Bangladesh Medical Research Council Bulletin* 23(2), 42–46.

Hornick, R.B., Greisman, S.E., Woodward, T.E. et al. (1970) Typhoid fever: pathogenesis and immunologic control. *New England Journal of Medicine* 283(14), 739–46.

Isenberg, H., Washington, J., Balows, A. et al. (1985) Collection, handling and processing of specimens. In Lennette, E., Balows, A., Hausler Jr, W., Shadomy, H. (eds.) *Manual of Clinical Microbiology.* American Society for Microbiology; Washington DC

Katafuchi, R. (2005) Remember typhoid fever as a cause of acute nephritic syndrome even in Japan. *Internal Medicine* 44(12), 1207–88.

Kawano, R.L., Leano, S.A., Agdamag, D.M. (2007) A comparison of serological test kits for the diagnosis of typhoid fever in the Philippines. *Journal of Clinical Microbiology* 45(1), 246–47.

Kelly, M., Brenner, D., Farmer III, J. (1985) Enterobacteriaceae. In Lennette, E., Balows, A., Hausler Jr, W., Shadomy, H. (eds.) *Manual of Clinical Microbiology*. American Society for Microbiology; Washington DC

Klotz, S.A., Jorgensen, J.H., Buckwold, F. J. et al. (1984) Typhoid fever. An epidemic with remarkably few clinical signs and symptoms. *Archives Internal Medicine* 144(3), 533–37.

Lakshmi, V., Ashok, R., Susmit, A. J. et al. (2006) Changing trends in the antibioGrams of *Salmonella* isolates at a tertiary care hospital in Hyderabad. *Indian Journal of Medical Microbiology* 24(1), 45–48.

Lang, L.H. (2006) FDA approves use of bacteriophages to be added to meat and poultry products. *Gastroenterology* 131(5), 1370.

Liu, Y., Lee, M. A., Ooi, E.E. et al. (2003) Molecular typing of *Salmonella* enterica serovar typhi isolates from various countries in Asia by a multiplex PCR assay on variable-number tandem repeats. *Journal of Clinical Microbiology* 41(9), 4388–94.

National Health and Medical Research Council (2003) *Australian Immunisation Handbook. 8th Edition.* National Health and Medical Research Council; Canberra. Available from www9.health.gov.au/immhandbook (Accessed 25 January, 2007)

Nsutebu, E.F., Martins, P., Adiogo, D. (2003) Prevalence of typhoid fever in febrile patients with symptoms clinically compatible with typhoid fever in Cameroon. *Tropical Medicine & International Health* 8(6), 575–78.

NSW Health (2004) *Typhoid Response Protocol for NSW Public Health Units.* NSW Health. Available from http://www.health.nsw.gov.au/infect/pdf/typhoid.pdf (Accessed 25 January, 2007)

Olopoenia, L.A., King, A.L. (2000) Widal agglutination test 100 years later: still plagued by controversy. *Postgraduate Medical Journal* 76(892), 80–84.

Parfitt, T. (2005) Georgia: an unlikely stronghold for bacteriophage therapy. *Lancet* 365(9478), 2166–67.

Parry, C.M. (2004) The treatment of multidrug-resistant and nalidixic acid-resistant typhoid fever in Viet Nam. *Transactions of the Royal Society of Tropical Medicine and Hygiene* 98(7), 413–22.

Parry, C.M., Hien, T.T., Dougan, G. et al. (2002) Typhoid fever. *New England Journal of Medicine* 347(22), 1770–82.

Pegues, D., Ohl, M., Miller, S. (2005) *Salmonella* species, including *Salmonella typhi*. In Mandell, G.L., Bennett, J.E., Dolin, R. (eds) *Principles and Practice of Infectious Diseases*. Churchill Livingstone; Philadelphia

Reller, M.E., Olsen, S.J., Kressel, A.B. et al. (2003) Sexual transmission of typhoid fever: a multistate outbreak among men who have sex with men. *Clinical Infectious Diseases* 37(1), 141–44.

Ryan, E.T., Kain, K.C. (2000) Health advice and immunizations for travelers. *New England Journal of Medicine* 342(23), 1716–25.

Saab, M., Doshi, D. (2006) A case of pyrexia from abroad. *European Journal of Emergency Medicine* 13(6), 366–68.

Skull, S.A., Tallis, G. (2001) An evidence-based review of current guidelines for the public health control of typhoid in Australia: a case for simplification and

resource savings. *Australian and New Zealand Journal of Public Health* 25(6), 539–42.
Steinberg, E.B., Bishop, R., Haber, P. et al. (2004) Typhoid fever in travelers: who should be targeted for prevention? *Clinical Infectious Diseases* 39(2), 186–91.
Thaver, D., Zaidi, A.K., Critchley, J. et al. (2005) Fluoroquinolones for treating typhoid and paratyphoid fever (enteric fever). Cochrane Database of Systematic Reviews (2), CD004530.
Thisyakorn, U., Mansuwan, P., Taylor, D.N. (1987) Typhoid and paratyphoid fever in 192 hospitalized children in Thailand. *American Journal of Diseases of Children* 141(8), 862–65.
Thomas, H.L., Addiman, S., Mellanby, A. (2006) Evaluation of the effectiveness and efficiency of the public health management of cases of infection due to *Salmonella typhi/paratyphi* in North East London. *Public Health* 120(12), 1188–93.
Tran, T.H., Bethell, D.B., Nguyen, T.T. et al. (1995) Short course of ofloxacin for treatment of multidrug-resistant typhoid. *Clinical Infectious Diseases* 20(4), 917–23.
Vollaard, A.M., Ali, S., Widjaja, S. et al. (2005) Identification of typhoid fever and paratyphoid fever cases at presentation in outpatient clinics in Jakarta, Indonesia. *Transactions of the Royal Society of Tropical Medicine and Hygiene* 99(6), 440–50.
Walia, M., Gaind, R., Mehta, R. et al. (2005) Current perspectives of enteric fever: a hospital-based study from India. *Annals of Tropical Paediatrics* 25(3), 161–74.
Wani, T., Kakru, D.K., Shaheen, R. et al. (2004) Infective endocarditis due to *Salmonella typhi*—a case report. *Indian Journal of Pathology & Microbiology* 47(1), 76–77.

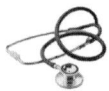

Case 8 Hepatitis A
Malini has jaundice …

Hepatitis A at a glance …

- **Agent:** family Picornaviridae; genus *Hepatovirus*; species hepatitis A virus
- **Geographical distribution:** worldwide
- **Main modes of transmission:** faeco-oral (mainly) and parenteral
- **Person-to-person transmission:** yes
- **Animal-to-person transmission:** yes (non-human primates to humans)
- **Incubation period:** 28 days (15–50 days)
- **Infectious period:** in immunocompetent adults, usually from 2 weeks before to 1 week after the onset of illness (no longer considered infectious 1 week after the onset of jaundice); young children and immunocompromised hosts can shed virus in faeces for up to 6 months
- **Clinical features:** typically, a short prodrome of non-specific features before jaundice supervenes; young children are usually asymptomatic and rarely jaundiced
- **Identification:** test serum for IgM against hepatitis A virus; polymerase chain reaction (PCR) of faeces and serum can be performed but rarely has clinical applications
- **Treatment:** supportive
- **Post-exposure prophylaxis:** primarily normal human immunoglobulin; however, vaccination may be used in certain circumstances
- **Vaccine:** a highly efficacious inactivated vaccine exists, which has been combined with other vaccines (e.g. hepatitis B, cholera and typhoid)

Main characters

Dr Manthri Pandit	infectious diseases registrar
Mr Victor Oldman	medical student doing an infectious diseases rotation
Dr Tikiri Fern	gastroenterology registrar
Ms Malini Udu	a woman with jaundice
Dr Sarath Sen	infectious diseases consultant
Dr Sunil Hailey	public health physician

Dr Manthri Pandit is an infectious diseases registrar in a busy hospital. She and her medical student, Mr Victor Oldman, are called to the emergency department by the gastroenterology registrar, Dr Tikiri Fern, to see a woman with jaundice.

Ms Malini Udu is a 42-year-old married woman with two children. She has no other health problems and takes no medications. She became sick seven days ago. After she experienced lethargy, anorexia and nausea for four days, her husband noticed she was slightly yellow. Today she became bright yellow and was rushed to hospital.

Examination reveals that she is jaundiced, slightly dehydrated and bradycardic with a normal blood pressure. She has posterior cervical lymphadenopathy and tender hepatomegaly. Blood tests show an elevated ALT of 4000 U/L (normal <40) and a bilirubin of 100 μmol/L (normal <20).

Tikiri says to Manthri, 'I am sure that this is hepatitis A, so she should be admitted under Infectious Diseases rather than Gastroenterology. Could you please look after her?'

What is hepatitis A?

Hepatitis A virus (HAV) is a non-enveloped RNA virus from the family Picornaviridae. The virus was first identified on electron microscopy in 1973 but outbreaks consistent with hepatitis A infection have been documented since the seventeenth century. This virus is responsible for hepatitis A infection, previously known as infectious hepatitis, epidemic hepatitis, epidemic jaundice and catarrhal jaundice (Wasley et al., 2006; World Health Organization, 2000).

CASE 8 HEPATITIS A

Worldwide there are approximately 1.5 million clinical cases of hepatitis A infection annually. However, this is a gross underestimate of the true prevalence because many cases are mild or subclinical. The cost of these infections is anywhere from US$1.5–3 billion annually (World Health Organization, 2000).

Although often regarded as a disease of the developing world, it is still a relatively common infection in many developed nations: some US states have a high enough prevalence to justify routine HAV vaccination (Wasley et al., 2006). In general, the main epidemiological difference between developed and developing nations is that the risk of infection and age of infection is inversely proportional to the level of hygiene. In developing countries, most children have been infected with HAV before the age of nine years. As sanitation improves, transmission shifts to older age groups (World Health Organization, 2000).

HAV is a hardy virus that survives in fresh or salt water and soil for long periods. While chlorine, bleach and formalin inactivate HAV, it is resistant to the effects of acid, detergent and freezing. Heating at 85°C for at least one minute also inactivates the virus (Brundage and Fitzpatrick, 2006; Wasley, 2006).

Malini's description of a prodromal illness preceding jaundice would be consistent with hepatitis A infection. The prodromal phase lasts 5–7 days and consists of a variable combination of non-specific symptoms including malaise, lethargy, fevers, abdominal pain, headache, nausea and vomiting. This is followed by the icteric phase which lasts 4–30 days and is associated with pale stool and tea-coloured urine (Brundage and Fitzpatrick, 2006).

Differential diagnoses

Tikiri cannot be sure that this illness is due to hepatitis A because the clinical features of infection are so non-specific and there is a long list of differential diagnoses (Table 8.1). Even the raised bilirubin and marked elevation of ALT are merely indicative of acute hepatocellular injury, the cause of which is uncertain. She may, however, be able to rule out some diagnoses by taking a thorough travel, recreational, animal contact, drug and sexual history.

Manthri challenges Tikiri, 'You can't be sure that this is hepatitis A. Why don't Gastroenterology look after her till we get a definitive diagnosis? If it does turn out to be HAV, then transfer her to us in Infectious Diseases.'

Tikiri agrees to this. 'So what is the definitive test for HAV?'

Table 8.1 Some differential diagnoses of hepatitis A infection

Infections	hepatitis B, C, D, E
	Q fever
	enteric fever
	HIV seroconversion illness
	Epstein-Barr virus
	cytomegalovirus
	primary herpes simplex infection
	primary varicella infection
	dengue
	leptospirosis
	parvovirus
	secondary syphilis
	disseminated gonococcal infection
	parasitic infestation
Drugs and toxins	wide variety
Autoimmune hepatitis	
Malignancy	A very uncommon cause of acute hepatitis. Aetiologies include non-Hodgkin's lymphoma and adult T-cell leukaemia (a complication of HTLV infection) (Powell et al., 2006).

SOURCE Adapted from Bhat et al., 1986; Bramkamp et al,. 1999; Brundage and Fitzpatrick, 2006

Investigations

Acute hepatitis A infection is routinely diagnosed around the world through serology with an anti-HAV IgM. The IgM can be detected through a variety of methods such as enzyme immunoassay (EIA), enzyme-linked immunosorbent assay (ELISA) and radioimmunoassay (RIA)(World Health Organization, 2000).

CASE 8 HEPATITIS A

It turns out that Malini's GP ordered anti-HAV IgM yesterday and the result will be available in a few hours.
Victor is concerned. He says, 'During my respiratory term, I saw a case of *Legionella* pneumonia. The patient seroconverted four weeks after they became sick. Isn't it too early in Malini's illness for her to be IgM-positive?'

The disadvantage of serology for many infections is that seroconversion takes place days after the onset of illness, resulting in a late diagnosis. However, this is not the case for hepatitis A infection. Anti-HAV IgM will be positive as early as 5–10 days before the onset of symptoms (Fiore, 2004).

Victor now asks, 'Is it a sensitive and specific test?'

Anti-HAV IgM is extremely sensitive and specific for diagnosing hepatitis A. Nevertheless, it is highly specific only for those with a high pre-test probability of disease, namely, patients with acute hepatitis. In people without the typical clinical syndrome of acute hepatitis, false-positive results have been commonly documented (Centers for Disease Control and Prevention, 2005).
Other situations where false-positive anti-HAV IgM results can occur are when testing people who have recovered from acute hepatitis A, where the IgM can sometimes take a year to disappear (Wasley et al., 2006), and testing in the month following vaccination against HAV (Fiore, 2004).

'But why has she got posterior cervical lymphadenopathy and bradycardia if she has hepatitis A infection?' Victor asks.

Posterior cervical lymphadenopathy and bradycardia are features of HAV infection (Brundage and Fitzpatrick, 2006). Cardiovascular instability with hypotension and dysrhythmias is an uncommon but serious complication (Atabek and Pirgon, 2007). Although Malini's blood pressure is stable, it would be prudent to commence cardiac monitoring.

Uncommonly, HAV causes an extensive number of extrahepatic manifestations, including neurological, haematological, vasculitic, renal, and other gastrointestinal findings (pancreatitis, acalculous cholecystitis) (Brundage and Fitzpatrick, 2006).

Malini is admitted to the infectious diseases ward. 'Does she need to be isolated?' the nurse unit manager asks.

Isolation measures

HAV is transmissible through the faeco-oral route; Malini should therefore be placed in a single room with a bathroom exclusively for her. Staff and visitors should gown and glove when entering the room and continue to practise good hand washing. In developing nations with limited resources, these measures may not be possible.

A few hours later, Malini's anti-HAV IgM result returns positive: the diagnosis is confirmed. Malini is shocked. She immediately asks, 'Am I going to die, Doctor?'

Prognosis

Death from acute hepatitis A infection is very unlikely. Death occurs when the infection is complicated by acute liver failure, which is extremely uncommon. The overall mortality rate is 0.6%, although it is over 2% in those aged ≥40 years old. The presence of chronic liver disease, for example, due to chronic hepatitis B or C infection, increases the risk of complications (Wasley et al., 2006; World Health Organization, 2000).

'Can you cure me?'

Treatment

There is no cure: management is purely supportive. Antivirals and corticosteroids have no role in the management of this infection (World Health Organization, 2000), although there is a case report of corticosteroid use for cardiovascular complications (Atabek and Pirgon, 2006). Supportive measures include antiemetics for nausea and vomiting, intravenous fluids to maintain hydration in patients too unwell to drink adequately, and avoiding potentially hepatotoxic agents such as alcohol (Brundage and Fitzpatrick, 2006). Nevertheless, more than 99% of patients fully recover.

'That's good news. How long will it take me to get over this Doctor, and will I ever get it again?'

Most people will have recovered after two months of illness. However, a prolonged or relapsing course occurs in 10–15% of individuals and lasts for up to six months (Wasley et al., 2006). Infection with HAV produces lifelong immunity (Wasley at al., 2006).

'There's no chance of getting cirrhosis from this is there?'

Unlike infection from hepatitis B and C, HAV is not associated with chronic hepatitis and cirrhosis (World Health Organization, 2000).

Manthri is approached by one of the blood collectors. 'Doctor, I just took blood from Malini. I don't know how but I ended up pricking myself with the needle. The syringe was full of blood. Am I at risk of infection?' Manthri isn't sure and asks her boss, Dr Sarath Sen.

According to Nainan et al. (2006) and Cuthbert (2001), HAV is transmitted predominantly through the faeco-oral route, typically in the following settings:

Personal contact, especially household contacts
Foodborne transmission through contaminated seafood or when an infected food-handler contaminates food at a restaurant or in the processing stage
Waterborne transmission through contaminated well water and

swimming pools (HAV is an occupational hazard for sewage workers in some parts of the world)
Sexual transmission, mainly through oral–anal contact and predominantly associated with homosexual men, although other groups are susceptible

Nevertheless, parenteral transmission is also well documented. According to Cuthbert (2001) this has occurred in the setting of:

Blood transfusion or transfusion of blood products
Injecting drug use, either through injection of blood containing HAV or through injecting drugs that have been carried in the rectum

> Given that Malini is only in her eighth day of illness, it is quite possible that a needlestick injury could result in parenteral transmission of the virus. Manthri therefore organises post-exposure prophylaxis (PEP) for the blood collector.
> 'Does the public health unit (PHU) need to be informed?' she asks Sarath.

Public health notification and response

In many parts of the world, hepatitis A infection is a notifiable disease, although it may be laboratory-notifiable only (i.e. laboratory staff inform the PHU of any positive anti-HAV IgM). This is because infection can be influenced by public health actions, namely, identifying the source of the infection to prevent further new cases occurring and providing PEP for contacts of the index case. In addition, public health officials are always interested in any disease that is potentially vaccine preventable, such as hepatitis A infection.

> Manthri speaks to the public health physician, Dr Sunil Hailey. Sunil says the lab has called him with the IgM result and that he was about to contact the clinical team for more details.
> Manthri fills him in, then asks, 'Is this an isolated case or have there been others?'
> Sunil says that they normally expect about three cases per month of HAV but this was the seventh case in the last two weeks. It appears that there is an outbreak.

> Sunil's first priority is to provide PEP to Malini's close contacts. 'Who would be a close contact of someone with HAV?' Manthri asks.

The definition of a close contact may vary between public health jurisdictions but according to Brundage and Fitzpatrick (2006) it generally includes:

- household/family contacts
- intimate/sexual contacts
- those who received a meal prepared by the case if it was not subject to further cooking
- other food-handlers in a restaurant/eating venue if the case was a food-handler
- attendees or employees of childcare centres

They all should receive PEP if less than two weeks has passed since their exposure to the case (National Health and Medical Research Council, 2003).

The infectious period for HAV depends on age. In immunocompetent adults, it is usually two weeks before the onset of illness to one week afterwards. In practical terms, cases should be considered infectious till one week after the onset of jaundice (National Health and Medical Research Council, 2003). Infants, young children and the immunocompromised, however, can shed HAV in their faeces for many months (Wasley et al., 2006; World Health Organization, 2000).

> Sunil calls Malini in hospital and determines which people require PEP.
> 'What will you give them?' she asks.

Passive immunisation with intramuscular normal human immunoglobulin (NHIG) should be used if it is available. Active immunisation with HAV vaccine is generally not recommended as PEP (National Health and Medical Research Council, 2003), despite one study demonstrating a protective efficacy of 79% among household/personal contacts (Sagliocca et al., 1999). The major limitation of the trial was that there was no comparison arm using NHIG.

UK guidelines recommend using HAV vaccine for PEP if the time of exposure is within one week (Centre for Protections and Health

Protection Agency, 2007) but Australian and US guidelines prefer NHIG (Brundage and Fitzpatrick 2006; National Health and Medical Research Council, 2003).

Malini is now in Day 10 of her illness (four prodromal days and six days of jaundice). After tomorrow, she will no longer be considered infectious. Sunil compiles a list of contacts and gets his staff to contact them over the next few hours about the need for NHIG. A few of the contacts have questions.
'How effective is this injection in preventing infection?'

NHIG is >85% effective if administered within two weeks of exposure to HAV. The efficacy is higher the sooner it is administered after exposure (Fiore, 2004). NHIG will either prevent HAV infection completely or attenuate the clinical presentation.

'So I could still get hepatitis A infection despite getting this injection?'

NHIG is not 100% efficacious, so it is important to educate contacts about the symptoms of breakthrough infection. They must contact the PHU or their GP immediately if such symptoms occur (NSW Health, 2004).

'I'm going to India for a month in three weeks. If I get this NHIG stuff, will I still need to be vaccinated against hepatitis A?'

One hundred units of NHIG will provide up to six months protection from hepatitis A infection (World Health Organization, 2000), so technically this contact will be immune to hepatitis A infection during the trip to India. Someone who plans to continue travelling to areas of high endemicity for HAV is better off getting a course of HAV vaccination.

'I have IgA deficiency. Can I still get NHIG?'

NHIG is not recommended for people with selective IgA deficiency because they are more likely to suffer anaphylaxis (Brundage and Fitzpatrick, 2006).

> 'Can I safely have the hepatitis A vaccine at the same time as the NHIG?'

NHIG and HAV vaccination can be given together. However, this does not apply to all vaccines. Due to interference with the immune response, mumps/measles/rubella vaccine should not be given within three months and varicella within five months of NHIG administration. Conversely, NHIG should not be given within two weeks of receiving a live attenuated vaccine (World Health Organization, 2000).

> 'I received two doses of hepatitis A vaccine last year just prior to travelling to China. Do I need the NHIG injection?'

Active immunisation with the two doses of HAV vaccine should provide long-term immunity against HAV.

The vaccine is an inactivated vaccine. Two doses are recommended, with the first causing more than 90% of recipients to seroconvert by four weeks and the second providing long-term protection. The vaccine has an excellent efficacy rate of 94–100%. It should provide at least 20 years of protection from hepatitis A infection (Fiore, 2004).

In the US, there has been a reduction in cases of HAV out of proportion to the modest vaccine uptake. This suggests herd immunity may develop (Wasley et al., 2006).

> 'I've been told I couldn't have the NHIG because my last contact with the person with hepatitis A was more than two weeks ago. Is this correct?'

Nothing is gained in administering NHIG at this late stage. The contact needs to be educated about the symptoms of infection and the importance of seeking medical attention if they occur.

> Sarath calls Malini in hospital a few days later to let her know that all her contacts have received PEP. Malini asks, 'Are you likely to find out where I contracted this infection from?'

Sarath will certainly look for a source but in a large proportion of cases one is never found. US researchers examined risk factors for hepatitis A infection and found that nearly half of cases (48%) had no clear source (Fiore, 2004). The risk factors that were identified were household or sexual contact (14%), men who have sex with men (10%), day care (8%), other contact (8%), international travel (5%), injecting drug use (5%) and a common source outbreak (4%).

> 'By the way, Doctor, my husband hasn't been feeling well for the past seven days. He has been tired and achy and probably has fevers. We forgot to mention this earlier because everyone was focussed on my illness.
>
> 'He hasn't become jaundiced like I did, so I assume he can't have hepatitis. Is that right?'

Nearly all adults with hepatitis A infection will be symptomatic and >70% will be jaundiced. This means that up to 30% of symptomatic adults with hepatitis A infection will not be jaundiced (Wasley et al., 2006). Malini's husband needs to be tested for acute hepatitis A infection.

> 'Oh no. Is there anything that he shouldn't do if he has hepatitis A?'

Restrictions vary from jurisdiction to jurisdiction but people with HAV are generally advised to not work in childcare facilities, prepare food for others or work as a food-handler or in healthcare facilities during the infectious period (National Health and Medical Research Council, 2003).

> Soon Malini's husband is confirmed as being anti-HAV IgM-positive. There have now been eight cases of hepatitis A infection in just over two weeks. Sunil forms an outbreak team and informs hospitals and GPs in the area of the outbreak.
>
> Using a hypothesis-generating questionnaire, the outbreak team work tirelessly to find clues to the source of the outbreak before the media find out about it. After exhaustive questioning, the only common thread appears to be that six of the eight cases all have children attending the Happy Titus Kindergarten.

> The outbreak team then conducts a case-control study. The results are summarised in Table 8.2.

Table 8.2 Two-by-two table from the case-control study examining the risk of hepatitis A infection in people whose children attend the Happy Titus Kindergarten

	Disease	No disease
Child attends the Kindergarten	6	2
Child doesn't attend	2	18
Odds ratio 27 (95% CI 2.3, 534.3)		

The study shows a strong association between cases of HAV and attendance at the Kindergarten. The lack of precision of the odds ratio, as evidenced by the wide range of the confidence intervals, reflects the small sample size.

> The outbreak team conduct further investigations at the Kindergarten and determine the source of the outbreak.
> Sunil fills Manthri in. 'It appears that a three-year-old girl from an African nation was the source of the outbreak. She had arrived in the country about eight weeks earlier and immediately started attending the kindergarten. She is anti-HAV IgM positive.
> 'I think she was infected in Kenya and was still in her infectious period when she started kindergarten. She then infected a number of other children, who in turn infected family members.'
> Manthri isn't convinced. 'But if you're right, shouldn't the other children have been clinically unwell? You told me that all your notifications were in adults.'

Seventy per cent of children under the age of six years with hepatitis A are asymptomatic and even the symptomatic ones do not get jaundice. Furthermore, young children have the highest rates of infection.

Since no one realises that they have an active infection, children are very efficient transmitters of HAV and are often the source of infection in regions with sustained transmission of the disease (Wasley et al., 2006). In this case, both the index case and the children she infected would have been asymptomatic or minimally symptomatic.

> 'There's good epidemiologic evidence, but it would be nice if you had some molecular evidence too,' Manthri says.
> 'But we have,' Sunil replies. 'All the cases linked to the Kindergarten are of the same genotype. Furthermore, it is a genotype never previously isolated here.'
> Manthri is surprised. 'I always thought there was only one serotype of HAV. Am I wrong?'

There is only one serotype of HAV but there are seven genotypes. Four genotypes are human, with genotypes I and III causing the bulk of human disease, and three are simian. Antibodies to particular genotypes seem to provide protection from the others (Nainan et al., 2006).

Various non-human primates are susceptible to infection with human genotypes of HAV. Infected animals can then transmit these human genotypes to susceptible humans. It is still unknown whether humans are susceptible to the simian genotypes (World Health Organization, 2000).

PCR techniques for detecting HAV RNA exist. They can be used on clinical or environmental specimens but given that the usefulness of serology lies in detecting acute infection, the need for PCR is not great. Nevertheless, molecular techniques may be useful in identifying an outbreak strain.

> 'What about the two hepatitis A cases that you can't link to the Kindergarten?'

There is always a background level of HAV activity and the cases not linked to the kindergarten may reflect that.

References

Atabek, M.E., Pirgon, O. (2007) Unusual cardiac features in cholestatic hepatitis A in an adolescent: improvement with corticosteroid treatment. *Journal of Infection* 54(2), 91–93.

Bhat, A., Kumar, A., Garg, A. et al. (1986) Disseminated gonococcaemia with arthritis, tenosynovitis and moderately severe jaundice. *Journal of the Association of Physicians of India* 34(7), 519–20.

CASE 8 HEPATITIS A

Bramkamp, G.R., Holt, R.I., Bending, J.J. et al. (1999) Hepatitis as the presenting feature of an HIV seroconversion illness. *International Journal of STD & AIDS* 10(10), 687–88.

Brundage, S.C., Fitzpatrick, A.N. (2006) Hepatitis A. *American Family Physician* 73(12), 2162–68, 2169–70.

Centre for Protections and Health Protection Agency (2007) *Immunoglobulin Handbook*. Available at www.hpa.org.uk/infections/topics_az/immunoglobulin/pdfs/ig_handbookJan2007.pdf (Accessed 23 April, 2007)

Centers for Disease Control and Prevention (2005) Positive tests results for acute hepatitis A virus infection among persons with no recent history of acute hepatitis—USA, 2002–4. *Morbidity and Mortality Weekly Report* 54(18), 453–56.

Cuthbert, J.A. (2001) Hepatitis A: old and new. *Clinical Microbiology Reviews* 14(1), 38–58.

Fiore, A.E. (2004) Hepatitis A transmitted by food. *Clinical Infectious Diseases* 38(5), 705–15.

Nainan, O.V., Xia, G., Vaughan, G. et al. (2006) Diagnosis of hepatitis A virus infection: a molecular approach. *Clinical Microbiology Reviews* 19(1), 63–79.

National Health and Medical Research Council (2003) *Australian Immunisation Handbook. 8th Edition*. National Health and Medical Research Council; Canberra. Available at www9.health.gov.au/immhandbook (Accessed 24 April, 2007)

NSW Health (2004) *Hepatitis A Response Protocol for NSW Public Health Units*. Available at http://www.health.nsw.gov.au/infect/pdf/hepA.pdf (Accessed 24 April, 2007)

Powell, N., Rusli, F., Hubscher, F.G. et al. (2006) Adult T-cell leukemia presenting with acute liver failure. *Leukemia Research* 30(10), 1315–17.

Sagliocca, L., Amoroso, P., Stroffolini, T. et al. (1999) Efficacy of hepatitis A vaccine in prevention of secondary hepatitis A infection: a randomised trial. *Lancet* 353(9159), 1136–39.

Wasley, A., Fiore, A., Bell, B.P. (2006) Hepatitis A in the era of vaccination. *Epidemiologic Reviews* 28, 101–11.

World Health Organization (2000) WHO/CDS/CSR/EDC/2000.7 *Hepatitis A*. World Health Organization Department of Communicable Disease Surveillance and Response, World Health Organization; Geneva. Available at www.who.int/csr/disease/hepatitis/HepatitisA_whocdscsredc2000_7.pdf (Accessed 20 April, 2007)

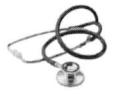

Case 9 Influenza
Toby's got the flu …

Influenza at a glance …

- **Agent:** family Orthomyxoviridae; genus *Influenzavirus* A and B; species influenza A virus, influenza B virus
- **Geographical distribution:** worldwide
- **Main mode of transmission:** droplet transmission
- **Person-to-person transmission:** yes
- **Animal-to-person transmission:** yes
- **Incubation period:** 2–3 days (1–7 days)
- **Infectious period:** 1 day before onset of symptoms to 7 days after onset of symptoms (possibly up to 21 days for very young children)
- **Clinical features:** an influenza-like illness (ILI) with abrupt onset of fevers, cough, headaches, myalgias and sore throat; less commonly, other respiratory and extra-respiratory manifestations
- **Identification:** serology, immunofluorescence, culture, 'rapid tests' [immunochromatographic tests (ICT), enzyme immunoassays (EIA), optical immunoassays (OIA)] reverse transcriptase polymerase chain reaction (RT-PCR)
- **Treatment:** M2 protein inhibitors (amantadine, rimantadine); neuraminidase inhibitors (oseltamivir, zanamivir)
- **Prophylaxis:** yes, with the above agents
- **Vaccine:** inactivated vaccine mostly used; vaccine for avian influenza still being developed

Main characters

Dr Didier Boden	general practitioner
Mr Toby Lam	man with a flu-like illness
Dr Kathleen Peters	general practice registrar
Ms Harriet Goodman	woman with cough and fevers
Dr Kiana Shaw	infectious diseases physician
Mr Greg Smith	infectious diseases nurse
Dr Tim Waters	general practitioner
Mr Neville Thomasson	patient with suspected avian influenza

'I had a little bird
Its name was Enza
I opened the window
And in flu Enza'

Children's nursery rhyme during the 1918 influenza pandemic, which killed at least 40 million people (Crawford, 1995).

> It is the height of winter and the influenza season in a big city. In one general practice, the waiting room is full of people sneezing and coughing. Dr Didier Boden calls in the next patient, 45-year-old Mr Toby Lam. With Toby's permission, a GP registrar, Dr Kathleen Peters, sits in.
>
> Toby is an otherwise healthy accountant who became suddenly unwell three days ago. He first noticed becoming hot and then cold. Soon after, he developed a headache, non-productive cough, generalised muscle aches and a runny nose. He has felt too run down to attend work. His physical examination is unremarkable, apart from a fever of 38.1°C.
> 'Is this influenza, Doctor?'

What is influenza?

Toby certainly has an influenza-like illness (ILI), which is characterised by the abrupt onset of symptoms with fevers, cough, sore throat, headaches and myalgias. However, the differential diagnosis for an ILI is not limited to influenza but includes other viral (parainfluenza, adenoviruses, coronaviruses, rhinoviruses and respiratory syncytial virus) and bacterial illnesses.

One study showed that a fever and cough developing within 48 hours of the onset of illness during an influenza outbreak had a positive predictive value of 79% (p <0.001) of correctly identifying patients with influenza (Monto et al., 2000). This leaves room for error when diagnosing influenza on clinical grounds alone. Still, it would be reasonable to tell Toby that influenza is probably the most likely diagnosis, given his symptoms and that it is influenza season.

Influenza tends to occur seasonally, maximally over a six-week period in temperate climates in the northern hemisphere (peaking between December and April) and southern hemisphere (peaking between June and September). However, it can occur throughout the year in tropical areas (Li et al,. 2005).

Toby wants to know how quickly a diagnosis of influenza can be made. Kathleen says, 'Can't we do a rapid test?'

Investigations

'Rapid test' is a non-specific term for several tests that can be used to diagnose influenza quickly, particularly those which can be used in the community setting, give a result in under 30 minutes and do not require the technical expertise of a scientist.

In general, influenza can be diagnosed from serum, using serology, or from respiratory secretions (nasopharyngeal swabs and aspirates, throat swabs, bronchoalveolar lavage samples and sputum specimens) using:

- viral culture
- reverse transcriptase polymerase chain reaction (RT-PCR)
- immunofluorescence
- rapid tests

Serology involves detecting a four-fold rise in antibodies between paired acute and convalescent sera. This may take up to two weeks. Viral culture often takes a week or more (even the most rapid culture techniques may still take 48 hours); RT-PCR can take 24 to 48 hours; and immunofluorescence may only take two hours but typically needs to be performed in a microbiology laboratory. Commercially-produced rapid tests differ with regard to:

- the principle behind the test (e.g. immunochromatographic tests [ICT], optical immunoassays [OIA] and enzyme immunoassays [EIA])
- the types of specimens that can be used (e.g. certain kits may only be effective with nasopharyngeal specimens)

- their ability to differentiate between influenza A and B

  A useful table which summarises the features of the different rapid tests can be found at www.cdc.gov/flu/professionals/labdiagnosis.htm.

Didier's practice does keep a rapid test kit. He collects a nasopharyngeal swab and asks Toby to sit in the consultation room. He then processes the specimen. While they wait, Kathleen asks, 'How reliable are rapid tests?'

Alexander et al. (2005) compared one commercially-available rapid test against established laboratory tests and found it was highly specific (100%) but had a sensitivity of only 80.8% (specificity refers to the probability of the test being negative in people without the disease and sensitivity is the probability of the test being positive in people with the disease).

Kathleen looks puzzled. 'So how can we use a test like this that has good specificity but poor sensitivity?'

There are two reasons why a test with good specificity but poor sensitivity can still be useful, usually known by their acronyms SnNOUT and SpPIN:

SnNOUT Sn = sensitivity, N = negative, OUT = out. This means that when a test is highly sensitive, a negative result is likely to rule out the disease. However, this particular rapid test was not very sensitive (only 80%).

SpPIN Sp = specificity, P = positive, IN = in. This means that when a test is highly specific, a positive result indicates that the person is likely to have the disease. This rapid test was extremely specific (100%).

Another statistical way of reflecting this is through positive and negative predictive values (PPV and NPV, respectively). The PPV is the probability of the person having the disease when the test is positive. The NPV is the probability of the person not having the disease when the test is negative. This rapid test had a PPV of 100% and NPV of 83%.

In conclusion, a positive test means the person is very likely to have influenza but a negative test does not exclude it and calls for testing at a microbiology laboratory.

Twenty minutes later, Didier calls Toby back in—the test is positive. Toby asks, 'Doctor, can you treat this?'

Treatment

There are two groups of medications that can be used not only for the treatment of influenza but also for chemoprophylaxis:

- M2 protein ion channel inhibitors (amantadine, rimantadine)
- neuraminidase inhibitors (NIs) (zanamivir, oseltamivir)

Detailed guidelines for the use of these antiviral agents in the treatment and chemoprophylaxis of influenza have been developed by the National Institute of Clinical Excellence (NICE) and the Centers for Disease Control and Prevention (CDC) (Centers for Disease Control and Prevention 2006, 2005 and 2003; National Institute of Clinical Excellence, 2003). See Teo et al. (2004) for a summary. The key points are:

1. M2 protein inhibitors only treat influenza A while the NIs have activity against influenza A and B.
2. Antiviral agents can reduce the duration of illness by one day if used within 48 hours of the onset of symptoms. Data are lacking on whether antivirals reduce the rate of influenza-related complications.
3. Antiviral agents are generally recommended for people at high risk of complications of influenza. This is more an issue of limited supply; if adequate supplies of antivirals are available, even low-risk individuals can be treated (Harper et al., 2004).
4. Zanamivir comes as a dry powder, which is inhaled orally, and oseltamivir and the M2 protein inhibitors are taken orally.
5. Major adverse reactions include gastrointestinal symptoms (oseltamivir, M2 protein inhibitors), central nervous system toxicity (M2 protein inhibitors) and a reduction in lung function (zanamivir).
6. Use NIs for five days and M protein inhibitors for 3–5 days in total or cease 24–48 hours after the symptoms and signs have disappeared.
7. Chemoprophylaxis can be considered for:

- an acute outbreak in an institution
- a household outbreak, especially where there are high-risk contacts
- high-risk individuals who are not likely to benefit from vaccination
- throughout influenza season (around two months)

8. Neither the NICE nor the CDC guidelines recommend amantadine or rimantadine for treatment or chemoprophylaxis of influenza A virus.

Didier's local guidelines recommend the use of antivirals for influenza only in high-risk individuals who have been symptomatic for under 48 hours. Didier tells Toby that there are antiviral medications for influenza, but he does not meet the guidelines for eligibility (because he has had symptoms for over 48 hours and has a low risk of complications) and therefore cannot get government-subsidised medication.

Toby asks, 'If I am low risk, then who are the high risk individuals?'

The NICE guidelines (2003) identify the following risk factors for complications:

- chronic obstructive pulmonary diseases (COPD)
- age ≥65 years
- chronic renal disease
- immunocompromise
- significant cardiovascular disease

Toby leaves the practice, satisfied with the diagnosis. Didier's next patient is Ms Harriet Goodman. She is a 54-year-old woman who presented one week ago with a two-day ILI. At that time, Didier diagnosed her with influenza using the rapid test kit. Since she also did not meet the criteria for treatment, he did not prescribe antivirals.

She tells Didier she was definitely feeling much better, albeit tired, three days after seeing him and continued to feel that way till two days ago. Now she is experiencing fevers, shivers, a dry cough and shortness of breath.

> On examination, the left lower lobe is dull to percussion, with bronchial breath sounds and inspiratory crackles: she has left lower lobe pneumonia.
>
> Didier is concerned about Harriet and phones the infectious diseases (ID) physician, Dr Kiana Shaw, for advice. He describes the history and examination findings and asks, 'What could be causing her pneumonia?'

Influenza can be complicated by pneumonia. Classically, there are two types of pneumonia: primary influenza pneumonia and secondary bacterial pneumonia (Table 9.1).

Sometimes a mixed bacterial and viral pneumonia can occur, which can have features of each.

Table 9.1 How to differentiate between primary influenza pneumonia and secondary bacterial pneumonia

	Primary viral pneumonia	**Secondary bacterial pneumonia**
History	ILI continues to worsen	Biphasic illness: ILI gets better but after 4–7 days patients become unwell again
Examination	Bilateral lung findings	Unilateral lung findings
Chest X-ray	Bilateral changes	Unilateral changes, often lobar consolidation
Isolation of influenza virus	Yes	No
Response to antibiotics	No response	Improves

SOURCE Adapted from Treanor, 2005

> Kiana suggests that the biphasic illness and unilateral focal signs suggest a secondary bacterial pneumonia complicating influenza.
>
> Didier says, 'So I guess *Streptococcus pneumoniae* is the most common cause of this?'

S. pneumoniae and Haemophilus influenzae—the most common causes of community-acquired pneumonia—are also two of the major pathogens in secondary bacterial pneumonia complicating influenza. However, there is also an increased risk of *Staphylococcus aureus* infection (Schwarzmann et al., 1971); unlike the other two organisms, *S. aureus* is an uncommon cause of community-acquired pneumonia. Any antibiotic regimen for bacterial pneumonia complicating influenza should therefore include anti-staphylococcal therapy as well as conventional therapy for *S. pneumoniae* and *H. influenzae*.

> The two doctors agree that Harriet should be assessed in hospital. She is admitted under Kiana, who commences an empiric regimen of intravenous (IV) ceftriaxone and flucloxacillin. A sputum sample from admission later isolates *S. aureus*. She recovers well and is discharged home.

Prognosis

Influenza has a number of complications apart from pneumonia, outlined in Table 9.2.

Table 9.2 Respiratory and non-respiratory complications of influenza

Respiratory	Non-respiratory
Otitis media	pericarditis/myocarditis
Croup	myositis/rhabdomyolysis
Tracheobronchitis	Reye's syndrome[†]
Pneumonia	toxic shock syndrome
Worsening of pre-existing chronic obstructive pulmonary disease	transverse myelitis
	encephalitis
	Guillain-Barré syndrome (GBS)[‡]

[†]Reye's syndrome is an encephalopathy commonly associated with elevated blood ammonia and typically seen in children using aspirin to control fevers during a viral illness.
[‡]A definitive causative association between influenza and GBS has not been established, although cases of GBS have been reported following influenza.
SOURCE Adapted from Treanor, 2005

Meanwhile an infectious diseases nurse at the local public health unit, Mr Greg Smith, receives a call from a worried GP, Dr Tim Waters.

'Hello. I'm a GP in the area. I am worried that one of my patients may have avian influenza (AI). What should I do?'

Greg will need to determine whether the patient meets the case definition for AI. A case definition is an epidemiologic description used to decide whether an individual has the disease or not. It consists of clinical criteria, laboratory criteria (sometimes) and criteria for time, place and person. Case definitions can be further classified into possible and confirmed. Particularly with emerging infectious diseases, it is not uncommon for the case definition to be modified as more is learnt about the disease or as the disease changes.

The current case definitions used in Australia by the Department of Health and Ageing (2004) for AI are:

Possible case Person with an acute respiratory illness characterised by fever (temperature >38°C), cough and fatigue beginning within seven days of:

- contact with a confirmed case of influenza A(H5) during the infectious period OR
- a visit to a poultry farm or other poultry contact in an area known to have outbreaks of influenza A(H5) OR
- work in a laboratory processing samples from persons or animals suspected to have influenza A(H5) infection

Confirmed case A possible case becomes a confirmed case when there is microbiologic confirmation of H5N1 infection.

The incubation period of influenza is typically 2–3 days but can be 1–7 days (National Institute for Clinical Excellence, 2003). The infectious period in children ≤12 years old is from one day before the start of a H5 illness to seven days after symptom onset, with a maximum of 21 days.

At the time of writing, avian influenza due to the H5N1 virus had caused human illness and deaths in South-East Asia. [Note: There have been 194 deaths from 321 lab-confirmed cases of AI, giving a disturbing mortality rate of over 60% (World Health Organization, 2007).] The first avian cases of H5N1, but no human cases, had only recently been discovered in a number of European countries.

CASE 9 INFLUENZA

Greg goes over the case definition for AI as he talks to Tim. The patient, Mr Neville Thomasson, is a 39-year-old man who returned from Vietnam six days ago. He was in Vietnam for a fortnight and went to a number of rural areas. He recalls passing through a village market with live poultry eight days ago and spending some time there talking to the locals. He became ill with an ILI with high fevers (>39°C) two days ago.

Tim performed a rapid test for influenza yesterday using a nasopharyngeal swab: the result was negative, but he sent another specimen on to the hospital laboratory. Today he spoke to the lab's microbiologist, who told him the immunofluorescence assay was positive for influenza A.

Neville meets the clinical criteria for possible AI: he has high fevers and an ILI; has had poultry contact in a region known to have cases of AI; and became ill within seven days of contact with the poultry market.

'How is AI spread? I am worried that everyone in my practice was exposed,' Tim says.

Greg first needs to reassure Tim that his patient may not have AI at all. The only certainty is that he has an influenza A virus, of which H5N1 is only a single subtype. With regard to transmission of AI, Beigel et al. (2005) outline three modes:

Poultry-to-person A well-established mode of transmission.
Person-to-person There have been reports suggesting person-to-person transmission in certain clusters. However, these occurrences appear to have been limited. Authorities have not discovered cases of person-to-person transmission by small-particle aerosol.
Environment-to-person This is theoretically possible through oral ingestion or conjunctival or intranasal transmission of infected water, fomites or chicken manure.

Even if Dr Water's patient has H5N1, person-to-person transmission within the practice is not certain by any means.

> Greg says the priority is to confirm whether the patient's influenza virus is H5N1 or not. He speaks to the microbiologist who has the original specimen. 'Can we find out if this virus is H5N1?'

Specific tests have been developed to identify H5 strains of the influenza. They include immunofluorescence, RT-PCR, serology and culture (World Health Organization, 2005). RT-PCR tests for H5 are more sensitive than other rapid tests for H5 (Beigel et al, 2005). However, respiratory specimens generally have to be sent to special reference laboratories.

> The microbiologist agrees that the specimen should be tested for H5. In Tim's country, there is one reference laboratory; fortunately, it is close by. She promises to speak to the reference laboratory and send the specimen across today for RT-PCR testing.
> Tim asks Greg what he should tell the patient, who is currently resting at home.

Isolation measures

Guidelines for management of a possible case of AI vary somewhat from country to country. For example, Australia's policy (Department of Health and Ageing, 2004) is in line with a number of other countries in suggesting that, for public health risk management, cases stay in isolation until they are no longer a risk to others. They can be released:

- after a plausible alternative diagnosis for the illness is confirmed OR
- after viral culture or PCR on NPA or throat swab is negative on two consecutive days OR
- seven days after the onset of fever ($\geq 38°C$) for adults or 21 days for a child aged ≤ 12 years *unless* fever continues up to the seventh day after onset. In these cases, a decision has to be made by the responsible treating medical doctor.

A strategy for managing household contacts of individual cases is discussed by Beigel et al. (2005).

> Greg recommends Neville remain in isolation at home; hopefully the RT-PCR will show that he does not have H5N1. Luckily, Neville lives alone, so Greg doesn't have to worry about managing household contacts.
> 'If he does turn out to have H5N1, are anti-influenza medications effective?' Tim asks.

Beigel et al. (2005) discuss this. M2 protein inhibitors (amantadine, rimantadine) are not recommended because of high-level resistance. NIs can be used in the treatment and chemoprophylaxis of AI, although oseltamivir resistance has developed in cases who received oseltamivir. This resistance is due to the H274Y mutation and has not been associated with cross-resistance to zanamivir (De Clercq, 2006).

Resistance to NIs can occur among 'normal' (non-AI) influenza viruses, for example, with H3N2. Mutations such as R292K and E119V have been identified as causes of NI resistance (De Clercq, 2006).

> The microbiologist from the national influenza reference laboratory calls the next morning: thankfully, the patient does not have H5N1 on RT-PCR testing. They will, however, culture the virus and type it.
> Greg calls with the good news. 'How long will I be infectious for?' Neville asks.

Viral shedding begins one day before the onset of symptoms and is undetectable after 5–10 days (Treanor, 2005). Peak shedding occurs within the first 1–2 days. However, children can shed higher levels of virus for longer because they have less immunity.

> The patient is now at Day 3 of his illness, so Greg tells him that he is over the most infectious period of his illness, although he could still shed virus for up to six days. The national influenza reference laboratory cultures the virus and types it. Greg receives the final typing result two weeks later, which identifies the virus as A/New Caledonia/20/99 (H1N1)-like.
> Tim asks Greg what this means.

The reference laboratory is using the WHO nomenclature for influenza viruses. 'A' refers to influenza A (rather than influenza B); 'New Caledonia' refers to the place of origin of the virus; '20' refers to the isolate number; '99' refers to the year in which it was first isolated, i.e. 1999; '(H1N1)-like' refers to the haemagglutinin and neuraminidase subtypes of the strain (Cinti, 2005).

There are three broad groups of influenza viruses—A, B and C—divided on the basis of their serologic response to internal proteins. Aquatic birds are the natural host for influenza A but other mammals, including humans, can be hosts. Influenza B and C, on the other hand, are found exclusively in humans. Influenza B causes an ILI whereas influenza C tends to cause a far milder infection, similar to a cold (Zambon, 1999).

Influenza A is subtyped into combinations of its haemagglutinin (HA) and neuraminidase antigens (NA). There are 15 HA and nine NA subtypes, such as H5N1 or H2N2. Both HA and NA are important in the pathogenicity of the virus. Until recently, humans were susceptible only to infection with influenza A viruses that had combinations of H1-3 and N1-2 (Zambon, 1999). Recently, humans have become susceptible to a broader range of influenza A viruses, such as H5N1 and H7N7.

The different HA and NA combinations are the basis for antigenic drift and antigenic shift. Antigenic drift refers to minor antigenic point mutations in the HA, NA or both, which can occur annually. The new virus has some relationship to the previous one. This results in some immunity but difference is enough to cause disease.

Antigenic shift means that major antigenic changes have occurred, resulting in a new virus which has never infected humans before. Since the human population has no immunity whatsoever to this new strain, a pandemic can result. There were three pandemics in the twentieth century: in 1918 (H1N1), 1957 (H2N2) and 1968 (H3N2). There are concerns that the current H5N1 avian influenza virus will cause a pandemic if sufficient reassortment results in a virus that can effectively be transmitted from person-to-person.

> The following day, Greg receives a call from a member of the public asking about influenza vaccination.
> 'My partner has got HIV. He is worried about bird flu and all that stuff. Is it safe for him to get the influenza vaccine?'

HIV is a condition associated with impaired immunity. Since most countries use an influenza vaccine with inactivated virus rather than live virus, it is safe to use in people with HIV. It is also effective in reducing influenza rates in HIV positive people (Tasker et al., 1999). In fact, influenza vaccine is recommended for all people with immunodeficiency. This is not just because of their risk of influenza but also because many of them have an increased susceptibility to the pneumococcal pneumonia that can complicate the influenza.

> 'So he can definitely go ahead and have the vaccine?'

HIV is no reason for him to not have the vaccine. However, there are contraindications to or precautions when having the vaccine. The National Health and Medical Research Council (2003) lists:

- anaphylactic allergy to eggs
- anaphylactic allergy to any of the vaccine components
- acute febrile illness (≥38.5°C)
- history of GBS

> 'So will this be like his hepatitis B vaccination, where he only needs one course to last him for life?'

Antigenic drift means that new vaccines for the new viruses need to be given annually.

> The caller thanks Peter and hangs up. Brenda, one of the receptionists, also has some questions about the influenza vaccination.
> 'I am keen to get the influenza vaccine. But flu season has just started. Is it too late?'

Ideally, the influenza vaccine should be given in the autumn (fall) prior to the winter influenza season. However, the influenza season lasts about two months and the vaccine will provide protection within two weeks, so it can be effective if given in the early part of the influenza season.

> Brenda says, 'Oh good. And I assume that I won't get influenza once I've been vaccinated?'

In healthy young adults, the vaccine is 70% effective in reducing serologically-confirmed cases of influenza (Demicheli et al., 2004), so there are failures. However vaccinated people who develop influenza may have mild disease.

> Brenda has another question. 'My husband and I are going to Europe for a holiday in December, so it will be flu season there. He works in a hospital, so he's already been vaccinated. Will our shots protect us while we're over there?'

The virus strains for the annual influenza vaccines can vary between hemispheres. Therefore, Brenda and her husband will need to check with their GP that the local vaccine strains match the northern hemisphere vaccine strains; otherwise they may be well advised to receive the northern hemisphere vaccine prior to leaving.

> Brenda has a final question. 'After Europe we wanted to stopover in Indonesia. Is there a vaccine for avian influenza that we can take?'

Unfortunately there is still no H5NI vaccine available. Obstacles in the production of the vaccine have included limited immunogenicity, difficulties in producing enough antigen and lack of inter-clade cross-reactive immunity (H5NI occurs as 3 clades with further subclades among clade 2). However, the use of an oil-in-water vaccine adjunct may have brought us a step closer to overcoming these problems (Leroux-Roels et al., 2007; Sambhara and Poland, 2007).

> The final call for the day is from an airline steward. 'I just got off a four-hour flight. One of the passengers had a fever and was coughing. I don't know for sure what he had, but it is flu season so I'm sure influenza is a possibility. Could I get influenza from him?'

There have been a number of cases of influenza transmission during flights, possibly due to low cabin humidity facilitating the survival and transmission of respiratory droplets (Leder and Newman, 2005).

References

Alexander, R., Hurt, A.C., Lamb, D. et al. (2005) A comparison of a rapid test for influenza with laboratory-based diagnosis in a paediatric population. *Communicable Diseases Intelligence* 29(3), 272–76.

Beigel J.H., Farrar, J., Han, A.M. et al. (2005) Avian influenza A (H5N1) infection in humans. *New England Journal of Medicine* 353(13), 1374–85.

Centers for Disease Control and Prevention (2006) Prevention and control of influenza: recommendations of the Advisory Committee on Immunization Practices (ACIP). *Morbidity and Mortality Weekly Report Recommendations and Reports* 55(RR-10), 1–42.

Centers for Disease Control and Prevention (2005) *Influenza Antiviral Medications: 2005–6 Chemoprophylaxis (Prevention) And Treatment Guidelines* Available from www.cdc.gov/flu/professionals/treatment/pdf/0506antiviralguide.pdf (Accessed 24 October, 2005)

Centers for Disease Control and Prevention (2003) *Antiviral Agents For Influenza: Background Information For Clinicians.* Available from www.cdc.gov/flu/professionals/pdf/antiviralsbackground.pdf (Accessed 20 October, 2005)

Cinti, S. (2005) Pandemic influenza: are we ready? *Disaster Management and Response* 3(3), 61–7.

Crawford R. (1995) *'The Spanish Flu,' stranger than fiction: vignettes of San Diego history.* San Diego Historical Society; San Diego, CA.

De Clercq, E. (2006) Antiviral agents active against influenza A viruses. *Nature Reviews, Drug Discovery* 5(12), 1015–25.

Demicheli, V., Rivetti, D., Deeks, J.J. (2004) Vaccines for preventing influenza in healthy adults. Cochrane Database of Systematic Reviews CD001269.

Department of Health and Ageing (2004) *Interim Protocol For Public Health Management Of Possible/Confirmed Cases Of Avian Influenza.* Available from www.health.gov.au/internet/wcms/publishing.nsf/Content/health-avian_influenza-protocol.htm#1 (Accessed 25 October, 2005)

Harper, S.A., Fukuda, K., Uyeki, T.M. et al. (2004) Prevention and control of influenza: recommendations of the Advisory Committee on Immunization Practices (ACIP). *Morbidity and Mortality Weekly Report Recommendations and Reports* 53(RR-6), 1–40.

Leder, K., Newman, D. (2005) Respiratory infections during air travel. *Internal Medicine Journal* 35(1), 50–55.

Leroux-Roels, I., Borkowski, A., Vanwolleghem, T. et al (2007) Antigen sparing and cross-reactive immunity with an adjuvanted rH5NI prototype pandemic influenza vaccine: a randomised controlled trial. *Lancet* 370 (9587), 580–89.

Li, J., Hampson, A., Roche, P. et al. (2005) Report of the National Influenza Surveillance Scheme, 2004. *Communicable Diseases Intelligence* 29(2), 125–36.

Monto A.S., Gravenstein, S., Elliott, M. et al. (2000) Clinical signs and symptoms predicting influenza infection. *Archives of Internal Medicine* 160(21), 3243–47.

National Health and Medical Research Council (2003) *Australian Immunisation Handbook. 8th Edition.* National Health and Medical Research Council; Canberra. Available from www9.health.gov.au/immhandbook (Accessed 25 October, 2005)

National Institute for Clinical Excellence (2003) *Guidance On The Use Of Zanamivir, Oseltamivir And Amantadine For The Treatment Of Influenza.* Available from www.nice.org.uk/pdf/58_Flu_fullguidance.pdf (Accessed 24, October 2005)

Sambhara, S., Poland, G.A. (2007) Breaking the immunogenicity barrier of bird flu vaccines. *Lancet* 370 (9587), 544–45.

Schwarzmann, S.W., Adler, J.L., Sullivan, R.J. et al. (1971) Bacterial pneumonia during the Hong Kong influenza epidemic of 1968–69. *Archives of Internal Medicine* 127(6), 1037–41.

Tasker, S.A., Treanor, J.J., Paxton, W.B. et al. (1999) Efficacy of influenza vaccination in HIV-infected persons: a randomized, double-blind, placebo-controlled trial. *Annals of Internal Medicine* 131(6), 430–33.

Teo, S.S.S., Nguyen-Van-Tam, J.S., Booy R. (2004) Influenza burden of illness, diagnosis, treatment, and prevention: what is the evidence in children and where are the gaps? *Archives of Disease in Childhood* 90(5), 532–36.

Treanor, J. J. (2005). Influenza virus. In Mandell, G.L., Bennett, J.E., Dolin, R.(eds) *Principles and Practice of Infectious Diseases*. Churchill Livingstone; Philadelphia

World Health Organization (2007) WHO cumulative number of confirmed human cases of avian influenza A/(H5NI) reported to WHO. Available from www.who.int/csr/disease/avian_influenza/country/cases_table_2007_08_16/en/index.html (Accessed 20 August, 2007)

World Health Organization (2005) *Recommended Laboratory Tests To Identify Avian Influenza A Virus In Specimens From Humans*. World Health Organization; Geneva. Available from www.who.int/csr/disease/avian_influenza/guidelines/avian_labtests2.pdf (Accessed 25 October, 2005)

Zambon, M.C. (1999) Epidemiology and pathogenesis of influenza. *Journal of Antimicrobial Chemotherapy* 44(Suppl B), 3–9.

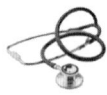

Case 10 Invasive pneumococcal disease
Maurice is very sick …

Invasive pneumococcal disease at a glance …

- **Agent:** family Streptococcaceae; genus *Streptococcus*; species *Streptococcus pneumoniae*
- **Geographical distribution:** worldwide, with higher rates in the developing world
- **Susceptible groups:** children (especially those <2 years); adults ≥65 years; indigenous peoples; immunocompromised individuals; individuals with cochlear implants
- **Main modes of transmission:** droplet spread; surfaces contaminated with respiratory secretions
- **Incubation period:** uncertain
- **Clinical features:** common presentations include septicaemia, meningitis, pneumonia with empyema, and pneumonia with bacteraemia
- **Identification:** cultures of blood, cerebrospinal fluid (if meningitis is suspected); immunochromatographic test for urinary or cerebrospinal fluid antigen; serotyping (commonly done by Quellung reaction, although molecular techniques are being used too)
- **Treatment:** antibiotic therapy (choice according to resistance patterns); adjunctive corticosteroid therapy in certain scenarios of meningitis
- **Post-exposure prophylaxis:** nil
- **Vaccine:** 23-valent polysaccharide vaccine; 7-valent conjugate vaccine (9-valent and 11-valent conjugate vaccines may become more widely used in the future)

Main characters

Dr Cindy Tan	infectious diseases physician
Dr Laura Rothschild	medical registrar
Mr Maurice Mendez	very sick patient
Dr Michael Mansfield	public health registrar

Dr Cindy Tan is the on-call infectious diseases physician at a large teaching hospital on a long weekend. She has just finished a ward round when she receives a call from Dr Laura Rothschild, her registrar in the emergency department.

'Hi. I'd be grateful if you could please review this patient urgently. He speaks a foreign language so I can't get a history from him, but he was found wandering aimlessly in front of the hospital a few minutes ago and brought here by the ambulance. He is about 50 years old, looks septic, and is febrile and tachycardic with a low blood pressure. He has extensive symmetrical ecchymoses on his legs consistent with purpura fulminans. He has features consistent with meningitis—a stiff neck and photophobia—but he has no papilloedema or focal neurological deficits.

'I think he has meningococcal meningitis and septicaemia. The intern has sent some blood tests, including two sets of blood cultures, for urgent analysis.'

Cindy rushes to see the patient. She makes her assessment within a few minutes, since time is of the essence. The only finding that Laura failed to mention is an old midline laparotomy scar. There is no otitis media. Cindy agrees this man is likely to have acute bacterial meningitis and septic shock with purpura fulminans.

Laura asks, 'Shall I do a lumbar puncture now to get a microbiological diagnosis?'

Investigations

A lumbar puncture is not advisable for a couple of reasons.

A pre-antibiotic cerebrospinal fluid (CSF) specimen is likely to identify the organism responsible for this acute presentation. However, the first priority is to keep the patient alive. A study has shown that the

CASE 10 INVASIVE PNEUMOCOCCAL DISEASE

delaying giving antibiotics in patients with acute bacterial meningitis is associated with increased mortality (Proulx et al., 2005). Specifically, a delay of >6 hours after presentation increased the risk of death by a factor of eight, with further delays associated with even higher risks. If this patient was stable, a short delay in antibiotic administration to allow a lumbar puncture may have been acceptable. However, he is haemodynamically unstable due to septic shock and needs antibiotics immediately.

Also, an extensive purpuric rash (purpura fulminans) is usually associated with a coagulopathy, increasing the risk of haemorrhagic complications from invasive procedures. Unless the results of his full blood count and coagulation studies suggest otherwise, a lumbar puncture should be avoided at this stage.

Just then, the laboratory calls through the blood tests taken earlier by an emergency department resident:

- white cell count: $25 \times 10^9/L$ (range 4–$11 \times 10^9/L$), 90% neutrophils
- platelet count: $75 \times 10^9/L$ (range 150–$400 \times 10^9/L$)
- prothrombin time: 20 seconds (range 9–15 seconds)
- APTT: 48 seconds (range 23–34 seconds)
- blood film: Howell-Jolly bodies, marked toxic changes
- sodium: 133 mmol/L (range 135–145 mmol/L)
- bicarbonate: 18 mmol/L (range 22–31 mmol/L)
- lactate: 3.2 mmol/L (range <2 mmol/L)

The raised white cell count, neutrophilia and lactic acidosis are all consistent with sepsis. The thrombocytopenia and prolonged prothrombin time and APTT are all consistent with a coagulopathy associated with severe sepsis and purpura fulminans.

Laura is very interested in the Howell-Jolly bodies described on the blood film. 'What could they mean?'

Howell-Jolly bodies are remnants of erythrocyte nuclei and can be seen on examination of the peripheral blood film. Their presence is often associated with asplenia. Asplenia predisposes patients to severe episodes of sepsis typically with encapsulated organisms, the so-called overwhelming post-splenectomy sepsis or infection (OPSS or OPSI). Pneumococcus, meningococcus, *Haemophilus influenzae* type b and *Capnocytophaga canimorsus* are typical organisms responsible for OPSS (Brigden and Pattullo, 1999).

However, pneumococcus is known to cause 60% of cases of OPSS (Taylor et al., 2005). Splenectomised patients are also more susceptible to infections from intra-erythrocytic parasites, such as malaria and babesiosis (Brigden et al., 2000).

The patient's midline laparotomy scar and the presence of Howell-Jolly bodies on his film probably represent a previous splenectomy. Splenectomy patients at greatest risk of severe infection include (Kyaw et al., 2006a):

- patients who had a splenectomy for haematological disorders (the risk is lowest for those who had splenectomy for trauma)
- patients in the first three years after splenectomy (the risk is potentially lifelong but declines after three years)
- young children, especially <5 years (they have the highest susceptibility and shortest time to infection, although one study showed increased risk with advancing age)

Cindy tells Laura to commence antibiotic therapy. 'Before you can start treatment, you need to know what you are likely to be treating.'

Laura replies, 'The most common causes of bacterial meningitis in adults in our community are *Streptococcus pneumoniae* (pneumococcus), *Neisseria meningitidis* (meningococcus) and *Listeria monocytogenes*.

'But let me see. He clearly has purpura fulminans over his legs, so *Listeria* and pneumococcus are unlikely. Is that right?'

Differential diagnosis

Meningococcus is the most common infective cause of purpura fulminans. However, there are reports of other organisms causing purpura fulminans, including pneumococcus (Noguera et al., 2004), *C. canimorsus* (Bryson et al., 2003) and even *Klebsiella* (Olowu, 2002).

Purpura fulminans in the setting of invasive pneumococcal disease (IPD) usually occurs in immunocompromised hosts; however rare cases in immunocompetent individuals have been described (Noguera et al., 2004). Given that the immune status of this patient is unknown, Cindy must include pneumococcus as part of the differential diagnosis.

C. canimorsus is a Gram negative bacillus typically associated with dog bites in immunocompromised hosts, although immuno-competent individuals can be affected. Again, since a history cannot be obtained from this patient, *C. canimorsus* must be included in the differential diagnosis.

'So what regimen would you use?' Cindy asks.

Laura replies, 'I've got our local guidelines here. They recommend empiric:

- ceftriaxone or cefotaxime (for meningococcus and pneumococcus) AND
- ampicillin or benzylpencillin (for *Listeria*) AND
- vancomycin (only if there are beta-lactam-resistant pneumococci in the region).

'Since meningococcus is the most common infective cause of purpura fulminans, I would use a third-generation cephalosporin such as ceftriaxone. If it does turn about to be *C. canimorsus*, he would still be covered.' Cindy chooses intravenous (IV) vancomycin 500 mg qid and ceftriaxone 2 g bd.

'Does he need corticosteroids prior to the antibiotics?' asks Laura.

Treatment

Using dexamethasone in adults with bacterial meningitis is controversial. It recently came into the limelight following a study suggesting that early use of dexamethasone led to better outcomes (de Gans et al., 2002). Tunkel et al. (2004) devised practice guidelines for the management of bacterial meningitis and concluded dexamethasone should be administered just prior to or with the first dose of IV antibiotics in all adults with proven or suspected pneumococcal meningitis. In animal studies, the use of dexamethasone has reduced the CSF penetration of vancomycin (the recommended antibiotic in beta-lactam-resistant pneumococcal infections,) so patients on vancomycin therapy need careful observation.

Although Weisfelt et al. (2006) agree adjunctive dexamethasone in adults with acute bacterial meningitis reduces mortality and neurological sequelae, they cite data showing that high-dose steroids can lead to an adverse outcome in patients with septic shock. There is also uncertainty about the impact of adjunctive dexamethasone on cognitive impairment after pneumococcal meningitis.

A systematic literature review by van de Beek et al. (2004) identified flaws in the methodology and design in some studies but still concluded that most adults with suspected acute bacterial meningitis should receive dexamethasone. They recommended a dose of 10 mg IV every six hours for four days with the first dose given before or with the first dose of parenteral antibiotics. They did not recommend adjunctive corticosteroids in patients with septic shock, those who had already received parenteral antibiotics, immunosuppressed patients and people with post-neurosurgical meningitis.

> This is a difficult decision for Cindy because the microbiology and infectious diseases communities have not reached a consensus. However, given the septic shock, she decides against steroids. The patient receives IV vancomycin and ceftriaxone within 10 minutes of Cindy seeing him.
>
> The intensive care unit (ICU) reviews him urgently and accepts him for management of his septic shock and coagulopathy. Ten hours later, his blood cultures are growing Gram positive diplococci. The organism is catalase negative, optochin sensitive, soluble in bile salts, and produces alpha-haemolysis. These findings are consistent with pneumococcal sepsis and meningitis.
>
> By this stage, the patient has clinical signs of left lower lobe consolidation. The intensivists wonder whether a CT brain would be useful, now that they have a microbiological diagnosis.

Once he is stable, the patient should have a CT brain looking for a focus of infection, such as mastoiditis or sinusitis, and any complications of pneumococcal meningitis requiring urgent intervention, such as cerebral oedema or hydrocephalus.

> A CT brain demonstrates some cerebral oedema; there is no mastoiditis. A bedside abdominal ultrasound confirms that he has no spleen. The ICU registrar asks Cindy, 'What is his source of meningitis?'

Sometimes the cause is never known. In one study, 42% of patients had no obvious focus, 30% had an otogenic focus, 18% had a lung focus and 8% had sinusitis as a focus; there were miscellaneous foci in 2% of cases (Ostergaard et al., 2005).

Given that this patient has no otogenic focus and has left lower lobe pneumonia, it is reasonable to assume that the pneumonia is the focus of infection.

> 'Pneumococcal pneumonia and meningitis—isn't that "Austrian's syndrome"?' asks the ICU registrar.

Austrian's syndrome refers to a triad of pneumococcal pneumonia, meningitis and endocarditis. It is also known as Osler's triad and is more commonly associated with alcoholic patients (du Cheyron et al., 2003). This patient does not have endocarditis.

> 'His prognosis isn't good. And I guess if he survives, he is likely to have complications, isn't he?'

Prognosis

Pneumococcal meningitis alone is a condition associated with terrible morbidity and mortality. Weisfelt et al. (2006) found that 16–37% of patients died during hospitalisation and 29–72% of surviving patients had neurological sequelae, such as cranial nerve palsies (16–28%), hearing loss (14–30%) or focal deficits (22–44%).

In addition, this patient has septic shock with purpura fulminans: digital gangrene requiring amputation is also a possibility, assuming he survives.

On the following day, Cindy asks the lab scientists if they have determined the antibiotic sensitivities to the organism. They have determined the minimum inhibitory concentrations (MIC):

- penicillin 1.0 mg/L
- ceftriaxone <1.0 mg/L

> Laura says, 'The organism is sensitive to ceftriaxone. But the MIC for penicillin represents only intermediate-level resistance (0.1–1.0 mg/L). I have treated patients with pneumonia due to penicillin-intermediate-resistant isolates with high doses of penicillin. Therefore, can't we use IV benzylpenicillin monotherapy?'

CSF penetration of penicillin is poor. When a pneumococcus with intermediate resistance to penicillin causes meningitis, IV penicillin must never be used. If the organism is sensitive to a third-generation cephalosporin, use appropriate doses of cefotaxime or ceftriaxone (Weisfelt et al., 2006).

> The team eventually learns from a distant relative that the name of the man is Mr Maurice Mendez. Unfortunately, Maurice's condition continues to deteriorate. He develops multi-organ failure, refractory coagulopathy, ischaemic feet, multiple cerebral infarcts and worsening hypotension despite maximum doses of inotropes. He dies on the fifth day of admission.
> Laura receives a call from Dr Michael Mansfield in the public health unit.
> 'Hi. The lab has notified us of a Mr Mendez with IPD. Could you please give me some more details for our database?'
> Laura is happy to oblige. She also asks, 'Michael, I also have another patient with pneumococcal pneumonia and pneumococcus isolated in the sputum. Do I need to notify you about him too?'

Public health notification and response

For public health data purposes, IPD refers to the isolation of pneumococcus from normally sterile sites. Sputum is not sterile; therefore, even though pneumococcus should not be found in the alveolar spaces of the lungs, pneumococcal pneumonia diagnosed on the basis of positive sputum cultures is not classified as IPD. However, pneumonia accompanied by microbiologically-proven bacteraemia, empyema or meningitis would be regarded as IPD.

CASE 10 INVASIVE PNEUMOCOCCAL DISEASE

> Laura also asks, 'Why do you collect notifications for every case of IPD?'

There are a number of reasons for notifying IPD:

- IPD is a condition with a high morbidity and mortality rates worldwide. It kills an estimated 1.2 million children in developing countries annually and is responsible for up to 40 000 deaths annually in the US. Also, pneumococci cause 30–50% of episodes of otitis media in children (Hausdorff et al., 2000).
- The highest incidence of age-related disease occurs in the two vulnerable groups, namely children <2 years old and the elderly. (The age distribution curve of IPD is therefore U-shaped, with peaks at the extremes of age).
- It is potentially a vaccine-preventable disease and surveillance for patterns of IPD can guide vaccination policy by identifying vulnerable groups and assessing the impact of vaccine introduction.

> Laura asks, 'I know quite a bit about treating cases of IPD in hospital. But I must admit that I don't know much about the vaccines. What types are available?'

For IPD, there are two types of vaccines:

- an older polysaccharide vaccine (with 23 serotypes)—23-valent pneumococcal polysaccharide vaccine (PPV-23)
- a newer conjugate vaccine (with 7 serotypes)— PCV-7

PPV-23 exclusively induces humoral immunity, which can limit its effectiveness. PCV-7, on the other hand, induces T-cell dependent immunity, with immunological memory and an enhanced immune response. The basis for this immune response to the conjugate vaccine is the presence of a protein antigen to which the polysaccharides are covalently conjugated (de Roux and Lode, 2005). Additionally, 9- and 11-serotype vaccines are available in experimental settings.

> 'So the 23-valent polysaccharide vaccine covers all the pneumococcal serotypes?'

There are 90 immunologically distinct serotypes of pneumococcus, each differentiated by the composition of their polysaccharide capsules, forming 46 serogroups (e.g. serotypes 19A and 19F belong to serogroup 19). PPV-23 covers only 23 serotypes.

Despite the presence of so many serogroups and serotypes, Hausdorff et al. (2000) found that most paediatric cases of IPD were due to 10 serogroups in each continent, with only an additional few causing disease in adults and older children. In countries such as Australia, PPV-23 contains the serotypes responsible for the majority of IPD in adults, regardless of ethnic origin. Also, 90% of healthy vaccinated adults will mount type-specific antibody responses within 2–3 weeks. Unfortunately, children <2 years old will only mount an effective antibody response to a small number of serotypes contained in the vaccine (National Health and Medical Research Council, 2003). This is important because these children form a peak age group for IPD.

Even though PCV-7 has only seven serotypes, compared to the 23 serotypes of PPV-23, its coverage is still quite far ranging. Rates of serogroup coverage for PCV-7 for young children were as high as 80–90% in Australia, the US and Canada but much lower (50%) in Asia. Overall, PCV-7 coverage for adults and older children was lower than for young children (30–60%), although again there was regional variation (Hausdorff et al., 2005).

However, in Australia there is disparity between indigenous and non-indigenous children <2 years when it comes to the proportion of serotypes covered by PCV-7 that cause IPD: two-thirds for indigenous children compared to five-sixths for non-indigenous children (National Health and Medical Research Council, 2003).

Laura asks Michael, 'Has the introduction of PCV-7 to childhood vaccination schedules reduced the incidence of IPD?'

In the US there have been statistically significant decreases in rates of IPD in infants since the introduction of PCV-7 vaccination (Poehling et al., 2006). There has also been success in the developing world using the conjugate pneumococcal vaccine. In Gambia, a trial with a 9-valent conjugate vaccine produced a significant reduction in rates of IPD and radiological pneumonia (Cutts et al., 2005).

Another, unexpected benefit from the US PCV-7 childhood vaccination program was a 55% reduction in the incidence of IPD due to the 7-conjugate vaccine serotypes in adults ≥50 years from 22.4 to

10.2 cases/100 000. This is an indirect effect because the adults never received the vaccine: childhood vaccination has resulted in herd immunity (Lexau et al., 2005). This can be partly explained by a reduction in nasopharyngeal carriage in vaccinated children, thereby reducing transmission to older adults. The same benefits have been seen in adults with HIV in the US who have not received the PCV-7 vaccine (Flannery et al., 2006).

Hopefully, this effect on herd immunity will also occur in developing nations that adopt childhood vaccination programs with a conjugate vaccine. However, a hurdle is the cost, since the PCV-7 is an expensive vaccine.

'What impact has the introduction of PCV-7 had on the incidence of IPD due to drug-resistant strains?'

The majority of drug-resistant pneumococcal infections are due to five serotypes contained in the PCV-7 vaccine (6B, 9V, 14, 19F, 23F) so it is not surprising that the rates of antibiotic-resistant invasive disease have dropped in the US since the introduction of the conjugate vaccine (Kyaw et al., 2006b).

'What about the impact of the conjugate vaccine on otitis media in children?'

There has been some benefit but not much. Healthy infants vaccinated with PCV-7 are less likely to get recurrent episodes of otitis media or need tympanoplasty tubes. However, there has been no significant reduction in the number of episodes in children with recurrent otitis media (McEllistrem et al., 2005).

'So why bother using the polysaccharide vaccine at all?'

PPV-23 is still a good vaccine, inducing an antibody response in 90% of adults. Controlled trials have shown that young adults who have received PPV-23 have reduced mortality from pneumonia. Observational studies have shown reduced rates of IPD in immunocompetent individuals vaccinated with PPV-23 (National Health and Medical Research Council, 2003).

Many countries recommend routine immunisation of people ≥65 years with PPV-23 and influenza vaccines because studies have shown that vaccine recipients have reduced hospitalisation rates for community-acquired pneumonia, reduced mortality rates from all causes (Christenson et al., 2001) and reduced mortality from pneumonia alone (Vila-Corcoles et al., 2005).

Laura, says, 'If expensive conjugate vaccines and expensive antibiotics for resistant strains are the answer, it's going to be difficult for the developing world to eradicate pneumococcal disease.'

These are challenges; however, it is important not to forget simple measures to reduce rates of infection. Since pneumococcus is a coloniser of the nasopharynx, hand washing and reducing crowding are valuable ways of preventing disease. Luby et al. (2005) conducted a trial in Pakistan looking at the value of using soap and encouraging hand washing in households and found that children <5 years from targeted households had a 50% lower incidence of pneumonia.

Michael now asks, 'Laura, do you know if Mr Mendez was vaccinated after his splenectomy?'

Certain groups have an increased susceptibility to IPD and should be vaccinated against pneumococcal disease (National Health and Medical Research Council, 2003). This includes immunocompromised individuals, such as those with functional or anatomical asplenia. Most countries recommend a single dose of the polysaccharide vaccine for asplenic adults, followed by one further booster five years later. With time, it is likely that the PCV-7 vaccine will also be recommended for these susceptible groups.

Patients undergoing elective splenectomy should be vaccinated at least two weeks before the operation. This is because it takes about nine days for IgM to be produced after exposure to antigen for the first time (Shatz, 2005).

Laura is uncertain about the patient's vaccination status. But she says, 'Presumably, if the organism from his blood is a serotype included in the PPV-23 vaccine, then he couldn't have been vaccinated.'

CASE 10   INVASIVE PNEUMOCOCCAL DISEASE

Breakthrough pneumococcal infection with a serotype contained in the polysaccharide vaccine can occur in vaccinated splenectomy patients, usually in those with an underlying immune disorder (Musher et al., 2005).

> Laura calls the lab and speaks to the microbiologist about how the serotyping is proceeding. 'We'll have the results of the Quellung reaction for you later today.'

The Quellung reaction is a widely used technique for serotyping pneumococci. Bacteria are added to specific antiserum; antibodies then bind to the capsule of the organism, leading to swelling, which can be visualised.

> The microbiologist calls Laura later that day. 'Your patient's isolate is serotype 19A. It could be replacement disease.'

One concern about the introduction of the PCV-7 vaccine was that other serotypes, not contained in the vaccine, would start to cause more IPD, even though immunity to the PVC-7 serotypes seemed to result in cross-reactive immunity with non-PVC-7 serotypes (e.g. the 6B vaccine component provides immunity against non-vaccine 6A). The expression for this phenomenon is replacement disease.

This does appear to happen. In the US, the incidence of IPD due to non-PCV-7 serotypes has risen in children <5 years and adults ≥40 years. However, the overall rates are still well below those prior to introduction of the PCV-7 vaccination program (Centers for Disease Control and Prevention, 2005). Serotype 19A is one serotype responsible for replacement disease (Kyaw et al., 2006b). Only time will tell if the incidence rates for non-vaccine serotypes will continue to rise or not.

> Later that day, Michael gets a call from the ear, nose and throat registrar.
> 'We just reviewed a child who is suitable for a cochlear implant. I just wanted to confirm with you that we should vaccinate the child against pneumococcal infection. Is that right?'

Cochlear implants have been a tremendous advance in correcting hearing impairment in young children. An implant lies in the mastoid and electrodes travel through the mastoid air cells, middle ear and inner ear to the cochlea. There is an external apparatus sitting behind the ear. Unfortunately, it was soon discovered in the US that implant recipients had rates of bacterial meningitis 30 times higher than similarly-aged children without implants. Pneumococcus was the commonest cause; other pathogens included *Acinetobacter*, *Enterococcus*, *Escherichia coli* and *H. influenzae*. Interestingly, there is no increased risk of meningitis of *Neisseria meningitidis* infection (meningococcus). Therefore, children with cochlear implants need to be immunised against pneumococcus (Whitney, 2004).

References

Brigden, M.L., Pattullo, A., Brown, G. (2000) Pneumococcal vaccine administration associated with splenectomy: the need for improved education, documentation, and the use of a practical checklist. *American Journal of Hematology* 65(1), 25–29.

Brigden, M.L., Pattullo, A.L. (1999) Prevention and management of overwhelming postsplenectomy infection—an update. *Critical Care Medicine* 27(4), 836–42.

Bryson, M.S., Neilly I., Rodger S. et al. (2003). Purpura fulminans associated with *Capnocytophaga canimorsus* infection. *British Journal of Haematology* 121(1), 1.

Centres for Disease Control and Prevention (2005) Direct and indirect effects of routine vaccination of children with 7-valent pneumococcal conjugate vaccine on incidence of invasive pneumococcal disease—United States, 1998–2003. *Morbidity and Mortality Weekly Report* 54(36), 893–97.

Christenson, B., Lundbergh, P., Hedlund, J. et al. (2001) Effects of a large-scale intervention with influenza and 23-valent pneumococcal vaccines in adults aged 65 years or older: a prospective study. *Lancet* 357(9261), 1008–11.

Cutts, F.T., Zaman, S.M., Enwere, G. et al. (2005) Efficacy of nine-valent pneumococcal conjugate vaccine against pneumonia and invasive pneumococcal disease in The Gambia: randomised, double-blind, placebo-controlled trial. *Lancet* 365(9465), 1139–46.

de Gans J., van de Beek, D. for the European Dexamethasone in Adulthood Bacterial Meningitis Study Investigators. (2002) Dexamethasone in adults with bacterial meningitis. *New England Journal of Medicine* 347(20), 1549–56.

de Roux, A., Lode, H. (2005) Pneumococcal vaccination. *European Respiratory Journal* 26(6), 982–83.

du Cheyron, D., Lesage, A., Le Page, O. et al. (2003) Corticosteroids as adjunctive treatment in Austrian's syndrome (pneumococcal endocarditis, meningitis, and pneumonia): report of two cases and review of the literature. *Journal of Clinical Pathology* 56(11), 879–81.

Flannery, B., Heffernan, R.T., Harrison, L.H. et al. (2006) Changes in invasive pneumococcal disease among HIV-infected adults living in the era of childhood pneumococcal immunization. *Annals of Internal Medicine* 144(1), 1–9.

Hausdorff, W.P., Feikin, D.R., Klugman, K.P. (2005) Epidemiological differences among pneumococcal serotypes. *Lancet Infectious Diseases* 5(2), 83–93.

Hausdorff, W.P., Bryant, J., Paradiso, P.R. et al. (2000) Which pneumococcal serogroups cause the most invasive disease: implications for conjugate vaccine formulation and use, part I. *Clinical Infectious Diseases* 30(1), 100–21.

Kyaw, M.H., Lynfield, R., Schaffner, W. et al. (2006a) Effect of introduction of the pneumococcal conjugate vaccine on drug-resistant *Streptococcus pneumoniae*. *New England Journal of Medicine* 354(14), 1455–63.

CASE 10 INVASIVE PNEUMOCOCCAL DISEASE

Kyaw, M.H., Holmes, E.M., Toolis, F. et al. (2006b) Evaluation of severe infection and survival after splenectomy. *American Journal of Medicine* 119(3), 276.e1–7.

Lexau, C.A., Lynfield, R., Danila, R. et al. (2005) Changing epidemiology of invasive pneumococcal disease among older adults in the era of pediatric pneumococcal conjugate vaccine. *Journal of the American Medical Association* 294(16), 2043–51.

Luby, S.P., Agboatwalla, M., Feikin, D.R. et al. (2005) Effect of handwashing on child health: a randomised controlled trial. *Lancet* 366(9481), 225–33.

McEllistrem, M.C., Adams, J.M., Patel, K. et al. (2005) Acute otitis media due to penicillin-nonsusceptible *Streptococcus pneumoniae* before and after the introduction of the pneumococcal conjugate vaccine. *Clinical Infectious Diseases* 40(12), 1738–44.

Musher, D.M., Caesar, H., Kojic, E.M. et al. (2005) Administration of protein-conjugate pneumococcal vaccine to patients who have invasive disease after splenectomy despite their having received 23-valent pneumococcal polysaccharide vaccine. *Journal of Infectious Diseases* 191(7), 1063–67.

National Health and Medical Research Council (2003) *Australian Immunisation Handbook. 8th Edition.* National Health and Medical Research Council; Canberra. Available from www9.health.gov.au/immhandbook (Accessed 12 April, 2006)

Noguera, A., Fortuny, C., Pons M. et al. (2004) Pneumococcal-associated purpura fulminans in a healthy infant. *Pediatric Emergency Care* 20(8), 528–30.

Olowu, W.A. (2002) *Klebsiella*-induced purpura fulminans in a Nigerian child: case report and a review of literature. *West African Journal of Medicine* 21(3), 252–55.

Ostergaard, C., Konradsen, H.B., Samuelsson, S. (2005) Clinical presentation and prognostic factors of *Streptococcus pneumoniae* meningitis according to the focus of infection. *BMC Infectious Diseases* 5, 93.

Poehling, K.A., Talbot, T.R., Griffin, M.R. et al. (2006) Invasive pneumococcal disease among infants before and after introduction of pneumococcal conjugate vaccine. *Journal of the American Medical Association* 295(14), 1668–74.

Proulx, N., Fréchette, D., Toye, B. et al. (2005) Delays in the administration of antibiotics are associated with mortality from adult acute bacterial meningitis. *Quarterly Journal of Medicine* 98(4), 291–98.

Shatz, D.V. (2005) Vaccination considerations in the asplenic patient. *Expert Review of Vaccines* 4(1), 27–34.

Taylor, M.D., Genuit, T., Napolitano, L.M. (2005) Overwhelming postsplenectomy sepsis and trauma: time to consider revaccination? *Journal of Trauma* 59(6), 1482–85.

Tunkel, A.R., Hartman, B.J., Kaplan, S.L. et al. (2004) Practice guidelines for the management of bacterial meningitis. *Clinical Infectious Diseases* 39(9), 1267–84.

van de Beek, D., de Gans, J., McIntyre, P. et al (2004) Steroids in adults with acute bacterial meningitis: a systematic review. *Lancet Infectious Diseases* 4(3), 139–43.

Vila-Corcoles, A., Ochoa-Gondar, O., Llor, C. et al. (2005) Protective effect of pneumococcal vaccine against death by pneumonia in elderly subjects. *European Respiratory Journal* 26(6), 1086–91.

Weisfelt M., de Gans J., van der Poll, T. et al. (2006) Pneumococcal meningitis in adults: new approaches to management and prevention. *Lancet Neurology* 5(4), 332–42.

Whitney, C.G. (2004) Cochlear implants and meningitis in children. *Pediatric Infectious Diseases* 23(8), 767–68.

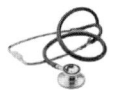

Case 11 Legionnaire's disease
Chris is drowsy and has a fever …

Legionnaire's disease at a glance …

- **Agent**: family Legionellaceae; genus *Legionella*; most common pathogenic species is *Legionella pneumophila*
- **Geographical distribution**: worldwide
- **Modes of transmission**: inhalation or aspiration of *Legionella*-containing aerosols
- **Person-to-person transmission**: no
- **Animal-to-person transmission**: no
- **Incubation period**: 4–6 days (2–18 days)
- **Clinical features**: most commonly, a pneumonia associated with a number of extrapulmonary features; Pontiac fever (a milder febrile illness with a shorter incubation period)
- **Identification**: urinary antigen; antibody testing of respiratory secretions and serum; cultures of respiratory secretions and serum
- **Treatment**: the best agents are fluoroquinolones and azithromycin
- **Post-exposure prophylaxis**: nil
- **Vaccine**: nil

CASE 11 LEGIONNAIRE'S DISEASE

Main characters

Dr Megan Day	infectious diseases registrar
Mr Chris Moss	80-year-old man with pneumonia
Professor Patrick Bayer	infectious diseases specialist
Mr Clint Easter	58-year-old man with pneumonia
Ms Dianne Potter	infection control nurse
Ms Wendy Smith	infection control nurse
Dr Lucy Nguyen	director, public health unit

An infectious diseases registrar, Dr Megan Day, receives a referral from the one of the internal medicine interns.

'Hi, could you please see Mr Chris Moss, an 80-year-old man with three days of fevers?

'He was admitted two weeks ago to optimise analgesia for vertebral compression fractures secondary to long-term corticosteroid use. He has polymyalgia rheumatica and has never been able to get below 15 mg/day of prednisolone. He also has a prosthetic heart valve.

'We don't know where this fever is coming from. Urine and blood cultures are negative. We wondered if he had aspirated his meals because he has been a bit drowsy since starting morphine for his back pain, but his chest X-ray from three days ago was normal. Also, he doesn't have a cough. The physical examination isn't helpful either, apart from crackles in the left base which we noticed today.'

Megan reviews Chris. From her preliminary assessment, it is obvious Chris has pneumonia: he is tachypnoeic (24 breaths/minute) with a low oxygen saturation on room air and has bronchial breathing and crackles in the left base and midzone of the lungs. He is slightly drowsy, due to the current infection, the morphine or both.

His blood tests only show a mild neutrophilia and elevated C-reactive protein.

'Did he pick up the infection here in the hospital?' the intern asks.

If Megan's assessment is correct, Chris has nosocomial pneumonia, which is defined as pneumonia occurring ≥48 hours after admission to hospital (Flanders et al., 2006).

In nosocomial pneumonia beginning ≥5 days into the hospital admission, Gram negative bacilli such as *Pseudomonas aeruginosa* and *Enterobacter* and *Acinetobacter* spp, as well as multiresistant methicillin-resistant *Staphylococcus aureus* (MRSA) are the usual culprits. Also, polymicrobial disease is not uncommon (Flanders et al., 2006).

According to his previous results, Chris has not been colonised with MRSA, so Megan does not prescribe vancomycin. She instead recommends a combination of piperacillin/tazobactam and gentamicin. She also suggests another chest X-ray, which now indeed shows patchy left lower lobe consolidation with a pleural effusion.

In 48 hours, she returns to see Chris with her boss, Professor Patrick Bayer. Chris does not look well. He is hypotensive and clearly in respiratory distress. The antibiotics clearly haven't worked and he will need to be transferred to the intensive care unit (ICU).

The intern clearly looks stressed. 'Thanks for coming back, Megan. You're not going to believe it, but we have another patient with nosocomial pneumonia. Mr Clint Easter is a 58-year-old man who was admitted three weeks ago with a delirium secondary to a new anticholinergic medication. He also has severe vascular dementia. Unlike Chris, he had diarrhoea before developing a cough and becoming hypoxic. But his stool cultures were negative for cells or pathogens. Can you see him too?'

Patrick and Megan review the new patient. They can't take a history from him because of his dementia but his wife is very helpful. Clint was doing well after recovering from his drug-induced delirium. Then three days ago, he developed non-bloody, semi-solid diarrhoea, up to six times a day. At the same time, his dementia worsened. Mrs Easter suspects the diarrhoea was accompanied by abdominal pain, given the way he was grimacing.

CASE 11 LEGIONNAIRE'S DISEASE

> Examination reveals a relative bradycardia (he is not on bradycardia-inducing medications), no pacemaker, tachypnoea, fever and right lower zone crackles.
> Megan says, 'Diarrhoea and abdominal pain preceding pneumonia with relative bradycardia. Hmm, if this were a case of community-acquired pneumonia, I would have suspected an atypical organism such as *Legionella*. But he has been in hospital for three weeks so I guess he is outside the incubation period for *Legionella*.'

What is *Legionella*?

The genus *Legionella* refers to a group of Gram negative bacilli which are the only member of the family Legionellaceae (Den Boer and Yzerman, 2004). There are over 40 species of *Legionella* and 60 serogroups. They are facultative intracellular pathogens that invade and replicate within free-living protozoa (e.g. amoebae) and mammalian cells (Plouffe and File, 1999). Under 50% of *Legionella* species have been associated with disease in humans; the remainder are avirulent environmental organisms (Stout and Yu, 1997).

Some species of *Legionella* can cause pneumonia in humans, known as Legionnaire's disease after the first recognised outbreak following a convention of the American Legions in Philadelphia in 1976 (Stout and Yu, 1997). Legionnaire's disease tends to peak in summer and autumn, in contrast to community-acquired pneumonia, which typically peaks in winter (Sopena et al., 2007). *Legionella* pneumonia in adults can be quite severe. It is the second most common cause of pneumonia requiring admission to the ICU after *Streptococcus pneumoniae* (Sopena et al., 1999). Legionnaire's disease can also occur in children (Greenberg et al., 2006).

The incubation period for *Legionella* infection (also known as legionellosis) is 2–18 days (median 4–6 days) (Edelstein, 2007). Since Clint has been hospitalised for three weeks, this could not be community-acquired *Legionella* infection.

> 'But Clint's infection isn't community acquired. Given that, can we dismiss *Legionella*?' the intern asks.

Legionella infection accounts for 2–5% of community-acquired pneumonia (Sopena et al., 1999) but up to 20% of notified cases of Legionnaire's disease are healthcare-associated infections. In fact, the healthcare-associated cases of Legionnaire's disease have a higher mortality (1–18%) than the community-acquired cases (4.8–11.2%) (Exner et al., 2005; Sopena et al., 2007). One study even found that *S. pneumoniae* and *Legionella* were two of the leading causes of nosocomial pneumonia in non-ICU patients where a microbiologic cause was identified (Sopena and Sabria, 2005). Nosocomial pneumonia due to *Legionella* can be sporadic or occur in the outbreak setting (Stout and Yu, 1997).

> 'What clinical features help point towards a diagnosis of *Legionella* pneumonia?'

Differential diagnoses

It is the extrapulmonary features of pneumonia due to *Legionella* infection that distinguish it from other causes of pneumonia, particularly other causes of community-acquired pneumonia (rather than nosocomial pneumonia). These extrapulmonary features include (Cunha, 2006):

- **Central nervous system (CNS) involvement** (confusion, prominent headache, encephalopathy) This makes *Mycoplasma* and *Chlamydia pneumoniae* unlikely, although *Mycoplasma* can rarely cause encephalitis.
- **Relative bradycardia** This excludes pneumonia due to *S. pneumoniae* and *Mycoplasma* as well as psittacosis; however, it isn't a particularly sensitive sign, so its absence should not exclude *Legionella* (Stout and Yu, 1997).
- **Gastrointestinal involvement** (loose stools rather than diarrhoea, abdominal pain) The combination of acute abdominal pain and community-acquired pneumonia is almost always only due to *Legionella* infection. The presence of abdominal tenderness, despite abdominal pain, argues against *Legionella* infection. *Mycoplasma* tends to cause watery diarrhoea rather than the loose stools seen in *Legionella* infection.
- **Absence of upper respiratory tract symptoms** (myringitis bullosa, otitis, sore throat) Their presence makes *Legionella* infection unlikely and favours other causes, particularly *Mycoplasma*.

CASE 11 LEGIONNAIRE'S DISEASE

'Good,' says Patrick. 'Clint has CNS symptoms (acute worsening of his dementia), relative bradycardia, loose stools and probable abdominal pain in addition to pneumonia. Everything would fit with *Legionella*. Here are his blood tests (bringing them up on the computer screen) (Table 11.1). Are they helpful too?'

Table 11.1 Blood results for Clint (* indicates abnormal result)

Test result	Normal range
Haemoglobin 140	130–180 g/L
Mean cell volume 82	80–100 Fl
White cell count 16*	3.5–11 × 10^9/L
Platelet count 200	150–450 × 10^9/L
Sodium 130*	135–145 mmol/L
Potassium 4.0	3.6–5.1 mmol/L
Chloride 98	95–107 mmol/L
Bicarbonate 25	22–32 mmol/L
Urea 6.2	2.9–7.1 mmol/L
Creatinine 100	60–110 μmol/L
Calcium 2.15	2.25–2.58 mmol/L
Phosphate 0.60*	0.80–1.50 mmol/L
Troponin <0.1	0–0.1 μg/L
Creatine kinase 350*	<175 U/L
Albumin 35	33–48 g/L
Bilirubin 20	0–25 μmol/L
ALP 110	38–126 U/L
GGT 30	0–30 U/L
AST 40	<45 U/L
ALT 80*	<45 U/L
Urinalysis	1+ blood, otherwise normal

Investigations

Clint's laboratory results consistent with *Legionella* infection. According to Cunha (2006), the laboratory features are:

- **Leukocytosis** While this is non-specific, the presence of leucopenia, thrombocytopenia or thrombocytosis would have made *Legionella* infection unlikely.
- **Hyponatraemia** Again, this is a non-specific finding which can be due to community-acquired pneumonia from other organisms but it tends to be more severe in *Legionella* infection.
- **Hypophosphataemia** Only community-acquired pneumonia due to *Legionella* infection is associated with hypophosphataemia.
- **Abnormal liver function tests** In the absence of epidemiological risk factors for psittacosis and Q fever, the main cause of abnormal serum transaminases and community-acquired pneumonia is Legionnaire's disease. It is uncommon for the transaminases to be elevated more than twice the upper limit of normal but this can occur.
- **Elevated creatine kinase** *Legionella* infection can be associated with rhabdomyolysis.
- **Microscopic haematuria** Although not a sensitive sign of Legionnaire's disease, the presence of microscopic haematuria excludes other causes of atypical pneumonia. Pyuria and haemoglobinuria exclude Legionnaire's disease, while proteinuria and myoglobinuria are uncommon.

The Winthrop-University Hospital Score was developed to identify cases of Legionnaire's disease. Calculations are based on a combination of clinical and laboratory criteria. An evaluation of the scoring system concluded that it is useful but that the sensitivity is not high enough to confidently exclude Legionnaire's disease (Gupta et al., 2001).

Patrick says, 'Okay Megan, you now have clinical and laboratory evidence for *Legionella*. How will a chest X-ray point you towards Legionnaire's disease?'

There is nothing remarkable about the radiographic changes of *Legionella* to distinguish it from other causes of pneumonia. About one-third of patients have a pleural effusion (Stout and Yu, 1997).

CASE 11　LEGIONNAIRE'S DISEASE

> 'So how are you going to confirm your diagnosis?'

The three tests most commonly used to diagnose Legionnaire's disease are urinary antigen testing, antibody testing and culture (Den Boer and Yzerman, 2004).

Urinary antigen testing has two advantages (Den Boer and Yzerman, 2004). It provides a rapid diagnosis, becoming positive within 1–3 days of the illness onset and possibly remaining positive for up to a year, and it is very specific (specificity >99%, sensitivity variable). However, there are disadvantages.

First, there are 15 serogroups of *L. pneumophila* (O'Neill and Humphreys, 2005). Urinary antigen testing primarily identifies *L. pneumophila* serogroup 1, which is good because this serogroup is responsible for the bulk of Legionnaire's disease notifications (91% of US isolates). However, this has also had a negative impact because it reduces the number of requests for culture, direct fluorescent antibody and serology for *Legionella*, the very tests that would identify the infections caused by *Legionella* from other serogroups. This is reflected in US data showing that increased use of the urinary antigen test in the 1980s was associated with an almost 90% reduction in the isolation of *Legionella* spp other than *pneumophila* serogroup 1 (Roig et al., 2003). This is even more of an issue in Australia and New Zealand, where 30% of *Legionella* notifications are due to *L. longbeachae*.

Second, although the overall sensitivity is 99%, this can vary considerably depending on the clinical picture (Table 11.2).

Table 11.2 Sensitivity of urinary antigen testing for *Legionella*

Mild disease	40–53%
Moderate-severe disease	88%
Travel-associated	94%
Community-acquired	76–87%
Nosocomial	44–46%
Serogroups other than serogroup 1	14–69% (the overall sensitivity for serogroup 1 is 70%)

Antibody testing on serum and respiratory specimens has the advantages of identifying different *Legionella* species and subclinical infection (Den Boer and Yzerman, 2004). However, it has a number of disadvantages including:

Poor sensitivity 41–75%

Late diagnosis Although 80% of patients seroconvert by four weeks after illness onset, seroconversion can take up to two months.

Poor specificity for recent infection Up to 33% of people with Legionnaire's disease remain seropositive for 48 months; therefore, demonstrating a rising titre between a baseline and convalescent specimen is preferable to making a diagnosis on a single high titre alone.

Also, acute infection can be represented by IgM alone, IgG alone or a mixture, which can further add to confusion.

Culture is the gold standard for identification of Legionnaire's disease and has 100% specificity (Den Boer and Yzerman, 2004). Blood and any respiratory specimen can be cultured. Nevertheless, it has poor sensitivity (25–75%), provides a late diagnosis (*L. pneumophila* takes three days while non-*pneumophila* spp can take up to 10 days to grow) and requires special culture media.

> Megan digests all this information. 'What about molecular testing?'

Polymerase chain reaction (PCR) is a promising test for the diagnosis of *Legionella* infections. It can be performed on respiratory specimens, urine and serum (Diederen et al., 2006). However, little data are available and it will initially only be available in reference laboratories, further delaying the diagnosis for those in more peripheral clinical settings.

> It appears that Clint could indeed have Legionnaire's disease, but one thing still bothers Megan. 'I thought Legionnaire's disease was an infection of the immunosuppressed. This patient has only got severe dementia. Isn't that odd?'

Immunosuppression from medications or illnesses, including diabetes, certainly do predispose to the infection. (One immunosuppressive illness where the incidence of Legionnaire's disease is low is in the acquired immune deficiency syndrome (Stout and Yu, 1997). This could be due to a combination of cotrimoxazole use for *Pneumocystis* prophylaxis plus cases not being recognised.) However, immunosuppression is only one of many risk factors, including severe dementia, which Clint has (Marston et al., 1994; O'Neill and Humphreys, 2005; Sopena et al., 2007). The others are:

- **Male sex**
- **Advanced age**   This may partly be because ageing is itself associated with immunosuppression (Bouree, 2003).
- **Chronic pulmonary disease**
- **Postoperative period**
- **Smoking**   2–7 times increased risk
- **Heavy alcohol use**
- **Cerebrovascular disease**
- **Neuromuscular disorders**

The association between Legionnaire's disease and dementia, cerebrovascular disease and neuromuscular disorders may partly be explained by an increased risk of aspiration, which is thought to be one of the modes of infection (Sopena et al., 2007).

Another important point to remember is that even healthy young people without risk factors can still develop Legionnaire's disease, even severe forms (Roig et al., 2003).

> Patrick decides to commence broad-spectrum antibiotic therapy, given that the provisional diagnosis of *Legionella* infection hasn't been confirmed. 'We'll also need an agent that covers *Legionella* specifically,' he says.

Treatment

A number of antibiotics have activity against *Legionella* (Stout and Yu, 1997) including:

- fluoroquinolones
- macrolides
- tetracyclines
- cotrimoxazole
- rifampicin

The uncommon, if not rare, occurrence of Legionnaire's disease in HIV infection may partly be explained by the use of cotrimoxazole for

Pneumocystis prophylaxis (Feldman, 2005). In clinical practice, however, the quinolones (such as levofloxacin and moxifloxacin) and macrolides (erythromycin, clarithromycin, azithromycin) are most commonly used. There are no randomised controlled trials examining which is best. It appears that the quinolones have the edge over macrolides when it comes to time to defervescence, time to achieve clinical stability and length of hospital stay but there are no trials involving azithromycin (a newer macrolide) (Pedro-Botet and Yu, 2006). In fact, research has shown a post-antibiotic effect: laboratory cell models that contain both azithromycin and the fluoroquinolones continue to have irreversible inhibition of *Legionella* growth even after these antibiotics have been physically removed from the cell models (Roig et al., 2003).

Another factor to consider is how much inflammation is caused by antibiotic use—too much inflammation can be detrimental. It appears that azithromycin causes the least inflammation, followed by the fluoroquinolones, with erythromycin causing the most (Roig et al., 2003).

In conclusion, fluoroquinolones or azithromycin should probably be given to the most severe cases but in immunocompetent individuals with mild–moderate illness even tetracyclines (doxycycline, minocycline) are reasonable (Roig et al., 2003).

Patrick decides to use moxifloxacin.

Megan then takes him to ICU to see Chris. 'I'm surprised he didn't improve,' she said. 'After all, I gave him such a broad-spectrum antibiotic combination—piperacillin, tazobactam and gentamicin.'

Patrick asks, 'What if his nosocomial pneumonia is due to *Legionella*? That would explain why the combination didn't work.'

Megan is taken by surprise. 'Okay, I now realise that *Legionella* can cause nosocomial pneumonia, Prof. But you just taught me the extrapulmonary features and laboratory tests that point towards a diagnosis of Legionnaire's disease, and Chris doesn't have any of those (apart from a mild hyponatraemia).'

Clinical and preliminary laboratory evidence in favour of Legionnaire's disease are not always present, especially in the elderly. A study comparing Legionnaire's disease in people <65 and ≥65 years old found that the older patients were less likely to present with fever, extrapulmonary symptoms, elevated transaminases, creatine kinase and hyponatraemia (Sopena et al., 2007).

Chris could have a non-*Legionella* pneumonia but could equally well have Legionnaire's disease. In particular, he has three risk factors for Legionnaire's disease (he is elderly, male and on corticosteroids).

> Patrick advises that Chris be placed on moxifloxacin and that both Chris and Clint be tested for *Legionella*.
>
> On the following day, the results of the urinary antigen return—both men are positive! It appears that the hospital has an outbreak of Legionnaire's disease.
>
> Megan is excited and concerned. 'The source of the outbreak must be the water cooling towers.'

Public health notification and response

Cooling towers have been implicated as the source of a number of outbreaks of Legionnaire's disease (Formica et al., 2000; Greig et al., 2004; Isozumi et al., 2005; Rota et al., 2005; Sabria et al., 2006). Colonisation of the cooling towers by *Legionella* allows aerosolisation of the bacterium, resulting in infection. When this happens, people as far away as 6 km from the towers can be infected (Nguyen et al., 2006).

But while cooling towers were originally considered to be the primary source for nosocomial cases of Legionnaire's disease, it was eventually recognised that the hospital's potable water supply was the main culprit (Stout et al., 1982). In fact, 95% of nosocomial outbreaks of Legionnaire's disease in the UK from 1982–90 were attributed to the hospital's potable water supply (O'Neill and Humphreys, 2005).

> Patrick and Megan meet urgently with the hospital infection control nurses, Dianne Potter and Wendy Smith. Megan immediately asks them whether recent samples from the potable water have grown *Legionella*. Dianne tells her that they never check the potable water system for *Legionella*.

There are arguments for and against a primary preventive surveillance system in hospitals, with no consensus (O'Neill and Humphreys, 2005).

Some studies have found no correlation between colonisation of the hospital water system with *Legionella* and nosocomial infections (Alary and Joly, 1992; Legnani et al., 2002); other studies have found a correlation (Kool et al., 1999; Yu et al., 1987). The results of one study (Marrie et al., 1991) have been used to support the views of both parties (O'Neill and Humphreys, 2005)!

However, the Centers for Disease Control and Prevention (CDC) does not recommend regular monitoring for *Legionella* in potable water in hospitals, except possibly in the setting of highly susceptible hosts, such as transplant units (Sehulster and Chinn, 2003).

'Okay then,' asks Megan, 'What about the cooling towers?'

Due to community outbreaks of Legionnaire's disease attributed to cooling towers, many health departments around the world enforce strict guidelines about maintenance of cooling towers and primary surveillance for *Legionella* colonisation. Therefore, hospital cooling towers are usually surveyed for *Legionella* regularly, for example, every 3–6 months. Guidelines also stipulate what levels of *Legionella* colonisation of cooling towers are acceptable, if at all; for example, NSW Health (2005) specifies that *Legionella* counts of >10 colony-forming units per millilitre (cfu/mL) or heterotrophic plate counts of >105 cfu/mL are unacceptable (2005).

Dianne and Wendy look up the most recent cultures from the hospital cooling towers. They had only been taken three weeks ago and found no *Legionella* whatsoever.

Patrick speaks to the public health unit director, Dr Lucy Nguyen. They form an outbreak team and begin an outbreak investigation.

Over the next four weeks, the outbreak team concentrates both on identifying cases of Legionnaire's disease in the hospital by testing all patients with nosocomial pneumonia for *Legionella* and on testing the water supply around the hospital (for a list of sites that should be sampled, see Sehulster and Chinn, 2003).

Nine cases of nosocomial pneumonia are identified over the four weeks. Two of these are proven to be Legionnaire's disease through positive urinary antigen tests. Pulsed field gel electrophoresis (PFGE) confirms that all four patients with Legionnaire's disease (including Chris and Clint) have the same strain of *L. pneumophila* serogroup 1.

The two latest patients are from a different ward. However, all the patients attended the hydrotherapy spa in the hospital. An environmental investigation identifies *L. pneumophila* serogroup 1 in the hydrotherapy spa water. PGFE confirms that the spa isolate and clinical isolates are all the same clone of *L. pneumophila* serogroup 1.

A showerhead from the geriatric ward and a tap in an adjacent ward also grow *Legionella*. However, these are from a different species and are at low concentrations; therefore, they are not thought to be related to the outbreak.

The outbreak team concludes that the hydrotherapy spa is the source of the outbreak. Megan is surprised. 'So how can spas cause nosocomial Legionnaire's disease?' she asks Lucy.

Outbreaks of Legionnaire's disease secondary to contaminated whirlpool spas can occur (Jernigan et al., 1996). The whirlpool jets create an aerosol that is inhaled, resulting in infection. Inhaling aerosols from sources such as nebulisers, showers and whirlpool spas is a well-recognised mode of infection in hospital settings (O'Neill and Humphreys, 2005). Micro-aspiration is also thought to be important in nosocomial infection (Yu, 1993).

'So how did the water system become contaminated with *Legionella*?'

Legionella can be introduced to hospital water supplies from a catch basin, raw water reservoirs or leaking into the distribution system (Exner et al., 2005). According to Exner et al. (2005) factors enhancing *Legionella* colonisation of hospital water systems include:

- temperature of 25–42°C
- water stagnation
- sediment and scale
- free-living aquatic amoebae that support the growth of *Legionella* intracellularly. In fact, some believe that only people who inhale amoebae

containing *Legionella*, rather than *Legionella* alone, develop Legionnaire's disease (O'Brien and Bhopal, 1993)

Apart from controlling the water temperature, there are a number of ways of preventing *Legionella* colonisation of hospital water distribution systems. O'Neill and Humphreys (2005) list these as:

- physical methods (heat, ultraviolet radiation, sonication, compressed air)
- chemical methods (sodium hypochlorite, ozone, charcoal filters)
- good plumbing practice in both the design and maintenance of the system

> 'But *Legionella* has also been isolated in other parts of the hospital's water system. How do we get rid of it there?'

There are a few methods for ridding water systems of *Legionella* (Darelid et al., 2002; Modol et al., 2007) including:

- a silver-copper ionisation system (bactericidal to *Legionella*)
- monochloramines, although they are not used everywhere because of concerns over toxicity (Exner et al., 2005)
- chlorine dioxide
- maintaining the hot water temperature above 55°C

> There is only one factor in the case that bothers Megan. A friend of Chris's visited him, just once, in hospital. He helped take Chris to the hydrotherapy spa. Within 36 hours of that visit, the friend became mildly unwell with fevers and myalgias but recovered within 24 hours.
>
> She asks, 'He couldn't have had Legionnaire's disease because the incubation period was too short (36 hours). Nevertheless, could his illness have been related to the Legionnaire's disease outbreak in the hospital?'
>
> Lucy replies, 'It is too difficult to say. The only illness that I can think of which could have such a short incubation period and be related to a Legionnaire's disease outbreak is Pontiac fever.'

Pontiac fever is a relatively mild, non-pneumonic, febrile illness with a high attack rate that is associated with *Legionella*. It is named after a city in Michigan where the first recognised outbreak of this illness occurred in 1968. It is unclear whether Pontiac fever is due to *Legionella* infection or is an allergic/inflammatory response to dead *Legionella* (Edelstein, 2007). Various species of *Legionella* have been associated with Pontiac fever, such as *L. pneumophila*, *L. micdadei*, *L. anisa* and *L. feeleii* (Tossa et al., 2006). A case definition has been proposed (Tossa et al., 2006) which includes:

- an incubation period of 24–72 hours
- ≥ 1 major symptom (headache, myalgias, fevers and shivers)
- duration of illness 2–8 days (adjust if antibiotics are used)
- detection of *Legionella* in the implicated environmental source

A recent study identified positive *Legionella* urinary antigen tests in cases of Pontiac fever (Burnsed et al., 2007).

> Once again Patrick and Megan go to the ICU where, unfortunately, Chris remains intubated and ventilated with persisting fevers and pulmonary infiltrates (thankfully Clint had recovered promptly and gone home quite a while ago). Despite the proven diagnosis of *Legionella* and use of moxifloxacin, Chris has improved very little.
> The intensivist asks Patrick whether there is any benefit in using corticosteroids or dual antibiotic therapy.

Immunosuppression caused by corticosteroids is a risk factor for Legionnaire's disease; however, if the infection is complicated by bronchiolitis obliterans with organising pneumonia (BOOP) or follicular bronchiolitis, corticosteroids may play a beneficial role. There may also be a beneficial role to combination antibiotic therapy, but the data for this are lacking (Roig et al., 2003).

> Patrick does not recommend corticosteroids because Chris does not have BOOP or follicular bronchiolitis. However, he sees no harm in adding azithromycin to the moxifloxacin, even though the supporting evidence isn't great. He also suggests a transoesophageal echocardiogram to exclude *Legionella* endocarditis, particularly because of Chris's prosthetic valve.

> 'I'd forgotten that *Legionella* could cause endocarditis,' the intensivist replies.

Although uncommon, extrapulmonary disease does occur. The heart is the most common site but syndromes as diverse as cellulitis (Waldor et al., 1993), pyelonephritis (Dorman et al., 1980), pancreatitis (Megarbane et al., 2000), sinusitis (Schlanger et al., 1984) and peritonitis (Arnouts et al., 1991) have been documented. Cardiovascular infection often occurs in the absence of pneumonia (Stout and Yu, 1997) but most of the other syndromes appear to occur in the context of *Legionella* pneumonia.

> A few weeks later, Patrick sees Clint in clinic for the first time since his discharge. He is doing extremely well and has clearly recovered. He has some questions, though. 'Professor, my friend told me that you can get Legionella from gardening. Is that right?'

Legionella is an environmental organism and not surprisingly has been found in potting mixes, compost (both animal and plant/vegetable) and soil. *L. longbeachae* is probably the best known species associated with Legionnaire's disease and gardening (O'Connor et al., 2007); however, even *L. pneumophila* serogroup 1 has been found in soil and linked to a case of Legionnaire's disease (Wallis and Robinson, 2005).

References

Alary, M., Joly, J.R. (1992) Factors contributing to the contamination of hospital water distribution systems by legionellae. *Journal of Infectious Diseases* 165(3), 565–69.

Arnouts, P.J., Ramael, M.R., Ysebaert, D.K. et al. (1991) *Legionella pneumophila* peritonitis in a kidney transplant patient. *Scandinavian Journal of Infectious Diseases* 23(1), 119–22.

Bouree, P. (2003) Immunity and immunization in elderly. *Pathologie Biologie (Paris)* 51(10), 581–85.

Burnsed, L.J., Hicks, L.A., Smithee, L.M. et al. (2007) A large, travel-associated outbreak of legionellosis among hotel guests: utility of the urine antigen assay in confirming Pontiac fever. *Clinical Infectious Diseases* 44(2), 222–28.

Cunha, B.A. (2006) The atypical pneumonias: clinical diagnosis and importance. *Clinical Microbiology and Infection* 12(Suppl 3), 12–24.

Darelid, J., Lofgren, S., Malmvall, B. E. (2002) Control of nosocomial Legionnaires disease by keeping the circulating hot water temperature above 55 degrees C:

experience from a 10-year surveillance programme in a district general hospital. *Journal of Hospital Infection* 50(3), 213–19.

Den Boer, J.W., Yzerman, E.P. (2004) Diagnosis of *Legionella* infection in Legionnaires' disease. *European Journal of Clinical Microbiology & Infectious Diseases* 23(12), 871–78.

Diederen, B.M., De Jong, C.M., Kluytmans, J.A. et al. (2006) Detection and quantification of *Legionella pneumophila* DNA in serum: case reports and review of the literature. *Journal of Medical Microbiology* 55(Pt 5), 639–42.

Dorman, S.A., Hardin, N.J., Winn Jr, W.C. (1980) Pyelonephritis associated with *Legionella pneumophila*, serogroup 4. *Annals of Internal Medicine* 93(6), 835–37.

Edelstein, P.H. (2007) Urine antigen tests positive for Pontiac fever: implications for diagnosis and pathogenesis. *Clinical Infectious Diseases* 44(2), 229–31.

Exner, M., Kramer, A., Lajoie, L. et al. (2005) Prevention and control of health care-associated waterborne infections in health care facilities. *American Journal of Infection Control* 33(5 Suppl 1), S26–40.

Feldman, C. (2005) Pneumonia associated with HIV infection. *Current Opinion in Infectious Diseases* 18(2), 165–70.

Flanders, S.A., Collard, H.R., Saint, S. (2006) Nosocomial pneumonia: state of the science. *American Journal of Infection Control* 34(2), 84–93.

Formica, N., Tallis, G., Zwolak, B. et al. (2000) Legionnaires' disease outbreak: Victoria's largest identified outbreak. *Communicable Diseases Intelligence* 24(7), 199–202.

Greenberg, D., Chiou, C.C., Famigilleti, R. et al. (2006) Problem pathogens: paediatric legionellosis—implications for improved diagnosis. *Lancet Infectious Diseases* 6(8), 529–35.

Greig, J.E., Carnie, J.A., Tallis, G.F. et al. (2004) An outbreak of Legionnaires' disease at the Melbourne Aquarium, April 2000: investigation and case-control studies. *Medical Journal of Australia* 180(11), 566–72.

Gupta, S.K., Imperiale, T.F., Sarosi, G.A. (2001) Evaluation of the Winthrop-University Hospital criteria to identify *Legionella* pneumonia. *Chest* 120(4), 1064–71.

Isozumi, R., Ito, Y., Ito, I. et al. (2005) An outbreak of *Legionella* pneumonia originating from a cooling tower. *Scandinavian Journal of Infectious Diseases* 37(10), 709–11.

Jernigan, D.B., Hofmann, J., Cetron, M.S. et al. (1996) Outbreak of Legionnaires' disease among cruise ship passengers exposed to a contaminated whirlpool spa. *Lancet* 347(9000), 494–99.

Kool, J.L., Bergmire-Sweat, D., Butler, E.W. et al. (1999) Hospital characteristics associated with colonization of water systems by *Legionella* and risk of nosocomial Legionnaires' disease: a cohort study of 15 hospitals. *Infection Control and Hospital Epidemiology* 20(12), 798–805.

Legnani, P.P., Leoni, E., Corradini, N. (2002) *Legionella* contamination of hospital water supplies: monitoring of private healthcare facilities in Bologna, Italy. *Journal of Hospital Infection* 50(3), 220–23.

Marrie, T.J., Macdonald, S., Clarke, K. et al. (1991) Nosocomial Legionnaires' disease: lessons from a four-year prospective study. *American Journal of Infection Control* 19(2), 79–85.

Marston, B.J., Lipman, H.B., Breiman, R.F. (1994) Surveillance for Legionnaires' disease. Risk factors for morbidity and mortality. *Archives of Internal Medicine* 154(21), 2417–22.
Megarbane, B., Montambault, S., Chary, I. et al. (2000) Acute pancreatitis caused by severe *Legionella pneumophila* infection. *Infection* 28(5), 329–31.
Modol, J., Sabria, M., Reynaga, E., et al. (2007) Hospital-acquired Legionnaires disease in a university hospital: impact of the copper-silver ionization system. *Clinical Infectious Diseases* 44(2), 263–65.
Nguyen, T.M., Ilef, D., Jarraud, S, et al. (2006) A community-wide outbreak of Legionnaires disease linked to industrial cooling towers—how far can contaminated aerosols spread? *Journal of Infectious Diseases* 193(1), 102–11.
NSW Health (2005) *Microbial control*. Available from www.health.nsw.gov.au/policies/PD/2005/pdf/PD2005_197.pdf (Accessed 20 February, 2007.)
O'Brien, S.J., Bhopal, R.S. (1993) Legionnaires' disease: the infective dose paradox. *Lancet* 342(8862), 5–6.
O'Connor, B.A., Carman, J., Eckert, K. et al. (2007) Does using potting mix make you sick? Results from a *Legionella longbeachae* case-control study in South Australia. *Epidemiology and Infection* 135(1), 34–39.
O'Neill, E., Humphreys, H. (2005) Surveillance of hospital water and primary prevention of nosocomial legionellosis: what is the evidence? *Journal of Hospital Infection* 59(4), 273–79.
Pedro-Botet, L., Yu, V. L. (2006) *Legionella*: macrolides or quinolones? *Clinical Microbiology and Infection* 12(Suppl 3), 25–30.
Plouffe Jr, J.F., File Jr, T.M. (1999) Update of *Legionella* infections. *Current Opinion in Infectious Diseases* 12(2), 127–32.
Roig, J., Sabria, M., Pedro-Botet, M.L. (2003) *Legionella* spp.: community acquired and nosocomial infections. *Current Opinion in Infectious Diseases* 16(2), 145–51.
Rota, M. C., Pontrelli, G., Scaturro, M. et al. (2005) Legionnaires' disease outbreak in Rome, Italy. *Epidemiology and Infection* 133(5), 853–59.
Sabria, M., Alvarez, J., Dominguez, A. et al. (2006) A community outbreak of Legionnaires' disease: evidence of a cooling tower as the source. *Clinical Microbiology and Infection* 12(7), 642–47.
Schlanger, G., Lutwick, L.I., Kurzman, M. et al. (1984) Sinusitis caused by *Legionella pneumophila* in a patient with the acquired immune deficiency syndrome. *American Journal of Medicine* 77(5), 957–60.
Sehulster, L., Chinn, R.Y. (2003) Guidelines for environmental infection control in health-care facilities. Recommendations of CDC and the Healthcare Infection Control Practices Advisory Committee (HICPAC). *Morbidity and Mortality Weekly Reports Recommendations and Reports* 52(RR-10), 1–42.
Sopena, N., Pedro-Botet, L., Mateu, L. et al. (2007) Community-acquired *Legionella* pneumonia in elderly patients: characteristics and outcome. *Journal of the American Geriatrics Society* 55(1), 114–19.
Sopena, N., Sabria, M. (2005) Multicenter study of hospital-acquired pneumonia in non-ICU patients. *Chest* 127(1), 213–19.
Sopena, N., Sabria, M., Pedro-Botet, M.L. et al. (1999) Prospective study of community-acquired pneumonia of bacterial etiology in adults. *European Journal of Clinical Microbiology & Infectious Diseases* 18(12), 852–58.

Stout, J.E., Yu, V.L. (1997) Legionellosis. *New England Journal of Medicine* 337(10), 682–87.

Stout, J., Yu, V.L., Vickers, R.M. et al. (1982) Ubiquitousness of *Legionella pneumophila* in the water supply of a hospital with endemic Legionnaires' disease. *New England Journal of Medicine* 306(8), 466–68.

Tossa, P., Deloge-Abarkan, M., Zmirou-Navier, D. et al. (2006) Pontiac fever: an operational definition for epidemiological studies. *BMC Public Health* 6, 112.

Waldor, M.K., Wilson, B., Swartz, M. (1993) Cellulitis caused by *Legionella pneumophila*. *Clinical Infectious Diseases* 16(1), 51–53.

Wallis, L., Robinson, P. (2005) Soil as a source of *Legionella pneumophila* serogroup 1 (Lp1). *Australian and New Zealand Journal of Public Health* 29(6), 518–20.

Yu, V.L. (1993) Could aspiration be the major mode of transmission for *Legionella*? *American Journal of Medicine* 95(1), 13–15.

Yu, V.L., Beam Jr, T.R., Lumish, R.M. et al. (1987) Routine culturing for *Legionella* in the hospital environment may be a good idea: a three-hospital prospective study. *American Journal of the Medical Sciences* 294(2), 97–99.

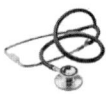

Case 12 Listeria
Ted is confused …

Listeria at a glance …

- **Agent:** family Corynebacteriaceae; genus *Listeria*; species *Listeria monocytogenes*; rarely other *Listeria* species have been implicated
- **Geographical distribution:** worldwide
- **Main mode of transmission:** foodborne; other modes much less common
- **Person-to-person transmission:** vertical transmission and cross-infection in the postnatal environment; adult-to-adult transmission is not documented but theoretically possible
- **Animal-to-person transmission:** yes
- **Incubation period:** 1 day–3 months
- **Clinical features:** adults—most commonly septicaemia and/or meningitis, although a wide variety of invasive sites of disease have been described; also gastroenteritis, rhombencephalitis and cutaneous disease; neonates—intrauterine infection can lead to spontaneous abortion, stillbirth or neonatal meningitis
- **Identification:** blood or cerebrospinal fluid (CSF) cultures; in gastroenteritis outbreaks, stools must be cultured in special media (e.g. PALCAM or Oxford agar)
- **Treatment:** antibiotics, usually a combination of ampicillin and trimethoprim/cotrimoxazole but other options are available
- **Prophylaxis:** none recommended, although trimethoprim/cotrimoxazole prophylaxis for *Pneumocystis jirovecii* infection in immunosuppressed patients might inadvertently provide some protection
- **Vaccine:** no, although *Listeria* is a commonly used vaccine vector in research

CASE 12 LISTERIA

Main characters

Mr Ted Wilkinson	patient with listeriosis
Dr Lisa Best	microbiology registrar
Dr Matthew Gregan	infectious diseases registrar
Dr David Porter	public health physician
Mr Brendon Jones	public health nurse
Mr Gary Wendell	food inspector

It is the daily microbiology laboratory round at a city hospital. The microbiologists, infectious diseases physicians and their registrars walk around the different benches (i.e. the 'blood culture' bench, the 'sterile site' bench and the 'poo' bench) looking at the interesting isolates. When they come to the sterile site bench, the scientist there shows them a cerebrospinal fluid (CSF) sample received in the last two hours from a Mr Ted Wilkinson. Under the microscope, they can see lots of polymorphonuclear cells with intracellular, Gram positive bacilli.

'But that's not all,' says Dr Lisa Best, the microbiology registrar. 'Have a look at the wet prep.'

Under the microscope, they examine a wet preparation slide of the CSF. They again can see the bacteria; however, now they are clearly mobile, with a tumbling motion.

Lisa adds, 'The same patient had blood cultures taken yesterday—they flagged positive about ten minutes ago; the Gram stain again shows a Gram positive bacillus.'

Lisa asks Dr Matthew Gregan, the infectious diseases registrar, what he concludes.

'Clearly, the patient has a bacteraemia associated with meningitis. However, the tumbling motion of the bacteria on the wet prep is strongly suggestive of *Listeria*.'

What is *Listeria*?

Listeria is an oxidase-positive, catalase-positive, Gram positive bacillus. The tumbling motion is due to the presence of polar flagella. It is named after Joseph Lister, the famous British doctor.

'Which species of *Listeria* is it likely to be?' Lisa asks.

Differential diagnoses

There are six species of bacteria in the genus *Listeria*: *L. monocytogenes*, *L. ivanovii*, *L. innocua*, *L. grayi*, *L. welshimeri* and *L. seeligeri*. However, virtually all human cases are due to *L. monocytogenes*. Human cases due to *L. ivanovii* and *L. seeligeri* have been described but are rare (Cummins et al., 1994; Lessing et al., 1994; Rocourt et al., 1987).

Lisa tells everyone that Ted is under the care of the geriatrics team. Earlier, Lisa had called the geriatrics intern to inform her of the result and get more information about the patient. However, the intern had just begun her rotation that day and didn't know much. Lisa suggested an antibiotic regimen and asked her to get a formal infectious diseases consultation immediately. Just then, Matthew's pager starts beeping.

'That must be her,' says Lisa. She's right—it is the geriatrics intern asking for a formal consult.

Matthew heads off to the ward immediately and meets the intern, who has now familiarised herself with the patient. Ted is an 84-year-old man whose wife of many years died earlier this year. He has well-controlled hypertension but is otherwise healthy. His son had brought him to hospital early yesterday morning after visiting and finding his father confused. He had last spoken to his father two days earlier, when Ted said he felt a bit odd but was otherwise okay.

In the emergency department, Ted was delirious, febrile to 39°C and tachycardic. At that time, there were no focal signs. He was placed on ceftriaxone and flucloxacillin empirically. Today, however, he developed neck stiffness and a lumbar puncture was performed.

'The microbiology registrar thought that the ceftriaxone and flucloxacillin wouldn't treat *Listeria*. Is that true?' asks the intern.

CASE 12 LISTERIA

Treatment

The best therapy would be intravenous ampicillin combined with trimethoprim/sulfamethoxazole; ceftriaxone and flucloxacillin would not be effective against *Listeria*.

> 'Why ampicillin instead of penicillin?' the intern asks. 'I'm sure I've seen someone given penicillin for *Listeria*. And do we really need combination therapy?'

Both ampicillin and penicillin have been used successfully to treat listeriosis, including meningitis (Hof et al., 1997). However, one study with a limited number of subjects demonstrated that ampicillin was more effective than penicillin. Ampicillin doses should be at least 6 g/day to be effective; doses as high as 18 g/day have been used (Lavetter et al., 1971).

The problem with beta-lactam antibiotics (e.g. ampicillin, penicillin) is that they are not bactericidal to *Listeria*. Both the aminoglycosides (killing time 1–2 hours) and trimethoprim/ sulfamethoxazole (killing time 6–24 hours) are bactericidal (Hof et al., 1997). In addition, Safdar et al. (2003) note that animal studies using combination therapy (gentamicin and ampicillin or penicillin) demonstrate 100-fold more effective killing (i.e. there is synergy).

But which combination is best? Another study compared combinations of ampicillin/amoxycillin with an aminoglycoside or trimethoprim/sulfamethoxazole (Merle-Melet et al., 1996). Although there were only 22 subjects, they showed a significantly higher success rate with the combination using trimethoprim/sulfamethoxazole.

Matthew examines Ted, who is still delirious. There are no findings to suggest other sites of invasive disease, apart from meningitis. He suggests combination therapy with ampicillin and trimethoprim/sulfamethoxazole, which Lisa had also suggested to the intern over the phone.

'What about cephalosporins and vancomycin?' the intern asks.

Cephalosporins should not be used to treat listeriosis. Although first-generation cephalosporins may show in vitro sensitivity or only intermediate resistance, there have been clinical failures. Although vancomycin may show in vitro sensitivity to *L. monocytogenes* and clinical success sometimes, there have also been treatment failures; this may be related to poor CSF penetration. Therefore it should be used with caution (Hof et al., 1997).

'What are his chances of recovering?'

Prognosis

The mortality rate from invasive listeriosis is 20–30% (often higher in neonatal disease). Long-term neurological sequelae, including psychiatric problems, are not uncommon in survivors (11% of neonates and 30% of adults) (Mead et al., 1999; World Health Organization and Food and Agriculture Organization, 2004).

Matthew returns the following day to see Ted. He is less delirious and his fever appears to be settling. The intern, however, looks a bit puzzled. 'I was telling my roommate about this case last night. She is an obstetric resident and said she recently looked after a pregnant woman with listeriosis. I always thought that it was just a disease of the immunosuppressed?'

Invasive listerial infection is mainly a disease of the immunosuppressed (including those on immunosuppressive medication and people with HIV/AIDS, malignancy, alcoholism or alcoholic liver disease). In fact, AIDS patients have a 100–500 higher rate of listeriosis than the general population (Schlech, 1996). However one-third of cases of meningitis and one-tenth of bacteraemias occur in immunocompetent individuals (McLauchlin et al., 2004).

Interestingly, certain clinical presentations of listeriosis are more common in immunocompetent people. An example of this is rhombencephalitis, which is a meningo-encephalitis of the posterior fossa associated with cranial nerve palsies and cerebellar signs.

Reduced gastric acidity may act as a risk factor for listeriosis. It appears that gastric acidity provides some degree of protection against the organism. A drug that reduces gastric acidity, cimetidine, reduced the ID_{50} for listeriosis (the dose at which 50% of people exposed to the organism become infected) in animals (Schlech, 1996).

> 'Interesting,' says the intern. 'But you still haven't explained why pregnant women are more prone to listeriosis. And is it dangerous to the mother and unborn child?'

Listeriosis is a mild illness for the pregnant woman. A review of 191 cases of listeriosis in pregnancy found that the pregnant women complained of fevers (65%), influenza-like illness (32%), back pain (21.5%) and headache (10.5%) or had asymptomatic infection (29%) (Wing and Gregory, 2002). However, it is a very dangerous infection for the unborn baby or neonates, with a mortality rate over 20% (stillbirth, perinatal death, spontaneous abortion).

Neonatal infection has two forms (Lorber, 2005), an early-onset sepsis picture (probably acquired in utero) and a meningitis syndrome at two weeks, postpartum (probably acquired around the time of birth). Granulomatosis infantiseptica is a terrible form of listeriosis in fetuses or neonates associated with multiple microabscesses in the liver and spleen.

Pregnancy is associated with 35% of cases of listeriosis globally and is the single most common risk factor (Drevets et al., 2004). The reason for this is not fully understood. A mild impairment of cell-mediated immunity occurs during pregnancy (Weinberg, 1984) and since cell-mediated immunity is an important defence against intracellular pathogens, such as *Listeria*, this reduction probably contributes to their susceptibility.

> The intern now asks, 'Well, why did an old man like Ted develop listeriosis?'

The mean age of adult infection of listeriosis is 55 years old. Therefore, it is commonly seen in older people. There are probably two reasons for this. First, ageing is associated with a global reduction in immunity, particularly cell-mediated immunity, which is so important for preventing listeriosis

(Bourée, 2003). Second, it is usually a foodborne disease; one study showed that elderly people were at increased risk of food poisoning because they did not meet the recommended food storage practices required to reduce cases (Johnson et al., 1998). Specific problems included refrigerators that were too warm and difficulty reading food labels.

> 'Okay, I understand. So it is purely a foodborne disease?'

The vast majority of cases of listeriosis are foodborne in origin. Rarely, *Listeria* can infect through other routes (McLauchlin and Low, 1994; McLauchlin et al., 2004), namely:

- cutaneously or through the eye by contact with naturally infected animals (so veterinarians and farmers are particularly at risk)
- environmental contamination (e.g. widespread contamination of the postnatal environment could potentially lead to additional neonatal cases due to cross-contamination)
- aerosols through the respiratory tract (this has been demonstrated in animal experiments but there was possibly one human case in 1981)
- listerial rhombencephalitis in sheep occurring through an ascending neuritis along the cranial nerves (since the human equivalent is anatomically and histologically similar, it may have a similar pathogenesis)

Interestingly, it has only been since the early 1980s that listeriosis has been shown to be a foodborne disease, although this had been suspected previously (Wing and Gregory, 2002). The turning point was an outbreak investigation in Canada in 1981, which demonstrated perseverance and good detective work by the investigators involved. They identified coleslaw as the vehicle of infection and were ultimately able to demonstrate that the manure used to fertilise the cabbage used in the coleslaw was the source of infection. The manure had come from a flock of sheep, among which there had been deaths from listeriosis (Schlech et al., 1983).

> 'A very nasty disease,' says the intern. 'Is there a vaccine against it?'

No vaccine is currently available. However, because it is one of the best-known intracellular organisms, *Listeria* is a commonly used vaccine vector for experimental DNA vaccines against infections such as HIV, TB, *Plasmodium* spp and Lyme disease (Schoen et al., 2004).

> 'Do I have to notify public health?' the intern asks.

Public health notification and response

Because of the association with contaminated food and serious illness, listeriosis is a notifiable disease in many parts of the world.

> The geriatrics intern contacts the public health unit and notifies one of the public heath doctors, Dr David Porter, of the case.
> Mr Brendon Jones, a new public health nurse in the unit looks on with interest. 'David, do you think that it is part of an outbreak?' he asks.

Because of the potentially long incubation period of listeriosis (up to three months), cases may be widespread in time and place, making it difficult to determine if a single case is part of a wider outbreak. Also, young immunocompetent individuals may have an asymptomatic infection, making it impossible to identify all infected individuals. For outbreaks and isolated cases, it may be difficult to work out what food was the vehicle of infection.

> 'So why even bother notifying us if we aren't going to find a source?'

While it will be impossible to investigate every meal and snack that Ted consumed in the last three months, the food contents of his refrigerator and cupboards can be examined.

For nosocomial infections, it is important to determine whether hospital food eaten during the incubation period was the source of infection. This is important for at least two reasons:

- Immunocompromised and pregnant patients in hospital may be exposed to contaminated food, so identifying and removing contaminated hospital food might prevent an outbreak of

> listeriosis among high-risk patients (hospitals often have special dietary requirements for patients known to be at risk of listeriosis, such as some renal and oncology patients).
> - Investigating hospital foods, food handling and storage is relatively easy in many countries because most health departments ensure that hospital kitchens and foods are routinely examined by food inspectors for *Listeria* counts (e.g. every six months).

'Isn't it just soft cheeses and salads that can carry listeria?'

> While soft cheeses and raw vegetables in salads are probably the best known food vehicles of *Listeria*, there are a wide variety of foods that have been associated with listeriosis including processed meats, apple cider, fresh meats and fish from delis, and most dairy products (Wing and Gregory, 2002).

Brendon says, 'Of course you are right. I now remember reading about *Listeria* being found in meat and poultry products. In fact, I think the US is using viruses to prevent *Listeria* infection from meat.'

> The US Food and Drug Administration has approved the use of a bacteriophage (a virus that infects bacteria) in meat and poultry products to combat *L. monocytogenes* contamination (Lang, 2006).

David and Brendon phone the ward to speak to Ted. Although he is improving, he is still not lucid enough to give an interview. However, his son confirms that his father has not been to hospital for more than two years. He is happy to let them into Ted's house to examine the kitchen. He believes that ever since his mother died, his father hasn't been looking after himself very well. He tries to help but his father is stubborn and tries to remain independent.

David, Brendon and Gary Wendell (a food inspector) are let inside Ted's house. They head for the refrigerator.

'Why are we looking in the refrigerator,' asks Brendon.

CASE 12 LISTERIA

One of the unusual features of *Listeria* is its ability to multiply at temperatures between 1–45°C. This allows it to proliferate in domestic refrigerators.

The refrigerator is set at 4°C. There is surprisingly little food: a meat pie, some beer, hard cheese, milk and an opened bottle of mussels. Gary collects specimens from each and sends them to the laboratory for culture. He calls David a few days later with the news that the mussels have high levels of *L. monocytogenes*, almost 1000 cfu/g. The other samples were culture negative.

Brendon is puzzled at this news. 'I'm surprised that mussels can be a source of *Listeria*. I assume it's cross-contamination from meats, cheeses and salads lying near them in the deli. I mean, you can't find *Listeria* in the sea, can you?'

Interestingly, *Listeria* has been isolated both from marine and freshwater environments. El Marrakchi et al. (2004) isolated *Listeria* spp from sea water, marine sediment and mussels. Colburn et al. (1990) found *Listeria* in fresh or low-salinity waters, sediment and oysters.

Food inspectors will need to investigate this further, looking for *Listeria* contamination of the factory that processed and packaged the mussels, as well as from the water from which they were originally taken. This may result in a product recall.

'Is a 1000 cfu/g of *Listeria* a lot?'

Although it may vary between countries, generally health or food authorities will recall a ready-to-eat (RTE) product if they find >100 cfu/g of *L. monocytogenes*. Some authorities, however, will have an even lower threshold or even a zero tolerance policy for certain high-risk RTE products such as soft cheeses. A count of 1000 cfu/g in the mussels is definitely too high and unacceptable (Food Standards Australia New Zealand, 2001).

Brendon now asks, 'Since listeriosis is a foodborne disease, do people get gastroenteritis?'

Listeria gastroenteritis is usually a non-invasive disease of immunocompetent individuals who consume large doses of the bacterium. The syndrome typically presents with fevers, myalgias, headache and diarrhoea (World Health Organization and Food and Agriculture Organization, 2004).

> 'Can *Listeria* be isolated from standard stool cultures?' asks Brendon. David is unsure and calls Lisa.

Investigations

It is difficult to identify *L. monocytogenes* from standard stool cultures because of all the other faecal bacteria present. Referring doctors need to let the laboratory know that *Listeria* is suspected so that special culture media such as the PALCAM (polymyxin-acriflavine-LiCl-ceftazidime-aesculin-mannitol) and Oxford agar can be used.

> 'Is culture the only way to identify *Listeria* spp?'

With human specimens, culture is the standard method of identifying the organism. In the food industry, however, other methods of identifying *Listeria* in food are being developed, for example, antibody-based tests and molecular tests such as polymerase chain reaction (PCR) (Gasanov et al., 2005).

> 'So why would *Listeria* be suspected as a cause of gastroenteritis in immunocompetent individuals if it hasn't been isolated from stool?'

Listeria gastroenteritis may only be suspected once other common causes of infectious diarrhoea have been excluded and/or a case's blood cultures become positive. A positive blood culture was what prompted investigators to test stool cultures for *L. monocytogenes* during a large *Listeria* gastroenteritis outbreak in two Italian primary schools (Aureli et al., 2000).

CASE 12 LISTERIA

> Brendon says, 'Gee, there must be many unrecognised sporadic cases of *Listeria* gastroenteritis because nobody specifically asks the lab to culture the stool for it.'

Investigators in Canada examined 7775 stool samples submitted for laboratory analysis for a diarrhoeal illness over a two-year period. All specimens were tested for *Listeria*; only 39/7775 tested positive, and of these only 17 were due to *L. monocytogenes*. They therefore concluded that sporadic gastroenteritis due to *L. monocytogenes* is uncommon and that routine screening of stool specimens is not necessary (Schlech et al., 2005).

> 'Does person-to-person transmission occur?'

Person-to-person transmission of listeriosis has not been documented (Lorber, 2005). However, *Listeria* can be found in the gastrointestinal tracts of up to 5% of healthy human adults (Wing and Gregory, 2002). Therefore, asymptomatic infection through faeco-oral or sexual routes from person-to-person is not implausible.

References

Aureli, P., Fiorucci, G.C., Caroli, D. et al. (2000) An outbreak of febrile gastroenteritis associated with corn contaminated by *Listeria monocytogenes*. *New England Journal of Medicine* 342(17), 1236–41.

Bourée, P. (2003) Immunity and immunization in elderly. *Pathologie Biologie* 51(10), 581–85.

Colburn, K.G., Kaysner, C.A., Abeyta Jr, C. et al. (1990) *Listeria* species in a California coast estuarine environment. *Applied and Environmental Microbiology* 56(7), 2007–11.

Cummins, A.J., Fielding, A.K., McLauchlin, J. (1994) *Listeria ivanovii* infection in a patient with AIDS. *Journal of Infection* 28(1), 89–91.

Drevets, D.A., Leenen, P.J., Greenfield, R.A. (2004) Invasion of the central nervous system by intracellular bacteria. *Clinical Microbiology Reviews* 17(2), 323–47.

El Marrakchi, A., Boum'handi, M., Hamama, A. (2004) Performance of a new chromogenic plating medium for the isolation of *Listeria monocytogenes* from marine environments. *Letters in Applied Microbiology* 40(2), 87–91.

Food Standards Australia New Zealand (2001) *Recall guidelines for packaged ready-to-eat foods found to contain* Listeria monocytogenes *at point of sale*. Available from www.foodstandards.gov.au/whatsinfood/listeria/listeriarecall-guidel1321.cfm (Accessed November 29, 2005)

Gasanov, U., Hughes, D., Hansbro, P.M. (2005) Methods for the isolation and identification of *Listeria* spp. and *Listeria monocytogenes*: a review. *FEMS Microbiology Reviews* 29(5), 851–75.

Hof, H., Nichterlein, T., Kretschmar, M. (1997) Management of listeriosis. *Clinical Microbiology Reviews* 10(2), 345–57.

Johnson, A.E., Donkin, A.J., Morgan, K. et al. (1998) Food safety knowledge and practice among elderly people living at home. *Journal of Epidemiology and Community Health* 52(11), 745–48.

Lang, L.H. (2006) FDA approves use of bacteriophages to be added to meat and poultry products. *Gastroenterology* 131(5), 1370.

Lavetter, A., Leedom, J.M., Mathies Jr, A.W. et al. (1971) Meningitis due to *Listeria monocytogenes*. A review of 25 cases. *New England Journal of Medicine* 285(11), 598–603.

Lessing, M.P., Curtis, G.D., Bowler, I.C. (1994) *Listeria ivanovii* infection. *Journal of Infection* 29(2), 230–31.

Lorber, B. (2005) *Listeria monocytogenes*. In Mandell G.L., Bennett, J.E., Dolin, R. (eds) *Principles and Practice of Infectious Diseases*. Churchill Livingstone; Philadelphia

McLauchlin, J., Mitchell, R.T., Smerdon, W.J. et al. (2004) *Listeria monocytogenes* and listeriosis: a review of hazard characterisation for use in microbiological risk assessment of foods. *International Journal of Food Microbiology* 92(1), 15–33.

McLauchlin, J., Low, J.C. (1994) Primary cutaneous listeriosis in adults: an occupational disease of veterinarians and farmers. *Veterinary Record* 135(26), 615–17.

Mead, P.S., Slutsker, L., Dietz, V. et al. (1999) Food-related illness and death in the United States. *Emerging Infectious Diseases* 5(5), 607–25.

Merle-Melet, M., Dossou-Gbete, L., Maurer, P. (1996) Is amoxicillin-cotrimoxazole the most appropriate antibiotic regimen for *Listeria* meningoencephalitis? Review of 22 cases and the literature. *Journal of Infection* 33(2), 79–85.

Rocourt, J., Schrettenbrunner, A., Hof, H. et al. (1987) New species of the genus Listeria: *Listeria seeligeri*. *Pathologie Biologie* 35(7), 1075–80.

Safdar, A., Armstrong, D. (2003) Listeriosis in patients at a comprehensive cancer center, 1955–1997. *Clinical Infectious Diseases* 37(3), 359–64.

Schlech, W.F. (1996) Overview of listeriosis. *Food Control* 7(4/5), 183–86.

Schlech 3rd, W.F., Schlech 4th, W.F., Haldane, H. et al. (2005) Does sporadic *Listeria* gastroenteritis exist? A 2-year population-based survey in Nova Scotia, Canada. *Clinical Infectious Diseases* 41(6), 778–84.

Schlech 3rd, W.F., Lavigne, P.M., Bortolussi, R.A. et al. (1983) Epidemic listeriosis—evidence for transmission by food. *New England Journal of Medicine* 308(4), 203–06.

Schoen, C., Stritzker, J., Goebel, W. et al. (2004) Bacteria as DNA vaccine carriers for genetic immunization. *International Journal of Medical Microbiology* 294(5), 319–35.

Weinberg, E.D. (1984) Pregnancy-associated depression of cell-mediated immunity. *Reviews of Infectious Diseases* 6(6), 814–31.

Wing, E.J., Gregory, S.H. (2002) *Listeria monocytogenes*: clinical and experimental update. *Journal of Infectious Diseases* 185(Suppl 1), S18–24.

World Health Organization and Food and Agriculture Organization of the United Nations (2004) *Risk assessment of Listeria monocytogenes in ready-to-eat food.* Available from www.who.int/foodsafety/publications/micro/en/mra4.pdf (Accessed 27 November, 2005)

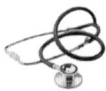

Case 13 Measles
Jean-Luc has a rash …

> **Measles at a glance …**
>
> - **Agent:** family Paramyxoviridae; genus *Morbillivirus*; species measles virus
> - **Geographical distribution:** worldwide
> - **Mode of transmission:** respiratory droplet transmission; infected surfaces
> - **Person-to-person transmission:** yes
> - **Incubation period:** 14 days (6–19 days)
> - **Infectious period:** 4 days before appearance of the rash to 4 days after
> - **Clinical features:** classical measles has a prodrome of fever, cough, conjunctivitis, coryza and Koplik's spots followed by a morbilliform rash that starts in the head and neck before becoming more generalised; complications in any organ system can occur, most commonly pneumonia, diarrhoea, hepatitis and otitis media; atypical measles is a rare and severe syndrome that usually occurs in those who have previously received killed measles vaccine; immunosuppressed individuals or those with partial immunity to measles may have a modified illness
> - **Identification:** serology (IgM or rise in IgG titres); immunofluorescence of nasopharyngeal and urinary specimens; reverse transcriptase polymerase chain reaction (RT-PCR) and culture of nasopharyngeal specimens, urine and blood; IgM in salivary specimens
> - **Treatment:** supportive for uncomplicated measles; antivirals may have some benefit in complicated measles; Vitamin A supplementation in certain circumstances
> - **Post-exposure prophylaxis:** vaccine within 3 days of exposure (the live vaccine is contraindicated in immunosuppression and pregnancy); normal human immunoglobulin 3–7 days after exposure
> - **Vaccine:** live attenuated vaccine usually found in combination with rubella and mumps (MMR vaccine)

Main characters

Dr Liam O'Donnell	infectious diseases registrar
Mr Lance Walker	medical student
Mr Jean-Luc Delauney	patient with a rash
Professor James Gorman	infectious diseases consultant
Dr Maria Zimmerman	public health specialist
Dr Chrissy Brooks	public health registrar

Dr Liam O'Donnell, an infectious diseases registrar, receives a page from the emergency department. He goes down there with Lance Walker, a medical student. There is a man with fever and a rash waiting in the isolation room for review.

Mr Jean-Luc Delauney is a 25-year-old who was previously well. Four days ago, he returned from a six-week holiday to India, Sri Lanka and Bangladesh. He became ill three days ago with fever, red eyes, a runny nose and a dry cough. He has been feeling a bit hot and cold. Today, he got worried when he noticed a rash on his face and neck.

On examination, Jean-Luc looks miserable. He has a fever, conjunctivitis and a runny nose. But the most striking feature is the rash. There are numerous discrete areas of erythema over the face and neck, as described by the patient, and Liam notices that the upper trunk is also now involved. He looks into Jean-Luc's mouth and nods to himself, apparently satisfied.

'This man has measles.'

Lance, however, looks sceptical: 'I've never seen measles. Isn't it a disease of the past?'

What is measles?

Measles has been familiar to the medical community for centuries. The first written descriptions came from Arabs writing in the tenth century AD but, unlike so many other communicable diseases, there are no earlier descriptions, such as in the writings of the ancient Greeks. Perhaps the populations were not large enough to sustain memorable epidemics (Rima and Duprex, 2006).

Measles is also a disease of the present. The World Health Organization (WHO) estimated that there were around half a million deaths due to measles worldwide in 2004 (World Health Organization, 2006).

CASE 13 MEASLES

It is caused by the measles virus, a single-stranded RNA virus from the genus *Morbillivirus* and family Paramyxoviridae (Ota et al., 2005).

> 'Okay, I didn't realise that measles was still around. But I would imagine that all the cases are found in developing countries, unlike ours?'

The majority of reported cases are from developing countries, but not all. The WHO estimated that almost 90% of the 33 million cases of reported measles in 2002 came from the African, South-East Asia and Western Pacific regions (Baringa and Skolnik, 2006a). This is probably due to a combination of limited public health resources in developing countries and relatively low vaccine uptake rates. In 2004, the regions with the three lowest rates for routine measles vaccine coverage were Sub-Saharan Africa, South Asia and the East Asia and Pacific regions (World Health Organization, 2006).

> Lance is still not happy. 'But with our immunisation program against measles, we shouldn't have susceptible people. How do you explain that?'

If a country maintains its immunisation program for measles, everyone may be completely immune to measles *eventually*. However, many countries brought in a two-dose immunisation program with a live attenuated measles vaccine relatively recently. This means some older individuals may not have been immunised, may have received only one dose of live attenuated vaccine or may have received inactivated vaccine, and these groups may still be susceptible. In Australia, for instance, individuals born between 1966–80 are a potentially susceptible group (National Health and Medical Research Council, 2003).

> In Liam's country, people aged 24–38 years may have received only one dose or never have been vaccinated, so a 25-year-old patient like Jean-Luc could well be susceptible.
> 'But wouldn't one dose of vaccine have been enough to provide immunity?'

The current mumps/measles/rubella (MMR) vaccine provides immunity to 95% of recipients who receive one dose and 99% of recipients who receive two doses (National Health and Medical Research Council, 2003). This means 5% of recipients of one dose of MMR vaccine will not be immune. With large populations, 5% can represent a large number of susceptible individuals.

> 'But where would he have caught it from? I haven't heard of any measles cases locally.'

Jean-Luc was almost certainly infected overseas. The incubation period of measles is 14 days (range 6–19 days) (Asaria and MacMahon, 2006). Jean-Luc returned from his six-week holiday to South Asia only four days ago and became ill the day after returning. Also, the burden of measles globally is mainly in the developing world, adding weight to this argument. A review of measles cases in the US 1993–2001 discovered that 17% of cases were imported (Vukshich Oster et al., 2004).

The important point is that measles should be in the differential diagnosis of an acute febrile illness with rash in the returning traveller.

> Lance grudgingly accepts that Jean-Luc may have measles. 'As I said before, I haven't seen measles previously and haven't learnt much about it. What makes you so sure that he has measles?'

Jean-Luc presents with a typical picture for measles. Additionally, the incubation period fits and places him geographically in countries where the burden of measles is highest.

The clinical illness of measles can be divided into three phases (Table 13.1).

Table 13.1 Clinical features of uncomplicated measles

Prodrome	Exanthem (rash)	Recovery
Lasts 2–3 days (up to eight days) Fevers Dry cough Conjunctivitis (which can be quite severe) Coryza (runny nose) Koplik's spots in most cases	Maculopapular Lasts about four days before starting to fade (turning brown) and possibly desquamating. Typically starts in the face and neck and moves inferiorly. Patients improve within 48 hours of the rash appearing.	Dry cough (which may persist for 1–2 weeks) In uncomplicated measles, fevers should not persist once the exanthem has been present for more than three days.

SOURCE Barinaga and Skolnik, 2006b

> Lance asks Liam, 'So why did you look in his mouth?'

Koplik's spots are an enanthem (an eruption of the mucous membrane) characterised by blue-white spots on an erythematous base on the buccal mucosa. They tend to occur in the prodrome period and persist for 2–3 days after the appearance of the rash (Asaria and MacMahon, 2006).

Koplik's spots are not always present but if found are pathognomonic of measles. They are classically located opposite the first molar but may also be present on the vagina, conjunctiva and soft palate (Perry and Halsey, 2004). Henry Koplik (1858–1927) was an American paediatrician who first recognised the significance of this sign of measles (Bass, 2005).

> Lance continues to play devil's advocate. 'Are you sure this couldn't be anything else?'

Differential diagnosis

In this particular case, the patient has so many epidemiological and clinical features to support a diagnosis of measles that anything else seems unlikely. However, as Barinaga and Skolnik (2006b) point out, there are differential diagnoses for the prodrome and exanthem phases of measles.

For the prodrome, these are:

- the common cold (although fevers and conjunctivitis are unusual);
- Fordyce spots (these occur in the buccal mucosa but are yellow-white rather than blue and do not have an erythematous base)

For the exanthem, these are:

- rubella
- parvovirus B19
- enteroviral infections
- human herpes virus 6 and 7 (HHV-6 and 7)
- Kawasaki's disease
- dengue fever
- human immunodeficiency virus (HIV)

- secondary syphilis
- meningococcal disease
- scarlet fever
- toxic shock syndrome
- drug reaction

> 'But the patient can't recall coming into contact with anyone with a rash. Wouldn't he have remembered something as obvious as the rash of measles?'

> Measles is infectious during both the prodrome and exanthem phases of the illness, from four days before the onset of the rash to four days after (Asaria and MacMahon, 2006). Consequently, the index case may have had only a runny nose and mild conjunctivitis at the time of infecting Jean-Luc.
>
> Additionally, the index case may not actually have been present when he infected Jean-Luc. Measles particles can remain infectious in the air and on surfaces for two hours after the infected case has left (Asaria and MacMahon, 2006). Imagine if the index case sat in the waiting lounge of an international airport—all susceptible people sitting in that lounge for the next two hours could potentially be infected and carry the virus overseas.

> Lance looks surprised. 'I didn't realise that measles was so infectious.'

Measles is one of the most infectious diseases of public health importance known to humanity. In a susceptible population, it has a reproductive number (R_0) of 15–20 (reproductive number is the number of secondary cases arising from a single case in a susceptible population): it is 5–6 times more infectious than SARS, which has a R_0 of 2.7. Measles also has an attack rate of 80% (attack rate refers to the proportion of people who become ill after being exposed to the infectious agent) (Mangili and Gendreau, 2005).

The potential for so many secondary cases makes controlling an outbreak of measles a real challenge for public health officials.

Liam knows that their laboratory can do IgM testing on serum in about 3–4 hours, so they will have a result later today. The specimens for antigen/virus testing, however, have to be sent to a larger laboratory, delaying the results.

Investigations

A laboratory diagnosis of measles can be made using tests by detecting IgM in serum or detecting antigen/virus from various tissues.

Later that afternoon, the laboratory calls back: the serum measles IgM from serum is negative.

Liam notifies his boss, infectious diseases consultant Professor James Gorman. 'I'm really surprised that the IgM serology is negative. I was sure he had measles.'

No test is perfect. The enzyme immunoassay (EIA) for measles has a fairly good sensitivity and specificity (83–89% and 95–100% respectively). However, it can still generate both false positive and false negative results (Bellini and Helfand, 2003). False positive results are due to:

Rheumatoid factor
Other infections For example, parvovirus B19 or rubella.
Measles immunisation The test detects measles IgM generated by vaccination, so this is a 'false positive' only in the sense that the IgM is in response to vaccine-strain measles rather than wild-type. The test may remain positive for 1–2 months post-immunisation (NSW Health, 2004).

In the case of false negative results the sensitivity of the IgM EIA drops to 70% if taken on Day 1 of the rash, so it is negative in 30% of true measles cases.

Jean-Luc probably does have measles but with the rash in its first day he probably has not produced IgM as yet.

'The lab can do a serum IgG for measles. Would that be useful?' Liam asks.

A serum IgG has two uses in the diagnosis of measles:

- A positive IgG within seven days of the appearance of the rash means that the diagnosis is unlikely to be acute measles.
- A four-fold rise in paired acute and convalescent sera for IgG can be used to diagnose measles (although this is not useful in the acute setting).

Are the antigen/viral assays likely to be positive this early into the infection?

Antigen/viral assays are positive early on. There are three methods usually used to identify measles virus or antigen: immunofluorescence (IF), culture or reverse transcriptase polymerase chain reaction (RT-PCR) (Bellini and Helfand, 2003). Some characteristics of each test are shown in Table 13.2.

In the acute setting, apart from serology, IF and RT-PCR are the most useful diagnostic tests. Unfortunately, RT-PCR and culture

Table 13.2 Some characteristics of tests to isolate measles virus or antigen

Test	Specimens	Days after the onset of the rash that the test remains positive	Time to perform the test
Immunofluorescence	NP aspirate/swab urine[†]	5	<2 hours
RT-PCR	NP aspirate/swab urine blood	14	1–2 days
Culture[‡]	NP aspirate/swab urine blood	5	5–7 days

NP = nasopharyngeal
[†]Urine specimens should be a morning 'first catch' with around 20–50 mL volume.
[‡]The sensitivity of cultures for measles varies according to the cell lines used. Examples of cell lines with good sensitivity include B95a and Vero/SLAM cell lines (Bellini and Helfand, 2003; Centers for Disease Control and Prevention, 2005). A diagnosis of measles from cultures can be made through IF of the cell lines or identifying typical cytopathic changes.
SOURCE Bellini and Helfand, 2003; Gershon, 2005; NSW Health, 2004

facilities are not available in smaller hospitals and some developing nations.

RT-PCR and culture of measles virus are also useful techniques for typing measles strains to determine whether epidemics are due to one or more strains and how extensively those strains have spread (e.g. to see if a single strain has caused multinational outbreaks).

Liam has already collected blood and a nasopharyngeal aspirate (NPA) from the patient for IF and RT-PCR. The reference laboratory assures him the results will be available tomorrow.

Liam also asks, 'Can we use saliva to diagnose measles?'

Saliva can be used to diagnose measles but the test is not performed everywhere. Saliva IgM can be tested for ≤6 weeks of onset and is quite sensitive (Brown et al., 1994; Oliveira et al., 1998). RT-PCR testing of salivary samples can also be performed (Asaria and MacMahon, 2006). In the UK, oral testing kits are sent to doctors or patients whenever there is a notification of measles.

Jean-Luc asks, 'Doctor, I feel terrible. Is there anything you can do to treat my measles?'

Treatment

Apart from symptomatic measures, there is no specific treatment for uncomplicated measles in an otherwise healthy adult from a developed nation.

In countries with measles mortality rates >1% or where vitamin A deficiency is an issue, UNICEF/WHO recommend that all children with measles receive vitamin A supplements. Children with measles in these settings appear to have a higher morbidity and mortality from the infection and measles increases the body's utilisation of vitamin A, depleting body stores (World Health Organization, 1987).

Antiviral agents such as ribavirin and interferon have been used in treating complication of measles (e.g. SSPE, pneumonitis) with varying success (Forni et al., 1994; Titomanlio et al., 2007).

Liam has admitted Jean-Luc under James for intravenous (IV) rehydration and symptomatic treatment. James wants the patient transferred to a single negative-pressure room to be nursed only by staff with a history of measles. Respiratory isolation measures are enforced.

James asks, 'So have you informed the public health unit?'

'No. I thought I should notify them when I have laboratory confirmation and right now my diagnosis is only clinical.'

Public health notification and response

Because measles is so infectious and potentially dangerous, many health departments require notification of suspected cases. This allows them to get basic demographic data on the patient and their movements during the infectious period and interview contacts about susceptibility to measles. If measles is confirmed, the outbreak team already have a head start for their investigation.

Positive laboratory findings are required to upgrade a patient's status from suspect to confirmed case, when a full-blown outbreak investigation is launched. This involves administering post-exposure prophylaxis (PEP) potentially to many susceptible contacts. This is a time-consuming and resource-consuming exercise, so it makes more sense to wait 24 hours to get laboratory confirmation. Also, studies show that doctors in developed nations are poor at differentiating measles from other fever and rash syndromes, so a clinical diagnosis has a low positive predictive value (Asaria and MacMahon, 2006; Lambert et al., 2000).

Liam calls the public health unit and gives the patient's details to Dr Maria Zimmerman, one of the public health specialists.

The next day, Jean-Luc still has fevers and the rash is more extensive; however, he isn't any worse and is possibly a bit better. He has developed diarrhoea, though, with three loose bowel motions overnight.

'Doctor, I just thought that measles gave you a rash,' he says. 'Why the diarrhoea?'

The rash is the most well-known feature of measles but it nevertheless is a systemic infection. Multinucleated giant cells typical of measles have been found in the respiratory and gastrointestinal tracts as well as in most lymphoid tissues, so it can affect a wide variety of organ systems (Table 13.3). The most common complications are pneumonia, diarrhoea, hepatitis and otitis media (mainly in children) (Asaria and MacMahon, 2006; Perry and Halsey, 2004).

Table 13.3 Some measles complications

System	Complication
Cardiovascular	myocarditis, pericarditis
Respiratory	pneumonia, otitis media, croup
Gastrointestinal	diarrhoea, hepatitis, appendicitis
Neurological	SSPE, ADEM, MIBE, febrile seizures
Ocular	blindness, keratitis
Haematological	TTP, DIC
Dermatological	cellulitis
Immunological	transient immunosuppression
Renal	nephritis, renal failure

SSPE = subacute sclerosing panencephalitis; ADEM = acute disseminated encephalomyelitis, occurring 3–10 days after acute measles; MIBE = measles inclusion body encephalitis, usually seen in immunocompromised hosts between five weeks and six months after acute measles; TTP = thrombotic thrombocytopenic purpura; DIC = disseminated intravascular coagulation
SOURCE Asaria and MacMahon, 2006; Perry and Halsey, 2004

> 'Doctor, am I going to die?'

Prognosis

The risk of death from measles is relatively low. Data from the US and UK estimate an overall mortality of 0.2–0.3%. The highest mortality occurs in infants, young children and adults; older children and adolescents seem to have a slightly lower mortality.

Pneumonia is the cause of most deaths (Department of Health, 2005; Perry and Halsey, 2004).

> Later that day, James receives a call from the reference laboratory: the RT-post-erposure prophylaxis (PCR) of the urine and NP specimens are positive for measles. Jean-Luc now meets the case definition for confirmed measles. He informs Maria at public health about this latest development.
> She officially launches an outbreak investigation. After forming an outbreak team, she needs to identify all susceptible contacts of Jean-Luc during his infectious period. 'Time is of the essence,' she says.

It is important to identify contacts and determine their susceptibility to measles as soon as possible. Measles can be prevented through the use of post-exposure prophylaxis (PEP) but only within days of exposure. National Health and Medical Research Council (2003) PEP protocols are determined by age:

Contacts <6 months of age If the mother is immune to measles, no PEP is required for the infant because of protective maternal antibodies. If the mother is susceptible, the infant should receive normal human immunoglobulin (NHIG) within seven days of exposure to the index case.

Contacts 6–9 months old who have not been immunised All infants should be offered NHIG within seven days of exposure to the index case. Maternal antibody levels will be waning and most children will not receive their first MMR immunisation till one year of age.

Contacts over 9 months of age Give MMR within 72 hours of exposure to the index case if there are no contraindications. Give NHIG if it is 3–7 days after exposure to the index case. Severely immunocompromised patients and susceptible pregnant women should receive only NHIG because MMR is a live attenuated vaccine.

Immunisation with MMR within 72 hours of exposure is effective at preventing measles because the incubation period for the vaccine strain is usually shorter than that for the wild-type virus (4–6 days versus 14 days) (National Health and Medical Research Council, 2003), allowing protective antibodies to develop in response to the vaccine before the infection appears.

CASE 13 MEASLES

After a detailed phone interview with the patient, Maria determines that Jean-Luc was infectious for four days prior to his hospital admission. His time line for the four days prior to the rash is as follows:

Day 4 before rash:

- airplane flight home from Singapore

Day 3 before rash:

- reunion at home with girlfriend
- romantic evening with girlfriend watching a movie at the local cinema followed by dinner at a fast food restaurant

Day 2 before rash:

- resting at home all day; visited by mother

Day 1 before rash:

- resting at home all day; visited by girlfriend

Day of rash onset:

- went from home to hospital
- spent 30 minutes in the waiting room of the emergency department
- triage nurse led him straight to a single room

Contacts that can be identified from this timeline are:

- hotel staff in his Singapore hotel, including staff cleaning his room after he checked out (if the cleaning took place within two hours of him departing), staff behind the checkout desk and staff serving breakfast
- the taxi driver who took him from the hotel to the airport
- people who were near Jean-Luc during his trip home, both in Singapore's international airport and Jean-Luc's home airport
- passengers on the flight
- the taxi driver who took him home from the airport
- his girlfriend
- staff working at the cinema and people attending the same movie session as Jean-Luc and his girlfriend
- staff and other people at the restaurant while Jean-Luc and his girlfriend were there

- his mother
- people (staff and patients) in the waiting room in the emergency department while Jean-Luc was seated there and for two hours afterwards

The Ministry of Health in Singapore need to be informed promptly that Jean-Luc would have been infectious on the day that he left his hotel and went to the airport. They will perform contact tracing according to their own guidelines.

Unfortunately, it will be impossible to identify most of the people at the hotel and both airports who were in close proximity to Jean-Luc prior to departure and after arriving home. Duty rosters at both airports may identify the immigration and customs officials who processed him. Similarly, rosters from the hotel might identify staff who had contact. A passenger manifesto from the airline will identify the other passengers on his flight.

> Maria's public health registrar, Dr Chrissy Brooks, asks, 'Which passengers on the flight are at risk of being infected?'

There have been only two publications of possible transmission of measles during a flight. It seemed that only those sitting within a few rows of the index cases were infected (Leder and Newman, 2005) but it may be that people further away were exposed but remained uninfected because they were already immune.

> Maria decides that passengers who were sitting two rows in front of and behind Jean-Luc, as well as those in the same row, should be classified as contacts and contacted as soon as possible to check their immunity. She also instructs the outbreak team to classify all flight crew working in the economy class as contacts.
>
> Over the next 12 hours, Maria and her team put all other work aside and tirelessly attempt to get in touch with as many contacts as possible. Due to their perseverance, they contact everyone by the end of that day. It turns out to be a staggering 81 people.
>
> Using immunisation records and documented measles serology from previously, the team can exclude 78 contacts. Only three have uncertain immunity. Contact 1 is a 28-year-old refugee who

> has no idea about his measles status. Contact 2 has AIDS with a very low CD4 count. Contact 3 is an elderly man who thinks he received a dose of measles vaccine about 70 years ago, a time when only killed measles vaccine was given.
>
> Contact 2 with AIDS definitely needs PEP. If blood can be taken from Contacts 1 and 3 tonight, the lab will be able to process the samples first thing in the morning to determine their measles immunity. This small delay won't affect the administration of PEP because Contact 1 will still be within the three-day window to receive MMR vaccine and Contact 3 in the seven-day window to receive NHIG.
>
> Contact 2 has some questions: 'First, could I get really sick with measles because of my advanced HIV infection?'

Data from patients with impaired cell-mediated immunity (e.g. HIV, some malignancies) show mortality rates a high as 70%, with serious complications occurring in 80% of patients. Furthermore, up to 40% of patients in these studies do not present with a rash, creating a diagnostic dilemma. This emphasises the importance of considering measles in the differential diagnoses in immunocompromised patients presenting with encephalitis or pneumonitis of unknown origin in the absence of a rash (Kaplan et al., 1992).

> 'Also, I've heard you can usually give two types of PEP for measles but only one type for people with AIDS. Is that true?'

Patients with advanced HIV/AIDS should not receive the MMR vaccine as it is a live attenuated vaccine. They should always receive passive immunisation with NHIG (National Health and Medical Research Council, 2003).

> On the following day, the measles IgG from the serum of the two contacts returns. Contact 1 is IgG negative but Contact 3 has an indeterminate IgG, which could mean low levels of IgG. Maria recommends PEP for both of them.
>
> 82-year-old Contact 3 refuses. 'Doctor, I am pretty sure I was immunised as a child. I thought that your blood test would

> show that. I really don't want your medicine. That's my final decision.'
>
> Contact 1 agrees to be vaccinated by his GP. However, he has a question. 'My wife is pregnant and I don't know if she is immune to measles. I have heard that pregnant women get really ill with measles. Is that true? Doesn't the MMR vaccine contain a live virus? If it does, I don't want my wife to get measles from the virus in the vaccine.'

Measles can be very severe in pregnant women. A case series of 13 pregnant women with measles found that more than 50% developed what was probably primary measles pneumonia; one woman died and a number required intensive care (Atmar et al., 1992). The fetus is at risk of premature birth and in utero death but not congenital deformities (Gershon, 2005).

While the MMR vaccine contains live virus, it is an attenuated strain and there is no risk of transmission to others (National Health and Medical Research Council, 2003), so the contact should not be worried about infecting his wife.

> Chrissy asks Maria, 'Do our susceptible contacts need to be educated about measles? After all, since they are receiving appropriate PEP (apart from Contact 3), measles infection shouldn't be an issue.'

Hopefully, administering timely PEP will prevent clinical infection. However, there are no guarantees so it is important to educate contacts about measles infection and the importance of seeking medical attention if they become unwell. Three specific points to mention are that:

- They should speak to their doctor over the phone if they become ill. This is to ensure that they do not turn up to a waiting room and infect other people. Their doctor can then make special arrangements to review them (NSW Health, 2004).
- Administering PEP might increase the incubation period of the illness (Gershon, 2005).
- Administering PEP might result in an atypical illness, so classical features might not occur (Gershon, 2005).

CASE 13 MEASLES

> Ten days pass with no new measles notifications. Before Maria can breathe a sigh of relief, she receives a call from James: 'I have an 82-year-old man in an isolation room in the emergency department. I believe you identified him as a susceptible contact in your measles investigation but he refused PEP.' (This sounds like Contact 3.)
> 'He is quite sick. The presentation is unusual for measles. He developed fevers yesterday and today noticed a maculopapular rash on his arms and legs. Clinically, he is short of breath and hypoxic with pulmonary infiltrates bilaterally on chest X-ray. He is quite oedematous and his blood tests show hepatitis. I am wondering if this man has atypical measles.'

Atypical measles is a syndrome that usually occurs in people who have received killed vaccine previously. It is thought that the immune response to the killed vaccine results in some type of hypersensitivity reaction when that person is exposed to wild-type measles virus (Gershon, 2005). Contact 3 would have been immunised with a killed form of the vaccine, so he could well have atypical measles.

The rash begins peripherally, rather than in the head and neck, after a short febrile prodrome. The rash itself does not have to be maculopapular. Oedema, severe pneumonitis, hepatitis and prolonged fever can also occur (Asaria and MacMahon, 2006). Other conditions need to be excluded but this clinical picture in a susceptible contact would make atypical measles highly likely.

Patients with this syndrome do not seem to be infectious and measles virus cannot be isolated from them (Gershon, 2005). However, a diagnosis can be made using serology (Henderson and Hammond, 1985).

> Chrissy knocks on Maria's door. She has a question.
> 'Last night I saw a TV medical drama where the patient was a teenager with encephalitis, the cause of which was a mystery. It turned out to be due to measles even though he had measles over a decade earlier. Could that be true?'

Subacute sclerosing panencephalitis (SSPE) is an uncommon complication of measles infection, with an estimated incidence of 1:10000–1:300000. The most unusual feature is the latent period between the original measles infection and the onset of SSPE: on average, this is eight years (9 months–30 years) (Rima and Duprex, 2005).

The disease itself tends to progress over years. It typically presents with behavioural problems and reduced academic performance before progressing to myoclonic seizures, a vegetative state and death (Perry and Halsey, 2004). The highest risk group is children <2 years (Rima and Duprex, 2005). There is no cure although a number of antiviral agents—including ribavirin and interferon (alpha and beta)—have been associated with prolonging life (Titomanlio et al., 2007).

> 'Sounds nasty,' Chrissy says. 'I presume immunisation against measles is the best prevention—is there any risk of encephalitis with the MMR vaccine?'

MMR can cause encephalopathy but this occurs at much lower rates than that due to wild-type virus (National Health and Medical Research Council, 2003).

> Later that day, Chrissy receives a call from a GP: 'I have a one-year-old baby due for her first MMR immunisation this week. The problem is that the mother read that MMR can cause autism and inflammatory bowel disease (IBD) and is worried about getting the child immunised. What should I tell her?'

There is no scientific evidence to demonstrate a causal link between MMR immunisation and IBD or autism (Demicheli et al., 2005; MacIntyre and McIntyre, 2001).

> Later that week, Contact 1 from the original measles investigation calls back. He received MMR vaccine within 72 hours of exposure to Jean-Luc but has another problem.
>
> 'Hi, Doc. I've been well since I got the vaccine but I really am having bad luck when it comes to infections. Yesterday, someone else from public health called me to say that someone at work had been diagnosed with tuberculosis and that I am a contact! Can you believe—first measles, then tuberculosis?'
>
> Chrissy agrees that it is indeed bad luck.

> 'The TB nurse told me I couldn't have the skin test for TB because I only received the MMR vaccine two weeks ago. Is that really true?'

The immunological basis for tuberculin skin testing is the induction of delayed-type hypersensitivity. An accurate result therefore requires a normal immune system. One of the remarkable features of the measles virus is that it induces immunosuppression for some weeks after acute infection. This could interfere with tuberculin skin testing and may cause remission of autoimmune/connective tissue diseases and reactivation of tuberculosis (Ota et al., 2005).

However, the tuberculin skin test should be accurate four weeks after administering MMR (National Health and Medical Research Council, 2003).

References

Asaria, P., MacMahon, E. (2006) Measles in the United Kingdom: can we eradicate it by 2010? *British Medical Journal* 333(7574), 890–95.

Atmar, R.L., Englund, J.A., Hammill, H. (1992) Complications of measles during pregnancy. *Clinical Infectious Diseases* 14(1), 217–26.

Barinaga, J., Skolnik, P. (2006a) *Epidemiology and transmission of measles.* UpToDate. Available from www.utdol.com (Accessed 11 January, 2007)

Barinaga, J., Skolnik, P. (2006b) *Clinical presentation and diagnosis of measles.* UpToDate. Available from www.utdol.com (Accessed 11 January, 2007)

Bass, M. H. (2005) Henry Koplik (1858–1927). *Seminars in Pediatric Infectious Diseases* 16(1), 66–69.

Bellini, W.J., Helfand, R.F. (2003) The challenges and strategies for laboratory diagnosis of measles in an international setting. *Journal of Infectious Diseases* 187(Suppl 1), S283–90.

Brown, D.W., Ramsay, M.E., Richards, A F. et al. (1994) Salivary diagnosis of measles: a study of notified cases in the United Kingdom, 1991–3. *British Medical Journal* 308(6935), 1015–17.

Centers For Disease Control And Prevention (2005) *Vero/SLAM cell line.* Available from www.cdc.gov/ncidod/dvrd/revb/measles/documents/vero_slam.pdf (Accessed 10 January, 2007)

Demicheli, V., Jefferson, T., Rivetti, A. et al. (2005) Vaccines for measles, mumps and rubella in children. *Cochrane Database of Systematic Reviews* (4), CD004407.

Department of Health (2005) *Measles. Immunisation against infectious diseases.* Available from www.dh.gov.uk/assetRoot/04/12/44/88/04124488.pdf (Accessed 8 December, 2006)

Forni, A.L., Schluger, N.W., Roberts, R.B. (1994) Severe measles pneumonitis in adults: evaluation of clinical characteristics and therapy with intravenous ribavirin. *Clinical Infectious Diseases* 19(3), 454–62.

Gershon A.A. (2005) Measles virus (Rubeola). In Mandell, G., Bennett, J., Dolin, R. (eds) *Principles and Practice of Infectious Diseases*. Churchill Livingstone; Philadelphia

Henderson, J.A., Hammond, D.I. (1985) Delayed diagnosis in atypical measles syndrome. *Canadian Medical Association Journal* 133(3), 211–13.

Kaplan, L.J., Daum, R.S., Smaron, M. et al. (1992) Severe measles in immunocompromised patients. *Journal of the American Medical Association* 267(9), 1237–41.

Lambert, S. B., Kelly, H. A., Andrews, R. M. et al. (2000) Enhanced measles surveillance during an interepidemic period in Victoria. *Medical Journal of Australia* 172 (3), 114–18.

Leder, K., Newman, D. (2005) Respiratory infections during air travel. *Internal Medicine Journal* 35(1), 50–55.

MacIntyre, C.R., Mcintyre, P.B. (2001) MMR, autism and inflammatory bowel disease: responding to patient concerns using an evidence-based framework. *Medical Journal of Australia* 175(3), 127–28.

Mangili, A., Gendreau, M. A. (2005) Transmission of infectious diseases during commercial air travel. *Lancet* 365(9463), 989–96.

National Health and Medical Research Council (2003) *Australian Immunisation Handbook. 8th Edition*. National Health and Medical Research Council; Canberra. Available from www9.health.gov.au/immhandbook (Accessed 8 December, 2006)

NSW Health. (2004) *Measles: Response Protocol for NSW Public Health Units*. Available from www.health.nsw.gov.au/infect/pdf/measles.pdf (Accessed 8 December, 2006)

Oliveira, S.A., Siqueira, M.M., Brown, D.W. et al. (1998) Salivary diagnosis of measles for surveillance: a clinic-based study in Niteroi, state of Rio de Janeiro, Brazil. *Transactions of the Royal Society of Tropical Medicine and Hygiene* 92(6), 636–38.

Ota, M.O., Moss, W.J., Griffin, D.E. (2005) Emerging diseases: measles. *Journal of Neurovirology* 11 (5), 447–54.

Perry, R.T., Halsey, N.A. (2004) The clinical significance of measles: a review. *Journal of Infectious Diseases* 189(Suppl 1), S4–16.

Rima, B.K., Duprex, W.P. (2006) Morbilliviruses and human disease. *Journal of Pathology* 208(2), 199–214.

Rima, B.K., Duprex, W.P. (2005) Molecular mechanisms of measles virus persistence. *Virus Research* 111(2), 132–47.

Titomanlio, L., Soyah, N., Guerin, V. et al. (2007) Rituximab in subacute sclerosing panencephalitis. *European Journal of Paediatric Neurology* 11(1), 43–45.

Vukshich Oster, N., Hopean Arpaz, R., Redd, S.B. et al. (2004) International importation of measles virus—United States, 1993–2001. *Journal of Infectious Diseases* 189(Suppl 1), S48–53.

World Health Organization (2006) Progress in reducing global measles deaths: 1999–2004. *Weekly Epidemiological Record* 81(10), 90–94.

World Health Organization (1987) Expanded programme on immunization programme for the prevention of blindness nutrition. *Weekly Epidemiological Record* 62(19), 133–34.

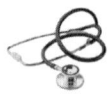

Case 14 Meningococcal disease
Victoria has a sore throat and a rash …

Meningococcal disease at a glance …

- **Agent:** family Neisseriaceae; genus *Neisseria*; species *Neisseria meningitidis* with 13 serogroups of which 5 (A, B, C, W135, Y) cause most disease
- **Geographical distribution:** worldwide; serogroup A is more commonly associated with the developing world and serogroup B is the most common cause of meningococcal disease in the developed world
- **Susceptible groups:** ages <5 years and between 15–24 years; immunocompromise; situations of crowding; smokers
- **Main modes of transmission:** droplet spread
- **Incubation period:** 3–5 days
- **Clinical features:** the most common presentations are meningitis with or without bacteraemia and meningococcal septicaemia
- **Identification:** cultures of blood, cerebrospinal fluid (CSF) (if meningitis suspected), pharynx and skin lesions; polymerase chain reaction (PCR) of blood or CSF; serology
- **Treatment:** IV benzylpenicillin but also third-generation cephalosporins or chloramphenicol
- **Post-exposure prophylaxis:** rifampicin, ciprofloxacin or ceftriaxone
- **Vaccine:** polysaccharide vaccines; conjugate vaccines (either C or quadrivalent)

Main characters

Dr Rachel Beck	general practitioner
Dr Anders Erikson	general practice registrar
Ms Victoria Low	young woman with fevers and a rash
Dr Diego Sanchez	infectious diseases physician
Dr Rick Zane	public health physician
Mr Owen Smith	Diego's intern
Zico	one of Victoria's flatmates

> Dr Rachel Beck is a general practitioner (GP) in a suburban city practice. Her registrar, Dr Anders Erikson, has just seen a young woman, Ms Victoria Low. Victoria dislikes seeing doctors but today is feeling sufficiently unwell that she asked her flatmate to drive her in for an urgent appointment.
>
> Anders says, 'This is a previously well 18-year-old college student who has been unwell for 12 hours. Her friend was watching a documentary on meningococcal disease last night and is convinced that's what Victoria has. She is sick, but I wonder if it is just a viral infection.'
>
> Rachel asks Anders to describe the illness and examination findings.
>
> 'In the early hours of this morning, Victoria woke up shivering. She also had a sore throat. Despite taking paracetamol (acetaminophen), she kept shivering and sweating. She has generalised aches and pains.
>
> 'The examination is unremarkable apart from a tachycardia, fever, a fine maculopapular rash on the trunk and limbs and cool peripheries. The rash blanches with pressure and is not haemorrhagic. Could it be meningococcal disease?'

What is meningococcal disease?

Meningococcal disease—also known as meningococcus—is caused by the bacterium *Neisseria meningitidis*. Its diagnosis in the community can be a real challenge because the early clinical picture is non-specific. Previous studies have found that doctors initially misdiagnosed around 50% of children with meningococcal disease (Riordan et al., 1996). The situation is often much easier for hospital-based physicians because, even in the absence of a clear microbiological diagnosis, patients are usually sick enough by the time they reach hospital to warrant empiric antibiotic therapy.

Thompson et al. (2006) attempted to identify early clinical features that might guide GPs towards a diagnosis of meningococcal disease. They performed a retrospective analysis of children under 16 years old with a diagnosis of microbiologically-confirmed or presumed meningococcal disease. They concluded that 72% of patients with meningococcal disease have one or more of the following eight hours after the onset of illness:

- leg pain
- cold hands and feet
- abnormal skin colour

These are signs associated with sepsis and poor perfusion. However, the study had limitations including the absence of a control group, such as children with proven viral upper respiratory tract infections (URTIs), and the potential for recall bias affecting the timing of symptoms. The absence of a control group is unfortunate because it would have been very helpful to see if there was a significant difference in the frequency of these symptoms in children with viral URTIs. One reply noted that almost 40% of healthy babies under six months of age were reported as having cold peripheries in one study (Gupta and Chadha, 2006). This does not mean, however, that the authors' findings are wrong: they may well be accurate but have to be viewed in the context of the limitations of the study.

With regard to an early diagnosis, Yung and McDonald (2003) note that:

- Meningococcal meningitis should be fairly straightforward to diagnose when it presents with the typical features of an acute meningitis—it is the septicaemia without meningitis that is a diagnostic challenge.
- A rash developing 12–24 hours of illness onset should alert clinicians to the possibility of meningococcal disease.
- The presence of true rigors suggests a serious bacterial illness. A rigor is an episode of uncontrolled and severe shaking related to fever, which the patient cannot voluntarily terminate. It tends to last minutes rather than seconds. A rigor is quite different to the mild 'shivers' or 'chills' which patients may describe.
- Severe muscular pain anywhere (particularly anterior thigh pain and tenderness) can point to bacteraemia; in fact, the authors recommend that any patient with severe generalised myalgias or bilateral anterior thigh pain should be referred to hospital.
- Rapid evolution of an illness within 24 hours suggests the presence of a very serious condition.

- With regard to paediatric patients, the level of anxiety or concern of parents can be a very useful indicator of how sick the child truly is (e.g. 'He normally doesn't look this sick when he has a bit of fever—I am really worried').
- Although it seems obvious, recent contact with another meningococcal case should increase a clinician's suspicion of meningococcal disease.

> Rachel concludes that the features in this girl favouring meningococcal disease or a serious bacterial illness are that:
> - her illness has evolved quickly;
> - she has had true rigors;
> - the rash has appeared within 24 hours of the onset of the illness;
> - she hates coming to see doctors but actually asked her flatmate to bring her here;
> - her generalised myalgias have been severe enough to make her take analgesia;
> - her peripheries are cool.
>
> 'But Victoria's rash isn't the classic haemorrhagic rash of meningococcal disease. How does that fit in to the picture?' Anders asks.

A haemorrhagic rash that does not blanch with pressure is the classic sign of meningococcal disease and one most clinicians would be familiar with. However, meningococcal disease can also cause the blanching maculopapular rash usually associated with viral illnesses. The maculopapular rash of meningococcal disease may evolve into the haemorrhagic rash or it may simply resolve spontaneously. While the presence of a maculopapular rash seems to make the diagnosis of meningococcal disease more difficult, its presence within 24 hours of the onset of illness can help point towards a diagnosis of meningococcal disease. Therefore, Victoria's rash could well be due to meningococcal disease.

> 'I always thought that meningococcal disease meant meningitis,' says Anders. 'But this patient clearly has no features of meningitis. So what's going on?'

CASE 14 MENINGOCOCCAL DISEASE

Lay people in particular—but also some health professionals—assume meningococcus is synonymous with meningitis, presumably because of the similarity of the names. This is actually a very reasonable assumption due the organism, *N. meningitidis*, was probably originally named because of its association with epidemics of meningitis (Apicella, 2005) and the most common syndrome associated with meningococcal disease is, in fact, meningitis (50–85% of cases: Rosenstein et al., 2001; Yung and McDonald, 2003).

Nevertheless, meningococcus can cause a wide variety of clinical syndromes, such as urethritis, endocarditis, meningoencephalitis, otitis media, conjunctivitis, pneumonia, cellulitis, pericarditis, epiglottitis and septic arthritis (Benes et al., 2003; Kennedy et al., 2006; Rosenstein et al., 2001). However, the most commonly encountered syndromes are:

- meningitis with or without bacteraemia
- meningococcaemia/meningococcal septicaemia without meningitis

> Rachel also talks to and examines Victoria. While her flatmate is out of the room, she takes the opportunity to get a sexual history, which gives no further clues. Rachel learns that Victoria smokes 20 cigarettes/day. She concludes that a diagnosis of meningococcal disease must be considered.
> Anders wants to send Victoria to hospital immediately.
> 'Are you sure you haven't forgotten anything?' Rachel asks him.

Victoria should be given a dose of benzylpenicillin immediately, before going to hospital. Many countries have guidelines which recommend that GPs administer a single dose of intramuscular or, ideally, intravenous (IV) benzylpenicillin. This would be consistent with both Australian and UK guidelines (Communicable Diseases Network Australia, 2001; Public Health Laboratory Service et al., 2002).

Interestingly, the data on the benefits of pre-hospital antibiotics for meningococcal disease are conflicting. Some studies have shown that pre-hospital antibiotics reduce mortality and/or complications from meningococcal disease (Cartwright et al., 1992; Strang and Pugh, 1992; Wang et al., 2000). Other, more recent studies have suggested the opposite, namely a higher mortality with pre-hospital antibiotics (Harnden et al., 2006; Norgard et al., 2002; Sorensen et al., 1998). These conflicting results probably represent the limitations of retrospective analyses of data, rather than prospective randomised controlled trials (RCTs). However, a RCT consisting of a control group of people with suspected meningococcal disease from whom antibiotics are deliberately withheld raises major ethical issues.

Other possible explanations for studies showing an adverse outcome with pre-hospital antibiotics are that:

- sicker patients are likely to receive pre-hospital antibiotics but are also more likely to have a poor outcome because they were sicker to begin with
- early antibiotics might cause a more severe inflammatory response through release of breakdown products of the bacteria, although Harnden et al. (2006) found no evidence of this.

Local guidelines on meningococcal disease recommend the immediate administration of parenteral benzylpenicillin in suspected cases before hospitalisation. Rachel gives an IV dose of 1.2 g benzylpenicillin and calls an ambulance to take Victoria to hospital. Anders rings the emergency department (ED) of the local teaching hospital to make them aware of Victoria's impending arrival and, at Victoria's request, calls her family.

In the half-hour it takes Victoria to reach the ED, she deteriorates. On arrival, she is hypotensive and her maculopapular rash is now evolving into the classical haemorrhagic rash of meningococcal disease.

The infectious diseases physician, Dr Diego Sanchez, and the intensive care and emergency specialists are ready for her. While Victoria is being resuscitated, the issue of diagnosis is brought up by the emergency physician.

'Clinically, this woman has meningococcal disease. But since she received antibiotics from the GP, will we be able to isolate the organism?'

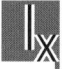

Investigations

A diagnosis of meningococcal disease can be made through a combination of culture, molecular and serological techniques.

Microscopy and culture can be performed on:

Blood The overall sensitivity for blood cultures is probably only about 50% for meningococcal disease; this is dramatically reduced to under 5% if antibiotics have been administered prior to collection (Cartwright et al., 1992; Hoyne and Brown, 1948).

Cerebrospinal fluid (CSF) Overall, for meningococcal meningitis the sensitivities of Gram staining and culture from untreated patients are around 65% and 70%, respectively (Cartwright et al., 1992; Public Health Laboratory Service et al., 2002).

Haemorrhagic skin lesions Gram staining from a needle aspirate of skin lesions can provide microbiological confirmation of meningococcal disease in suspected cases within an hour. The overall sensitivity of culture, Gram staining or both is over 60%, with higher rates in more severe sepsis. Another advantage of punch biopsies or needle aspirates of skin lesions is that both Gram staining and cultures will be positive up to 45 and 13 hours, respectively, after giving antibiotics (van Deuren et al., 1993).

Pharynx The advantage of throat/pharyngeal swabs for meningococcus is that its sensitivity (about 50%) is not greatly affected by prior antibiotic administration. The disadvantage of a positive throat culture, in the absence of identifying meningococcus from another site, is that it may be unclear whether the isolate is simply colonising the pharynx without causing invasive disease (Cartwright et al., 1992).

Polymerase chain reaction (PCR) can also be used. The advantage of molecular tests such as PCR is that they will remain positive for some days after antibiotic therapy has begun. Meningococcal PCR is usually performed on EDTA blood (sensitivity 62–76%, specificity 99–100%) or CSF (sensitivity 89%, specificity 100%) (Munro, 2002).

Serology may be performed. A single elevated titre of IgM based on enzyme immunoassay techniques can diagnose meningococcal disease. This has been shown to be positive on Days 5–18 of illness with a sensitivity of 100% and specificity of at least 93%. A serological diagnosis can also be made on the basis of rising acute and convalescent antibody titres (Munro, 2002; Robertson et al., 2001).

Victoria clinically does not have meningitis so collecting CSF will not help. However, two sets of blood cultures, a throat swab, blood PCR and a skin aspirate are rapidly collected.

One of the emergency registrars asks, 'Is there any point contacting public health without a microbiologically-confirmed diagnosis?'

Meningococcal disease is notifiable in many nations around the world. One purpose of notification is to identify contacts of the index case who may need post-exposure prophylaxis (PEP). This is considered such a serious condition that most health departments would initiate contact screening on suspicion of meningococcal disease alone.

> The on-call public health officer, Dr Rick Zane, is notified about Victoria while she continues to be stabilised in the resuscitation room.
> A call soon arrives from the microbiology lab. The Gram stain of the aspirate from the skin lesion demonstrates Gram negative diplococci: Victoria has meningococcal disease.
> Victoria receives IV ceftriaxone and is soon transported to the intensive care unit, where she is very unwell. The intensivist asks Diego, 'Do you want to give her rhAPC (recombinant human activated protein C)?'

Treatment

APC is an endogenous anticoagulant that prevents thrombosis, promotes fibrinolysis in sepsis and has anti-inflammatory properties (Jahan, 2006). However, in sepsis-induced disseminated intravascular coagulation (DIC), protein C cannot be activated; this is due to sepsis-induced inhibition of thrombomodulin and binding of protein C to other proteins (Belloni et al., 2006) (Bernard et al. 2001). In purpura fulminans due to meningococcal sepsis, the degree of protein C depletion is inversely proportional to mortality. Protein C levels ≤5% correlate with mortality rates over 90% in this setting (Weisel et al., 2002).

For these reasons, the use of recombinant human activated protein C (rhAPC) in sepsis has been studied. In 2001, the PROWESS study demonstrated an absolute risk reduction in death of 6% in those who received rhAPC (number needed to treat 16). Manns et al. (2002) demonstrated that the use of rhAPC in patients with severe sepsis was also a relatively cost-effective measure.

In 2004, guidelines from an international collaboration of intensivists and infectious diseases specialists (Dellinger et al., 2004) recommended that rhAPC be used in patients at high risk of death such as those with:

- an Acute Physiology and Chronic Health Evaluation (APACHE) II score ≥25

- sepsis-induced multi-organ failure
- septic shock
- sepsis-induced acute respiratory distress syndrome (ARDS)

There are absolute and relative contraindications to rhAPC in this setting, which are related to its anticoagulant effects and the risk of serious haemorrhage. rhAPC should not be used in paediatric cases of severe sepsis (Harrison, 2006).

The intensivist calculates Victoria's APACHE score as 26. She has no contraindications to rhAPC. Victoria is given rhAPC after a discussion of its potential benefits and the risk of serious bleeding with her family.
The intensivist now asks Diego about antibiotic choice.

In the developed world, third-generation cephalosporins (ceftriaxone, cefotaxime) and benzylpenicillin are the most commonly used agents. Though reduced susceptibility to penicillin has been reported, IV benzylpenicillin remains the treatment of choice for meningococcal disease (Munro, 2002). The main advantage of third-generation cephalosporins over benzylpenicillin therapy is that the they eradicate nasopharyngeal carriage of meningococcus as well as treating invasive disease; patients on benzylpenicillin therapy require additional medication to eradicate carriage.

IV chloramphenicol is also used but mainly in developing nations. Resistance to chloramphenicol, mediated by an enzyme (chloramphenicol acetyltransferase), has been reported but is rare (Shultz et al., 2003).

A frightening finding from India is the emergence of multiresistant strains of meningococcus, resistant to penicillin, third-generation cephalosporins and ciprofloxacin (Manchanda and Bhalla, 2006).

Victoria is placed on high-dose IV benzylpenicillin and receives a dose of IV ceftriaxone.
The intensivist now asks about duration of antibiotic therapy.

Australian Therapeutic Guidelines recommend 5–7 days of therapy in total (Expert Group, 2006). However, a New Zealand study examined the outcome of patients with meningococcal disease (including meningitis) who received only three days of IV benzylpenicillin and found that no patient relapsed—in fact, three patients received only one or two days of therapy without relapsing (Briggs et al., 2004).

In Africa, epidemics of meningococcal disease lead to already under-resourced medical facilities being overwhelmed. In such a situation, it is not always practical or possible to give multiple dose regimens such as four-hourly benzylpenicillin. The World Health Organization (1998) recommends a single daily intramuscular dose of chloramphenicol or ceftriaxone for one or two days.

Victoria's flatmate and family ask about her chances of survival.

Prognosis

Overall, the mortality rate for meningococcal disease has remained at around 10% (9–12%) (Rosenstein et al., 2001). Septicaemia has mortality rates as high as 40% but meningitis without septicaemia has a much lower mortality rate (1–5%) (Yung and McDonald, 2003).

An hour later, Rick arrives from the public health unit. He wants to commence contact tracing as soon as possible. Victoria is still too sick to provide a history, so he talks to her flatmate.

Victoria's flatmate asks, 'Is this contact tracing exercise to find out who infected Victoria?'

Public health notification and response

The objective of contact tracing for meningococcal disease is to identify contacts of the index case who are most likely to have meningococcal carriage in the nasopharynx. These contacts will receive chemoprophylaxis in a timely fashion to eradicate carriage. Eradicating carriage will not only prevent contacts developing invasive disease but also prevent them infecting others. It may well be that one of these contacts is the one who infected Victoria, but it is near impossible to establish this.

Another important aspect of contact tracing is education. All contacts, even those who do not need chemoprophylaxis, should be provided with information sheets that outline the disease, especially the symptoms and what to do if they become sick (Communicable Diseases Network Australia, 2001).

She says, 'I will certainly help you, Doctor. Please tell me how you decide who is a contact and I will provide you with a list.'

The definition of a contact who requires chemoprophylaxis is not universal and varies between countries. However, according to the Communicable Diseases Network Australia (2001) and the Public Health Laboratory Service et al. (2002), some principles are:

- Give chemoprophylaxis to contacts exposed to the index case in the seven days prior to the index case becoming ill. The average incubation period for meningococcal disease is 3–5 days.
- Give chemoprophylaxis as soon as possible. The risk of invasive disease to contacts is highest in the first week after exposure and, in particular, in the first 48 hours.
- The people at highest risk are household contacts. Although the estimated risk to household contacts of meningococcal disease is only 0.4%, this is still up to 800 times higher than in the general population (Meningococcal Disease Surveillance Group, 1976). Sexual contacts should be regarded as household contacts even if they are not living with the case.

Victoria's has another flatmate, who is bushwalking and cannot be contacted, and a boyfriend, who lives elsewhere. All are listed as contacts. Victoria's flatmate also is worried about other university students.

'What about the students in her tutorials and lectures? Should they be given medication?'

One approach is to only treat the household contacts or household-like contacts (e.g. sexual contacts) if there is only a single sporadic case. However, if a cluster of cases occurs among the tutorial group (i.e. ≥2 cases within four weeks of each other) and these are not otherwise linked through household or sexual contact, chemoprophylaxis should be considered for all students and staff involved (Communicable Diseases Network Australia, 2001).

Rick tells the flatmate that only household and household-like contacts require chemoprophylaxis because Victoria is the only case so far.
'But isn't it just easier to give everyone prophylaxis and put their minds at ease?'

There are good reasons to not indiscriminately provide chemoprophylaxis for meningococcal disease:

- the burden on public health resources
- the development of antibiotic-resistant strains of meningococci
- serious adverse drug reactions
- eradication of non-pathogenic *Neisseria* spp that may provide some level of cross-protective immunity against meningococcus. An example of this is *N. lactamica* in young children (Public Health Laboratory Service et al., 2002).

Rick also asks the flatmate whether Victoria travelled in the week prior to her illness. 'Actually, she returned from a trip to Fiji one week ago today,' she says. 'Will the passengers be okay?'

The US, Australia and Canada all recommend chemoprophylaxis to certain passengers if the index case was in the infectious period while flying (Centers for Disease Control and Prevention, 2001; Communicable Diseases Network Australia, 2001; Public Health Agency of Canada, 2005). Generally, chemoprophylaxis will be offered to those sitting adjacent to the index case in flights ≥8 hours duration. However, the UK does not offer chemoprophylaxis (Public Health Laboratory Service et al., 2002).

The main problem is that on-board transmission of meningococcal disease from an index case has not been definitively documented. O'Connor et al. (2005) provide a compelling argument for in-flight secondary transmission; however, the two cases identified in this study were sitting 12 rows apart with a galley between the two sections, suggesting that limiting chemoprophylaxis to passengers sitting adjacent to the index case may not be sufficient.

Local guidelines recommend chemoprophylaxis to passengers sitting adjacent to the index case. Rick asks one of his infection

CASE 14 MENINGOCOCCAL DISEASE

control officers to get the flight details and manifest. 'What chemoprophylaxis can we offer them?' she asks.

There are three commonly used agents for chemoprophylaxis of meningococcal disease:
- oral rifampicin twice daily for two days
- a single oral dose of ciprofloxacin
- a single intramuscular dose of ceftriaxone

In pregnant women, ceftriaxone is used because of concerns over possible teratogenic effects from ciprofloxacin and rifampicin. While these drugs are very useful in eradicating carriage, it is important to realise that none of them are 100% effective, with ceftriaxone 97% effective, ciprofloxacin 97% and rifampicin 75–95%, respectively (Communicable Diseases Network Australia, 2001; Schwartz, 1991). It is therefore important to reinforce to contacts that they must seek medical attention if they develop an illness compatible with meningococcal disease, despite having received chemoprophylaxis. Another reason to reinforce this message is that resistance to rifampicin and decreased susceptibility to ciprofloxacin have been documented, albeit rarely (Corso et al., 2005; Rainbow et al., 2005).

Limited studies suggest azithromycin may also be an effective alternative in children (Girgis et al., 1998; Gonzalez de Aledo Linos and Garcia Merino, 2000).

Rick prescribes rifampicin chemoprophylaxis. However, he finds out that Victoria's flatmate is taking the oral contraceptive pill. 'Is this a problem?' she asks.

Rifampicin can decrease the efficacy of the oral contraceptive pill, leading to an unexpected pregnancy. This is not a contraindication to rifampicin as long as barrier precautions are observed during and for up to four weeks after taking rifampicin; also contraceptive pill-free intervals should be omitted (Public Health Laboratory Service et al., 2002).

Hospital staff are relieved to find that Victoria rapidly improves over the next four days until she is completely out of danger and is transferred from intensive care to a general ward. On Day 5

> of her admission, the meningococcal reference laboratory sends Rick the final identification of her isolate: C:2a:P 1.5
> One of the infection control officers asks Rick, 'What on earth does that mean?'

The C means that the isolate is serogroup C; serogroups are determined on the basis of the composition of the capsule. 2a refers to the serotype; serotypes are based on the PorB outer membrane protein. P 1.5 refers to the subserotype; subserotypes are based on the PorA outer membrane protein.

This level of detail is not important for acute hospital management of cases. Its importance lies in providing important epidemiological data about epidemics and vaccine development and/or vaccine failure.

> 'Rick, there are 13 serogroups of encapsulated meningococci, aren't there?'

There are 13 serogroups of encapsulated meningococci but only five cause the majority of invasive disease: A, B, C, W135 and Y (Harrison, 2006; National Health and Medical Research Council, 2003):

- Serogroup A is typically associated with epidemic meningococcal disease, particularly in the developing world. The best known outbreaks are the devastating cyclical epidemics in Sub-Saharan Africa every 8–10 years in the dry season.
- Serogroup B is the major cause of sporadic meningococcal cases in the developed world but can also cause epidemics.
- Serogroup C is another strain endemic to many developed countries which can also cause outbreaks of disease.
- Serogroup W135 has only recently become a cause of outbreaks of meningococcal disease.
- Serogroup Y was classically associated with pneumonia and the military. It is now the main cause of invasive meningococcal disease in the elderly in the US.

> Diego has also received a copy of the final identification of the isolate and informs Victoria of the news.

CASE 14 MENINGOCOCCAL DISEASE

> Victoria now asks, 'Doctor, how could I have developed this infection?'

Victoria has three identifiable risk factors, namely that she is a university student and a smoker and it is winter. Booy et al. (2007), Harrison (2006) and the National Health and Medical Research Council (2003) outline other risk factors as including:

- lack of serum bactericidal antibody titres
- lower socioeconomic status
- immunocompromise (asplenia, HIV, terminal complement pathway deficiency, mannose-binding lectin deficiency, diabetes, malignancy)
- men up till the age of about 45 years, after which it is more common in women
- smoking, active or passive (it is contact with smokers rather than smoking itself which is an important risk factor for meningococcal disease. The basis for this may be increased carriage of meningococcus among smokers coupled with increased coughing.)
- concomitant upper respiratory tract infection
- crowding (the military, university students)
- winter and spring (when there are peaks in incidence in temperate regions)
- children <5 years and those aged 15–24 years
- laboratory workers handling meningococcal specimens

> Diego's intern, Owen Smith, listens to this with interest and adds, 'Obviously nasopharyngeal carriage is also a prerequisite for invasive disease with meningococcus, isn't it?'

As with certain serotypes of pneumococcus, some invasive strains of meningococcus are only rarely associated with nasopharyngeal carriage (e.g. ET-37/S-11 strains of group C meningococcus. ET stands for enzyme-type and ST for sequence-type. Strains can be classified according to their ET and ST, which are based on multi-locus enzyme electrophoresis and multi-locus sequence typing). However, other strains of invasive meningococci are well-known to be associated with nasopharyngeal carriage (Harrison, 2006; Kellerman et al., 2002).

> 'Are there vaccines to prevent this?' Owen asks.

Broadly speaking, there are two types of vaccine for meningococcal disease: polysaccharide and conjugate.

Polysaccharide vaccines exclusively induce humoral immunity, which can limit their effectiveness. In school-aged children and adults, the serogroups A and C components of the polysaccharide meningococcal vaccine can induce fairly good efficacy rates of 85–90% but only in the short term. Studies have shown that the polysaccharide vaccine's efficacy declines over time. In addition, the polysaccharide meningococcal vaccines are poorly immunogenic in infants and can cause hyporesponsiveness (a reduced antibody response with a subsequent dose of the polysaccharide vaccine compared to the first dose).

Conjugate vaccines, on the other hand, induce T-cell-dependent immunity, with immunological memory and an enhanced immune response. They can even overcome the hyporesponsiveness induced by the polysaccharide vaccines. The basis for this immune response to the conjugate vaccine is the presence of a protein antigen to which the polysaccharides are covalently conjugated (de Roux and Lode, 2005; Harrison, 2006).

A number of countries have recently introduced immunisation programs using conjugate meningococcal vaccines. They involve either a meningococcal C conjugate vaccine (Australia, UK) or a quadrivalent conjugate vaccine (A, C, W135, Y, introduced in the US in 2005). In the UK, the program has successfully reduced the nasopharyngeal carriage in adolescents by 67% (Maiden et al., 2002). In addition, a herd immunity effect has occurred, with a 67% reduction in meningococcal disease in unvaccinated children (Ramsay et al., 2003).

> 'Is it worth immunising me against the C strain now that I have had the disease?' Victoria asks.

According to UK guidelines, the immune response to the conjugate vaccine may be superior to that induced by natural infection, particularly in children. They therefore recommend giving the conjugate vaccine to all patients <25 years who have recovered from serogroup C infection (Public Health Laboratory Service et al., 2002). It is also possible that index cases will benefit from vaccination because they have an unrecognised immunodeficiency predisposing them to recurrent infections.

Australian guidelines also recommend administration of the conjugate C vaccine to people who have recovered from serogroup C infection (National Health and Medical Research Council, 2003).

> 'What about my friends who are getting the medication? Should they get the vaccine too?'

If the serogroup of meningococcus responsible for the index case's infection is identified, close contacts (i.e. the people who received chemoprophylaxis) should be vaccinated if it is a vaccine-preventable strain. In this case, Victoria's household contacts or household-like contacts should be offered the conjugate C vaccine (Public Health Agency of Canada, 2005; Public Health Laboratory Service et al., 2002).

> Victoria wants to know if her pet bird is safe.

Meningococcus is a purely human pathogen.

> Victoria again looks worried. 'I just remembered that I played basketball a few days before I got sick. All the players shared a bottle of water. Will the other players get it from sharing a drink with me?'

Saliva is inhibitory to meningococcus, so sharing drinks is not a source of transmission (Gordon, 1917; Orr et al,. 2003; Senanayake, 2007).

> Many weeks later, Rick receives a call from the bushwalking flatmate. 'Hi, my name is Zico. I have been bushwalking for the last three weeks. I've been fine but do I need medication?'

Early in the outbreak investigation, Zico would have received chemoprophylaxis for meningococcal disease because he was a household contact. However, nasopharyngeal colonisation is also an immunising process. Most newly colonised contacts would have developed immunity to the colonising strain by two weeks or so; therefore, after that time they would be protected from invasive disease by that strain (Harrison, 2006). This presumably is why the risk of invasive disease in contacts is highest in the first week after exposure and has returned to baseline by four weeks after exposure.

Consequently, many countries do not offer chemoprophylaxis to household or other close contacts if more than two weeks have elapsed since exposure.

> Rick explains to Zico that he doesn't need chemoprophylaxis because he either has developed natural immunity to the colonising strain or was never colonised in the first place.
>
> One of the public health officers is going through their meningococcal surveillance data for this year. He goes to Rick and asks, 'Almost 70% of meningococcal disease here is caused by serogroup B infection. So why haven't we got a vaccination program in place?'

The polysaccharide capsule of serogroup B meningococci cross-reacts with human neurological tissue, resulting in poor immunogenicity. That is why there is no meningococcal vaccine directed at all strains of serogroup B. A New Zealand vaccine is directed against a specific clone of serogroup B, using lipopolysaccharide PorA and PorB, but it is not effective against all B strains (Harrison, 2006).

> Rick explains that there is no vaccine which is effective against all B strains. 'And even if there was a universal B vaccine, the organism would capsular switch to escape the vaccine.'
>
> The public health officer replies, 'What do you mean?'

Capsular switching is a remarkable mechanism whereby meningococci can switch capsular serogroups; for example, a serogroup B strain can become a C strain. This is achieved through horizontal gene transfer, presumably for the purpose of escaping natural or vaccine-induced immunity. Scientists can identify capsular switching through molecular analysis demonstrating genetically similar species despite a different capsular serogroup.

CASE 14 MENINGOCOCCAL DISEASE

One concern was that the impact of the conjugate C vaccine would be dampened by capsular switching but so far this has not been an issue, as demonstrated by data from the UK (Harrison, 2006).

> Soon after, Rick gets a call from a GP.
> 'I saw a 15-year-old boy with conjunctivitis three days ago. I took a swab back then and the lab called me just now to say that they have isolated a pure growth of *N. meningitidis*. What should I do?'

Meningococcus is an uncommon cause of primary conjunctivitis, accounting for <2% of causes in some series. Research has shown that almost 20% of patients with primary meningococcal conjunctivitis (PMC) develop invasive disease and that patients receiving topical, instead of systemic therapy, for PMC are almost 20 times more likely to develop invasive disease. Health authorities therefore recommend intravenous antibiotic therapy for the index case (Communicable Diseases Network Australia, 2001; Poulos et al., 2002; Public Health Agency of Canada, 2005).

Chemoprophylaxis of close contacts with PMC is a controversial issue. Some health authorities recommend it (Communicable Diseases Network Australia, 2001), others do not (Public Health Agency of Canada, 2005) and still others recommend deciding on chemoprophylaxis on a case-by-case basis according to risk, such as the severity of the conjunctivitis and the serogroup involved (Poulos et al., 2002).

References

Apicella, M.A. (2005) *Neisseria meningitidis*. In Mandell, G.E., Bennett, J.E., Dolin, R. (eds) *Principles and Practice of Infectious Diseases*. Churchill Livingstone; Philadelphia

Belloni, G., Ramello, P., Salcuni, M.R. et al. (2006) Purpura fulminans during meningococcal sepsis treated with Drotrecogin alpha. A clinical case. *Minerva Anestesiologica* 72(4), 249–54.

Benes, J., Dzupova, O., Kabelkova, M. et al. (2003) Infective endocarditis due to *Neisseria meningitidis*: two case reports. *Clinical Microbiology and Infection* 9(10), 1062–64.

Bernard, G.R., Vincent J.L., Laterre, P.F. et al. (2001) Efficacy and safety of recombinant human activated protein C for severe sepsis. *New England Journal of Medicine* 344(10), 699–709.

Booy, R., Iskander, M., Viner, R. (2007) Prevention of meningococcal disease. *New England Journal of Medicine* 356(5), 524–25.

Briggs, S., Ellis-Pegler, R., Roberts, S. et al. (2004) Short course intravenous benzylpenicillin treatment of adults with meningococcal disease. *Internal Medicine Journal* 34 (7), 383–87.

Cartwright, K., Reilly, S., White, D. et al. (1992) Early treatment with parenteral penicillin in meningococcal disease. *British Medical Journal* 305(6846), 143–47.

Centers for Disease Control and Prevention (2001) Exposure to patients with meningococcal disease on aircrafts—United States 1999–2001. *Morbidity and Mortality Weekly Report* 50(23), 485–89.

Communicable Diseases Network Australia (2001) *Guidelines for the early clinical and public health management of meningococcal disease in Australia.* Commonwealth Department of Health and Ageing; Canberra. Available from www.health.gov.au/internet/wcms/publishing.nsf/Content/cda-pubs-other-mening.htm (Accessed 4 July, 2007)

Corso, A, Faccone, D, Miranda, M. et al. (2005) Emergence of *Neisseria meningitidis* with decreased susceptibility to ciprofloxacin in Argentina. *Journal of Antimicrobial Chemotherapy* 55(4), 596–97.

Dellinger, R.P., Carlet, J.M., Masur, H. et al. (2004) Surviving sepsis. Campaign guidelines for management of severe sepsis and septic shock. *Critical Care Medicine* 32(3), 858–73.

de Roux, A, Lode, H. (2005) Pneumococcal vaccination. *European Respiratory Journal* 26(6), 982–83.

Expert Group. (2006) *Therapeutic guidelines: antibiotic. Version 13.* Therapeutic Guidelines Limited; Melbourne

Girgis, N., Sultan, Y., Frenck Jr, R.W. et al. (1998) Azithromycin compared with rifampin for eradication of nasopharyngeal colonization by *Neisseria meningitidis*. *Pediatric Infectious Disease Journal* 17(9), 816–19.

Gonzalez de Aledo Linos, A, Garcia Merino, J. (2000) Control of a school outbreak of serogroup B meningococcal disease by chemoprophylaxis with azithromycin and ciprofloxacin. *Anales Espanoles de Pediatria* 53(5), 412–17.

Gordon, M.H. (1917) The inhibitory action of saliva on growth of the meningococcus. Great Britain Medical Research Committee, Special Report Series 3, 106–11.

Gupta, R.K., Chadha, A. (2006) Clinical recognition of meningococcal disease. *Lancet* 367(9520), 1395.

Harnden, A., Ninis, N., Thompson, M. et al. (2006) Parenteral penicillin for children with meningococcal disease before hospital admission: case-control study. *British Medical Journal* 332, 1295–98.

Harrison, L.H. (2006) Prospects for vaccine prevention of meningococcal infection. *Clinical Microbiology Reviews* 19(1), 142–64.

Hoyne, A.L., Brown, R.H. (1948) 727 Meningococcic cases, an analysis. *Annals of Internal Medicine* 28, 248–59.

Jahan, A. (2006) Septic shock in the postoperative patient: three important management decisions. *Cleveland Clinic Journal of Medicine* 73(Suppl 1), S67–71.

Kellerman, S.E., McCombs, K., Ray, M. et al. (2002) Genotype-specific carriage of *Neisseria meningitidis* in Georgia counties with hyper- and hyposporadic rates of meningococcal disease. *Journal of Infectious Diseases* 186(1), 40–48.

Kennedy, K.J., Roy, J., Lamberth, P. (2006) Invasive meningococcal disease presenting as cellulitis. *Medical Journal of Australia* 184(8), 421.

Maiden, M.C., Stuart, J.M., UK Meningococcal Carriage Group (2002) Carriage of serogroup C meningococci 1 year after meningococcal C conjugate polysaccharide vaccination. *Lancet* 359(9320), 1829–31.

Manchanda, V., Bhalla, P. (2006) Emergence of non-ceftriaxone-susceptible *Neisseria meningitidis* in India. *Journal of Clinical Microbiology* 44(11), 4290–91.

Manns, B.J., Lee, H., Doig, C.J. et al. (2002) An economic evaluation of activated protein C treatment for severe sepsis. *New England Journal of Medicine* 347(13), 993–1000.

Meningococcal Disease Surveillance Group (1976) Analysis of endemic meningococcal disease by serogroup and evaluation of chemoprophylaxis. *Journal of Infectious Diseases* 134(2), 201–04.

Munro, R. (2002) Meningococcal disease: treatable but still terrifying. *Internal Medicine Journal* 32(4), 165–69.

National Health and Medical Research Council (2003) *Australian Immunisation Handbook. 8th Edition.* National Health and Medical Research Council; Canberra. Available from www9.health.gov.au/immhandbook (Accessed 19 May, 2006)

Norgard, B. Sorensen, H.T., Jensen, E.S. (2002) Pre-hospital parenteral antibiotic treatment of meningococcal disease and case fatality: a Danish population-based cohort study. *Journal of Infection* 45(3), 144–51.

O'Connor, B.A., Chant, K.G., Binotto, E. et al. (2005) Meningococcal disease— probable transmission during an international flight. *Communicable Diseases Intelligence* 29(3), 312–14.

Orr, H.J., Gray, S.J., Macdonald, M. et al. (2003) Saliva and meningococcal transmission. *Emerging Infectious Diseases* 9(10), 1314–15.

Poulos, R.G., Smedley, E.J., Ferson, M.J. et al. (2002) Refining the public health response to primary meningococcal conjunctivitis. *Communicable Diseases Intelligence* 26(4), 592–95.

Public Health Agency of Canada. (2005) *Guidelines for the prevention and control of meningococcal disease.* Available from www.phac-aspc.gc.ca/publicat/ccdr-rmtc/05vol31/31s1/index.html (Accessed 21 May, 2006)

Public Health Laboratory Service, Public Health Medicine Environmental Group, Scottish Centre for Infection and Environmental Health (2002) Guidelines for public health management of meningococcal disease in the UK. *Communicable Disease and Public Health/PHLS* 5(3), 187–204.

Rainbow, J., Cebelinski, E., Bartkus, J. et al. (2005) Rifampin-resistant meningococcal disease. *Emerging Infectious Diseases* 11(6), 977–79.

Ramsay, M.E., Andrews, N.J., Trotter, C.L. et al. (2003) Herd immunity from meningococcal serogroup C conjugate vaccination in England: database analysis. *British Medical Journal* 326(7385), 365–66.

Riordan, F.A., Thomson, A.P., Sills, J.A. et al. (1996) Who spots the spots? Diagnosis and treatment of early meningococcal disease in children. *British Medical Journal* 313(7067), 1255–56.

Robertson, P.W., Reinbott, P., Duffy, Y. et al. (2001) Confirmation of invasive meningococcal disease by single point estimation of IgM antibody to outer membrane protein of *Neisseria meningitidis*. *Pathology* 33(3), 375–78.

Rosenstein, N.E., Perkins, B.A., Stephens, D.S. et al. (2001) Meningococcal disease. *New England Journal of Medicine* 344(18), 1378–88.

Schwartz, B. (1991) Chemoprophylaxis for bacterial infections: principles of and application to meningococcal infections. *Reviews of Infectious Diseases* 13(Suppl 2), S170–73.

Senanayake, S.N. (2007) Prevention of meningococcal disease. *New England Journal of Medicine* 356(5), 525.

Shultz, T.R., Tapsall, J.W., White, P.A. et al. (2003) Chloramphenicol-resistant *Neisseria meningitidis* containing catP isolated in Australia. *Journal of Antimicrobial Chemotherapy* 52(5), 856–59.

Sorensen, H.T., Nielsen, G.L., Schonheyder, H.C. et al. (1998) Outcome of pre-hospital antibiotic treatment of meningococcal disease. *Journal of Clinical Epidemiology* 51(9), 717–21.

Strang, J.R., Pugh, E.J. (1992) Meningococcal infections: reducing the case fatality rate by giving penicillin before admission to hospital. *British Medical Journal* 305(6846), 141–43.

Thompson, M.J., Ninis, N., Perera, R. et al. (2006) Clinical recognition of meningococcal disease in children and adolescents. *Lancet* 367(9508), 397–403.

Van Deuren, M., van Dijke, B.J., Koopman, R.J. et al. (1993) Rapid diagnosis of acute meningococcal infections by needle aspiration or biopsy of skin lesions. *British Medical Journal* 307(6896), 1229–32.

Wang, V.J., Malley, R., Fleisher, G.R. et al. (2000) Antibiotic treatment of children with unsuspected meningococcal disease. *Archives of Pediatrics & Adolescent Medicine* 154(6), 556–60.

Weisel, G., Joyce, D., Gudmundsdottir, A. et al. (2002) Human recombinant activated protein C in meningococcal sepsis. *Chest* 121(1), 292–95.

World Health Organization (1998) *Control of epidemic meningococcal disease. WHO practical guidelines. 2nd edition.* World Health Organization; Geneva. Available from www.who.int/csr/resources/publications/meningitis/WHO_EMC_BAC_98_3_EN/en/ (Accessed 17 May, 2006)

Yung, A.P., McDonald, M.I. (2003) Early clinical clues to meningococcaemia. *Medical Journal of Australia* 178(3), 134–37.

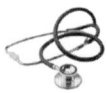

Case 15 Mumps
Kevin has a stiff neck …

Mumps at a glance …

- **Agents:** family Paramyxoviridae; genus *Rubulavirus*; species mumps virus
- **Geographical distribution:** worldwide
- **Main modes of transmission:** droplet spread; fomites; direct contact with saliva
- **Incubation period:** 16–18 days (12–25)
- **Infectious period:** from 2 days before symptom onset to 9 days after symptom onset
- **Clinical features:** typically, a febrile prodrome followed by parotitis but extra-salivary manifestations such as meningitis and orchitis can occur in the absence of parotitis
- **Identification:** serology (IgM and baseline and convalescent IgG); salivary IgM or reverse transcriptase polymerase chain reaction (RT-PCR); urinary culture or RT-PCR
- **Treatment:** supportive
- **Post-exposure prophylaxis:** nil
- **Vaccines:** live attenuated vaccine with 2 doses at least 28 days apart needed for maximal efficacy

Main characters

Dr Frank Byrd	infectious diseases registrar
Mr Kevin Peat	patient with meningitis
Professor Rosemary Ng	infectious diseases specialist
Ms Susan Finch	senior infectious diseases nurse at a public health unit

Dr Frank Byrd is the on-call infectious diseases registrar for a large teaching hospital. He has been asked by a resident medical officer in the emergency department to review a 26-year-old man with what sounds like viral meningitis.

The patient is Mr Kevin Peat. Two days ago, he developed a headache and neck stiffness which gradually worsened. He hasn't experienced fevers or chills but has been nauseated and describes photophobia. His physical examination is unremarkable, apart from the photophobia. Kevin has no risk factors for sexually transmitted infections with bloodborne viruses. He has never travelled outside the country. He works in the kitchen at a fast-food store. People at work have had the odd cough and cold in the last few weeks, but nothing more than usual.

While Frank talks to the patient, some pathology tests become available.

His lumbar puncture shows:

- clear, colourless fluid
- normal opening pressure
- cell count: 0 red blood cells, 200 white cells/mm^3 (95% lymphocytes)
- cerebrospinal fluid (CSF)/serum glucose ratio: 45%
- protein: 700 g/L (normal range 150–450 g/L)

His blood tests show:

- mild peripheral neutrophilia
- mildly elevated C-reactive protein (CRP) of 16 mg/L (normal range <10 mg/L)

'Is it viral meningitis?' the resident asks.

Kevin's clear colourless CSF with a mildly elevated protein and lymphocytic pleocytosis is consistent with viral meningitis. Even the slightly reduced

CASE 15 MUMPS

CSF/serum glucose ratio can still occur in viral infections, although it is typically associated with bacterial infections. The blood tests also are in keeping with a viral illness.

> Frank speaks to his consultant, Professor Rosemary Ng, who agrees that viral meningitis is the most likely scenario. They admit Kevin for observation and symptomatic relief. Despite the unremarkable history, Frank gets Kevin's consent for an HIV test. In addition, he orders serology for Epstein-Barr virus and cytomegalovirus and polymerase chain reaction (PCR) of CSF for enterovirus, varicella zoster and herpes simplex (the laboratory has a multiplex kit which can test the CSF for all these viruses at once).
>
> In 48 hours, Kevin is feeling much better with only minimal analgesia. The serological tests and multiplex PCR of CSF are all negative. Kevin is discharged with a diagnosis of viral meningitis.
>
> Just over two weeks later, Frank develops a mild headache, low-grade fevers and generalised myalgias. After 24 hours, he develops pain and swelling in his face bilaterally. Clinically he has bilateral parotitis.
>
> He calls up his boss and declares, 'Oh darn, I've got mumps!'

What is mumps?

Mumps is a purely human infection due to a single-stranded RNA virus belonging to the genus *Rubulavirus* and the family Paramyxoviridae. In susceptible populations, it is usually a disease of children with a peak incidence at 5–9 years of age, although adolescents and adults can be affected (National Health and Medical Research Council, 2003). It has an excellent prognosis (Falk et al., 1989).

It is an old infection, having been described by Hippocrates as early as the fifth century BC. There is one distinct mumps serotype, which has been further classified into genotypes A–J (and possibly K) (Muhlemann, 2004).

Its name may be related to an old word (mump) which meant grimace.

> 'Are you right to be so confident about the diagnosis?' Rosemary asks.

Case definitions vary in their details but are broadly similar (NSW Health, 2004). The Centers for Disease Control and Prevention (CDC, 2006a) use the following case definitions:

Probable case A case meeting the clinical case definition but where virologic or serologic test results are unavailable or unhelpful and where there is no epidemiological link to a probable or confirmed case. The clinical case definition is the acute onset of tender unilateral or bilateral parotid or other salivary gland swelling of ≥2 days duration with no other obvious cause.

Confirmed case A case that is laboratory-confirmed OR meets the clinical case definition and is epidemiologically linked to a confirmed or probable case.

A febrile prodrome with headache may or may not occur in mumps but its presence certainly supports a diagnosis.

In temperate climates, peak incidence is usually in winter and spring; in tropical climates, the incidence is fairly uniform throughout the year (World Health Organization, 2007).

Frank is puzzled. 'But what else causes parotid swelling other than mumps?'

Differential diagnoses

Although the best known cause of bilateral parotitis is mumps, there is a surprisingly broad list of differential diagnoses for parotitis (Gupta et al., 2005; Mandel and Surattanont, 2002) including:

- viral infection (influenza A, parainfluenza, adenovirus, coxsackie, Epstein-Barr virus, HIV)
- bacterial infection
- salivary calculi
- autoimmune disease (sarcoidosis, Sjögren's syndrome, Wegener's granulomatosis)
- neoplasia (Warthin's tumour, mucosal-associated lymphoid tissue lymphoma)
- iatrogenic/self-induced disease (iodide contrast, radioactive iodine, ingestion of starch or thiazide diuretics)
- polycystic parotid disease
- Kimura disease

> Frank wants to confirm that he has mumps but believes it is too early to demonstrate an IgM response in serum. 'Isn't that right?'

 Investigations

By the onset of the clinical illness, nearly every case of mumps should have positive serum IgM. However, false-negative tests can occur, with sensitivities being as low as 24–51% depending on the assay used (Krause et al., 2007). False-positive IgM tests can also occur due to parainfluenza viruses (Campos-Outcalt, 2006).

Additionally, positive mumps IgM or IgG seroconversion titres can be elevated by the mumps vaccine, so serology can be difficult to interpret in the context of recent immunisation (NSW, 2004). Conversely, previous immunisation can also lead to mumps cases having undetectable IgM, an absence of an IgG seroconversion or the presence of a single high IgG titre (Campos-Outcalt, 2006).

> 'Apart from a serum IgM, how else can I confirm my diagnosis?'

I There are a number of methods, outlined in Table 15.1.

Table 15.1 Tests for mumps

Test	Comment
Four-fold rise in serum IgG in the two weeks between an acute and convalescent serum	
Salivary IgM	Sensitivity 75% in the first week; thereafter, 100% Specificity 98%
Salivary reverse transcriptase polymerase chain reaction (RT-PCR)	Can be positive when salivary IgM is negative
Urinary RT-PCR for mumps virus	Positive within two weeks of the onset of symptoms
Urinary culture for mumps virus	Positive within two weeks of the onset of symptoms

SOURCE Gupta et al., 2005

> 'Would a peripheral blood count and film be helpful?'

A peripheral blood count and film would probably not be helpful because they are usually normal. Leukopenia with a relative lymphocytosis can occur. A left shift with leukocytosis may occur with the extra-salivary manifestations of mumps. Serum amylase may be elevated for 2–3 weeks due to Frank's parotitis but this is not specific for mumps parotitis (Litman and Baum, 2005).

> Frank decides to get a salivary and serum IgM taken for mumps. He is reluctant to go to the blood collection centre, concerned that he might infect others. He asks Rosemary for her opinion.

Isolation measures

Mumps is a highly contagious infection for susceptible populations, with a reproductive number (R_0) of 10–12 (reproductive number is the number of secondary cases arising from a single case in a susceptible population). Such populations have an incidence of 100–1000/100 000/year with epidemic peaks every 2–5 years (World Health Organization, 2007). It is transmitted through droplet spread, direct contact or fomites (Singh et al., 2006). The infectious period is quite long, from two days before the onset of symptoms to nine days after symptom onset (Campos-Outcalt, 2006), so Frank is definitely still infectious to susceptible people.

Frank should let the pathology collection centre know that he is coming in and that he may have mumps so they can put respiratory and contact precautions in place. Alternatively, he can arrange for a blood collector with known immunity to mumps to visit him at home.

> It is decided that the easiest option is for a blood collector with known immunity to mumps to come to Frank's place and take his blood, thereby eliminating the risk of infecting others. In the meantime, Frank recalls that even probable cases of mumps need to be notified to the public health unit (PHU). He therefore he calls Ms Sue Finch, the head infectious diseases nurse there.

CASE 15 MUMPS

> Frank tells Sue about his predicament, in particular stating that he isn't sure who infected him. 'I can't recall contact with anyone over the last three weeks with parotitis. So how could I have been infected?'

Not all cases of mumps have parotitis. Although 70–90% of mumps cases have parotitis, with up to 25% having unilateral involvement only, 10–30% of cases do not have parotitis. Also, 30% of mumps infections are asymptomatic (Gupta et al., 2005; Singh et al., 2006).

> Sue tries to get Frank to think about possible sources of infection during the incubation period, which is normally 16–18 days but can be anywhere from 12 to 25 days (Campos-Outcalt, 2006).
> His social and household contacts have all been well. Over the last few weeks most of his patients have had cellulitis, osteomyelitis or diarrhoea—he has seen very few people with respiratory illnesses. He does mention Kevin, who had aseptic meningitis.
> Sue gets excited, 'Maybe Kevin had mumps.'
> Frank is surprised. 'Does mumps cause central nervous system disease?'

The central nervous system (CNS) manifestations of mumps include (Bajaj et al., 2001; Duncan et al., 1990; Gupta et al., 2005; Singh et al., 2006; Unal et al., 2005):

- CSF pleocytosis in the absence of clinical features of meningitis (this occurs in half of all mumps cases)
- aseptic meningitis occurring 3–4 days after the parotitis begins (10–15% of all cases of mumps)
- seizures, which occur in 20–30% of children with neurological symptoms during their mumps illness
- encephalitis, which tends to be a mild, self-limiting illness without focal neurological deficits (however, 1/6 000 cases develop a far more serious condition, post-infectious immune-mediated encephalomyelitis, which is associated with focal neurological deficits and case fatality rates of 10%)
- Guillain-Barré syndrome (very uncommon)

According to Gupta et al. (2005), in cases of aseptic meningitis the CSF usually shows:

- normal opening pressure
- lymphocytic pleocytosis of around 250 cells/mm^3
- elevated protein in 60–70%
- reduced CSF/serum glucose ratio (<50% expected value) in up to 25% of cases

Kevin's LP was consistent with mumps, although the results are too non-specific to distinguish between mumps or another virus. Furthermore, up to 50% of patients with meningitis from mumps do not have parotitis (Singh et al., 2006).

> It's a long shot, but Kevin may be the source of Frank's infection. Frank knows that all CSF specimens are stored in the laboratory for one year, so his sample is still available for testing. They contact Kevin and get his permission to test his CSF for mumps. Kevin agrees. In fact, he would love to know the diagnosis.
> 'What tests should I order?' Frank asks Rosemary.

The following tests are useful for diagnosing mumps meningitis (Forsberg et al., 1986; Gupta et al., 2005; Poggio et al., 2000; Ukkonen et al., 1981):

- RT-PCR, with 96% sensitivity (may be positive for up to two years later)
- CSF IgM, with 50% sensitivity (may be positive for up to one year later)
- CSF IgG, with 33% sensitivity (may be positive for up to one year later)

> 'As you can tell, Rosemary, I haven't seen many cases of mumps. Can any other organs be affected, besides the salivary glands and CNS?'

Despite having a relatively benign course with a mortality of only 1/10 000 (World Health Organization, 2007), mumps can infect a number of organs outside the salivary glands and CSF. Syndromes include (Gupta et al., 2005; Singh et al., 2006):

- epididymo-orchitis (30% of cases in post-pubertal men)
- oophoritis (5% of cases in post-pubertal young women) which rarely can lead to secondary oligomenorrhoea, reduced fertility and premature menopause (Morrison et al., 1975; Taparelli et al., 1988)
- pancreatitis (5% of cases; a link with diabetes is uncertain)
- permanent unilateral deafness (1/15 000 cases)
- migratory polyarthritis, typically occurring 10–14 days after onset of parotitis and resolving within five weeks (an association with adult Still's disease has been reported: Caranasos and Felker, 1967; Gordon and Lauter, 1982)
- thyroiditis, mastitis, myocarditis hepatitis, interstitial nephritis and autoimmune thrombocytopenic purpura (Unal. S et al., 2005)

With regard to the parotitis itself, the swelling can result in speech and mastication difficulties and even cause trismus (Singh et al., 2006). The intra-oral entry point to the duct of the parotid gland (Stensen's duct at the level of the upper second molar) is often swollen and erythematous during the parotitis (Gupta et al., 2005). In 10% of cases, other salivary glands may be involved in addition to the parotid glands (Litman and Baum, 2005). Long-term complications from the parotitis are uncommon (it usually resolves within a week) but sialectasia with recurrent bouts of inflammation may occur (Singh et al., 2006).

> Within 48 hours Frank's serum and salivary IgM both return positive, confirming that he has mumps. Three days later, the lab calls to confirm that Kevin's CSF was RT-PCR and IgM negative.
> Frank calls Susan at the PHU. 'Do you have to start contact tracing in the hospital? Is there any post-exposure prophylaxis (PEP) to give?'

Public health notification and response

Given its relatively benign course, contact tracing is not usually recommended in mumps (NSW Health, 2004). There is no role for immunoglobulin or vaccination as PEP during a mumps outbreak (National Health and Medical Research Council, 2003).

The CDC recommends primary prophylaxis by screening and identifying susceptible staff, who should then be offered immunisation with one or two doses of vaccine. During a healthcare-related outbreak, vaccination can be offered to staff who are unlikely to be immune; however, this may be impractical or inefficient (CDC, 2006b). The difficulties of using vaccine as PEP in this setting are that:

- By the time that the vaccine generates enough immunity, the contact may already have developed an infection (i.e. it doesn't work).
- The recent use of mumps vaccine makes serology difficult to interpret because the vaccine alone can cause a serum IgM response or IgG seroconversion (NSW Health, 2004). Consequently, it can be difficult to identify subclinical cases or mildly symptomatic cases without parotitis.

> Frank remains at home till he is no longer contagious. When Rosemary calls him to see how he is feeling, Frank sounds quite anxious.
> 'Professor, I can't stop thinking about mumps orchitis—I'm too young to be sterile!'

Prognosis

Frank has been unwell for over a week now. Nearly 70% of cases of epididymo-orchitis occur during the first week of illness with another 25% occurring the second week, so his risk of developing orchitis is much lower at this stage of the illness. Sterility itself is rare but testicular atrophy occurs in 30–50% of cases and oligospermia or asthenospermia in 7–13% of cases (Singh et al., 2006).

> 'How does the virus get to the testicles?'

After entering the host through the upper respiratory tract, the virus multiplies in the respiratory lymphoid and reticuloendothelial system. A viraemia then ensues for 7–10 days, which can result in dissemination to various parts of the body (Singh et al., 2006). Histologically, the orchitis from mumps is almost identical to the parotitis, which is dominated by diffuse interstitial oedema and a predominantly mononuclear serofibrinous exudate. Unlike the parotitis, though, the orchitis may also demonstrate a relative increase in polymorphonuclear cells, interstitial haemorrhage and local infarction due to the effect of oedema on the vascular supply (Litman and Baum, 2005).

> 'Rosemary, my sister wants to see me. But she's pregnant. I've asked her to check her mumps serology before she visits. If it comes back negative, is it safe for her to come?'

Mumps may increase the risk of embryonic and fetal death; therefore, his sister should not visit if there is any uncertainty about her immunity. There appears to be no association between mumps and congenital deformities (Ornoy and Tenenbaum, 2006).

> 'I believe that there isn't any specific therapy for this and I just have to wait till the illness resolves. Is that right?'

Treatment

Treatment of mumps is purely supportive. Use of local measures, such as heat or cold packs, and a combination of antipyretics and analgesics is generally recommended (Litman and Baum, 2005). There are conflicting data on the subject of alpha-interferon-2B in preventing testicular atrophy in mumps orchitis (Erpenbach, 1991; Yeniyol et al., 2000).

> 'Rosemary, how did I get mumps? I am sure I was immunised as a child.'

If Frank had definitely been immunised, the possibilities are primary vaccine failure (failure to seroconvert after primary immunisation) or secondary vaccine failure (immunogenicity fails despite earlier seroconversion).

Primary vaccine failure appears to be more likely in those who received only one dose of mumps vaccine rather than two (Harling et al., 2005). Seroconversion rates of around 90% are achieved after a single dose (World Health Organization, 2007) with the second dose resulting in around 95% seroconversion with a slower decline in antibody titres over time compared to those vaccinated only once (Davidkin et al., 1995). These immunogenicity data are in conflict with calculation of vaccine efficacy during observational studies of mumps outbreaks, where the efficacy rates are consistently below 80% (Harling et al., 2005). Other factors that may contribute to primary vaccine failure include damaged vaccine due to improper storage and poor administration technique.

The use of avidity testing of IgG antibodies has been important in demonstrating secondary vaccine failure, where immunity from previous mumps immunisation wanes with time, resulting in populations becoming susceptible to mumps again (Campos-Outcalt, 2006; Cohen et al., 2007; Narita et al., 1998; Vandermeulen et al., 2004).

> 'Would I be more susceptible to infection if the vaccine genotype that I received as a child was different to the infecting genotype?'

There is cross-neutralisation between genotypes, which means that the antibodies generated by one genotype should provide protection against another genotype. However, reports have emerged where this cross-neutralisation has failed (Muhlemann, 2004; Watson-Creed et al., 2006).

> 'Do most countries use a two-dose vaccine regimen?'

Over 80% of the 110 countries that have a mumps immunisation program use a two-dose schedule. The first dose is given at 12–18 months, after which an interval of at least 28 days should elapse before the second dose is given (World Health Organization, 2007).

> Frank soon recovers completely and returns to work. Meanwhile, Susan receives a call from a GP.
> 'Hello. I have a patient with advanced HIV who is not immune to mumps. He is requesting a mumps vaccination. Is it okay?'

Mumps vaccine consists of a live attenuated virus, so it is not recommended in advanced immunosuppression and pregnancy (World Health Organization, 2007). Interestingly, there is little information on mumps infection and vaccine efficacy in the immunocompromised (Gupta et al., 2005). A killed vaccine would have been safe but these were abandoned a long time ago due to poor efficacy (World Health Organization, 2007).

Otherwise, it is a safe vaccine. The more common reactions are local reactions at the injection site, fever and parotitis. Less commonly, however, the following reactions occur (World Health Organization, 2007):

- orchitis
- sensorineural deafness
- aseptic meningitis. This usually occurs 2–3 weeks after immunisation at varying frequencies of 1/400–1/500000. Some mumps genotypes (C, D, H, J), including the vaccine strain Urabe Am9 (genotype B), are associated with enhanced neurovirulence (Muhlemann, 2004).

References

Bajaj, N.P., Rose, P., Clifford-Jones, R. et al. (2001). Acute transverse myelitis and Guillain-Barré overlap syndrome with serological evidence for mumps viraemia. *Acta Neurologica Scandinavica* 104(4), 239–42.

CDC (Centers for Disease Control and Prevention) (2006a) Mumps case definition and case classification. In Centers for Disease Control and Prevention *National Immunization Program*. Centers for Disease Control and Prevention; Atlanta. Available from www.cdc.gov/nip/diseases/mumps/case-def.htm (Accessed 20 January, 2007)

CDC (Centers for Disease Control and Prevention) (2006b) Notice to readers: updated recommendations of the Advisory Committee on Immunization Practices (ACIP) for the control and elimination of mumps. *Morbidity and Mortality Weekly Report* 55(22), 629–30.

Campos-Outcalt, D. (2006) Mumps epidemic in 2006: are you prepared to detect and prevent it? *Journal of Family Practice* 55(22), 500–02.

Caranasos, G.J, Felker, J.R. (1967) Mumps arthritis. *Archives of Internal Medicine* 119(4), 394–98.

Cohen, C., White, J. M., Savage, E. J. et al. (2007) Vaccine effectiveness estimates, 2004–2005 mumps outbreak, England. *Emerging Infectious Diseases* 13(1), 12–17.

Davidkin, I., Valle, M., Julkunen, I. (1995) Persistence of anti-mumps virus antibodies after a two-dose MMR vaccination. A nine-year follow up. *Vaccine* 13(16), 1617–22

Duncan, S., Will, R.G., Catnach, J. (1990) Mumps and Guillan-Barré syndrome. *Journal of Neurology, Neurosurgery, and Psychiatry* 53(8), 709.

Erpenbach, K.H. (1991) Systemic treatment with interferon-alpha 2B: an effective method to prevent sterility after bilateral mumps orchitis. *Journal of Urology* 146(1), 54–56.

Falk, W. A., Buchan, K., Dow, M. et al. (1989) The epidemiology of mumps in southern Alberta 1980–1982. *American Journal of Epidemiology* 130(4), 736–49.

Forsberg, P., Fryden, A., Link, H. et al. (1986) Viral IgM and IgG antibody synthesis within the central nervous system in mumps meningitis. *Acta Neurologica Scandinavica* 73(4), 374–80.

Gordon, S.C., Lauter, C.B. (1982) Mumps arthritis: unusual presentation as adult Still's disease. *Annals of Internal Medicine* 97(1), 45–47.

Gupta, R. K., Best, J., Macmahon, E. (2005) Mumps and the UK epidemic 2005. *British Medical Journal* 330(7500), 1132–35.

Harling, R., White, J.M., Ramsay, M.E. et al. (2005) The effectiveness of the mumps component of the MMR vaccine: a case control study. *Vaccine* 23(31), 4070–74.

Krause, C.H., Molyneaux, P.J., Ho-Yen, D.O. et al. (2007) Comparison of mumps-IgM ELISAs in acute infection. *Journal of Clinical Virology* 38(2), 153–56.

Litman, N., Baum, S.G. (2005) Mumps virus. In Mandell, G.L., Bennett, J.E., Dolin, R. (eds) *Principles and Practice of Infectious Diseases*. Churchill Livingstone; Philadelphia.

Mandel, L., Surattanont, F. (2002) Bilateral parotid swelling: a review. *Oral Surgery, Oral Medicine, Oral Pathology, Oral Radiology and Endodontics* 93(3), 221–37.

Morrison, J.C., Givens, J.R., Wiser, W.L. et al. (1975) Mumps oophoritis: a cause of premature menopause. *Fertility and Sterility* 26(7), 655–59.

Muhlemann, K. (2004) The molecular epidemiology of mumps virus. *Infection, Genetics and Evolution* 4(3), 215–19.

Narita, M., Matsuzono, Y., Takekoshi, Y. et al. (1998) Analysis of mumps vaccine failure by means of avidity testing for mumps virus-specific immunoglobulin G. *Clinical and Diagnostic Laboratory Immunology* 5(6), 799–803.

National Health and Medical Research Centre (2003) *Australian Immunisation Handbook. 8th Edition*. National Health and Medical Research Centre; Canberra. Available from www9.health.gov.au/immhandbook (Accessed 12 February, 2007)

NSW Health (2004) *Mumps Response Protocol for NSW Public Health Units*. Available from www.health.nsw.gov.au/infect/pdf/mumps.pdf (Accessed 12 February, 2007)

Ornoy, A., Tenenbaum, A. (2006) Pregnancy outcome following infections by coxsackie, echo, measles, mumps, hepatitis, polio and encephalitis viruses. *Reproductive Toxicology* 21(4), 446–57.

Poggio, G.P., Rodriguez, C., Cisterna, D. et al. (2000) Nested PCR for rapid detection of mumps virus in cerebrospinal fluid from patients with neurological diseases. *Journal of Clinical Microbiology* 38(1), 274–7–8.

Singh, R., Mostafid, H., Hindley, R. G. (2006) Measles, mumps and rubella—the urologist's perspective. *International Journal of Clinical Practice* 60(3), 335–39.

Taparelli, F., Squadrini, F., De Rienzo, B. et al. (1988) Isolation of mumps virus from vaginal secretions in association with oophoritis. *Journal of Infection* 17(3), 255–58.

Ukkonen, P., Granstrom, M.L., Rasanen, J. et al. (1981) Local production of mumps IgG and IgM antibodies in the cerebrospinal fluid of meningitis patients. *Journal of Medical Virology* 8(4), 257–65.

Unal, A., Emre, U., Atasoy, H.T. et al. (2005) Encephalomyelitis following mumps. *Spinal Cord* 43(7), 441–44.

Unal, S., Yetgin, S., Kara, A. et al. (2005) Autoimmune thrombocytopenic purpura after mumps infection. *Turkish Journal of Pediatrics* 47(3), 270–71.

Vandermeulen, C., Roelants, M., Vermoere, M. et al. (2004) Outbreak of mumps in a vaccinated child population: a question of vaccine failure? *Vaccine* 22(21–22), 2713–16.

Watson-Creed, G., Saunders, A., Scott, J. et al. (2006) Two successive outbreaks of mumps in Nova Scotia among vaccinated adolescents and young adults. *Canadian Medical Association Journal* 175(5), 483–88.

World Health Organization (2007) Mumps virus vaccines. *Weekly Epidemiological Record* 82(7), 51–60.

Yeniyol, C.O., Sorguc, S., Minareci, S. et al. (2000) Role of interferon-alpha-2B in prevention of testicular atrophy with unilateral mumps orchitis. *Urology* 55(6), 931–33.

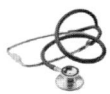

Case 16 Pertussis
Hilary has been coughing for weeks …

Pertussis at a glance …

- **Agent:** family Alcaligenaceae; genus *Bordetella*; species *Bordetella pertussis* (small minority of infections due to *B. parapertussis*)
- **Geographical distribution:** worldwide; although the burden of disease is in the developing world, pertussis in the developed world is an important emerging problem
- **Susceptible groups:** all age groups but infants under 6 months experience the most severe infections
- **Main modes of transmission:** droplet spread
- **Incubation period:** 7–10 days (5–21)
- **Infectious period:** untreated infants can be infectious for the first 6 weeks after the onset of cough; other untreated children, adolescents and adults are considered infectious for the first 21 days after onset of the cough; treated cases are no longer considered infectious after completing 5 days of therapy
- **Clinical features:** classically a chronic cough illness characterised by whooping and/or paroxysms of coughing and/or post-tussive vomiting
- **Identification:** culture of nasopharyngeal specimens; polymerase chain reaction (PCR) of nasopharyngeal or throat specimens; serology
- **Treatment:** standard therapy is with macrolides (erythromycin or clarithromycin for 7 days or azithromycin for 5 days); azithromycin may be preferable in infants <1 month to avoid infantile hypertrophic pyloric stenosis; people allergic to macrolides can have 14 days of trimethoprim/sulfamethoxazole
- **Post-exposure prophylaxis:** same antimicrobial agents as for treatment
- **Vaccines:** acellular or whole cell vaccines for pertussis are available in combination with other infection antigens (e.g. diphtheria/tetanus/pertussis vaccines)

CASE 16 PERTUSSIS

Main characters

Dr Lin Chan	general practitioner
Ms Hilary Benfold	woman with a chronic cough
Mr Tony Carter	medical student
Dr Kevin Minto	public health physician
Anne and Sarah	Hilary's sisters
Dr Kathleen Bell	public health registrar

> Dr Lin Chan is a general practitioner (GP) in an inner city practice in a major city. Her first patient is Ms Hilary Benfold, a 39-year-old woman who has been attending the practice for years. She is a fit and healthy and generally only comes in for sporting injuries or when her children are sick.
>
> Hilary tells Lin that she has been coughing for almost three weeks now and has aches and pains from all the coughing. It all started with a runny nose and teary eyes for a few days but no fevers; about a week later, these symptoms improved but a dry cough started.
>
> In her head, Lin runs through the causes of a chronic cough.

Chronic cough (cough lasting more than eight weeks) can be due to a wide variety of infective and non-infective conditions. Common non-infective causes include postnasal drip, gastro-oesophageal reflux disease and medications such as angiotensin converting enzyme inhibitors. Infective causes include *Bordetella pertussis*, other *Bordetella* spp, *Mycoplasma pneumoniae*, *Chlamydia pneumoniae*, adenovirus and other respiratory viruses (Mattoo and Cherry, 2005).

> Mr Tony Carter is a medical student doing a general practice rotation and sitting in on the consultation. He immediately wonders aloud, 'Could this be pertussis?'

What is pertussis?

Pertussis, also known as whooping cough, is an acute upper respiratory tract infection usually caused by *Bordetella pertussis*, a Gram negative bacterium.

The cough is the best known feature of this infection; in fact, 'pertussis' (coined by Sydenham in 1679) means a violent or strong cough. Other terms for pertussis also refer to the characteristic cough, such as 'tosse canina' (Italian for dog's bark), 'tos ferina' (Spanish for ferocious cough) and in Chinese the 'cough of a hundred days'.

'Bordetella' was named after Jules Bordet who, along with Gengou in 1906, first identified the organism now known as *B. pertussis*.

> Hilary says, 'But isn't pertussis something that only children get?'

Pertussis used to be regarded as a disease of young children. US data show that in the pre-vaccine era (before the 1940s), only 7% of reported cases of pertussis occurred in children >10 years but in 1997–2000 that proportion increased to over 50% (Cherry, 2005). This increased reporting by doctors may be partly attributable to an increased awareness of the infection in this age group, as well as the availability of more diagnostic tools. However, it is unlikely to account for the bulk of the increase. Increasing rates of pertussis amongst adolescents and adults has also been noted in a number of other countries (World Health Organization, 2005).

But it is important to understand that while adults may be the major reservoir of pertussis in vaccinating countries, it is the infected children (especially infants) who are prone to the greatest disease severity and highest mortality.

> Hilary asks (after a splutter of coughing), 'Okay, even if adults can get it, isn't it rare?'

The World Health Organization (WHO) reported that 17.6 million cases of pertussis occurred globally in 2003 and 90% were from developing countries (WHO, 2005). Nevertheless, even developed nations have notification rates for pertussis that are not insignificant, for example, about 40/100 000/year in Australia and 10–35/100 000/year in Canada over the last few years (Department of Health and Ageing, 2006; Galanis et al., 2006). In the US, pertussis is the only disease with recommended universal childhood vaccination that has had an increase in reported cases; also in the US, the number of reported cases has increased six-fold since 1980 (Hewlett and Edwards, 2005; Tiwari et al,. 2005).

The typical pattern has been one of a steady rate of cases interrupted by an epidemic every four years or so. Cherry (2005) notes that the time interval between epidemic cycles of pertussis in the pre-vaccine and post-vaccine eras has not changed. This is in contrast to other vaccine-preventable diseases, such as measles, where the interval between epidemic cycles has lengthened since the introduction of immunistion programs. This suggests that pertussis is circulating in the community in the post-vaccine era as in the pre-vaccine era but with adolescents and adults the main reservoir of infection.

The proportion of prolonged cough illnesses attributed to pertussis in adolescents and adults varies in different studies from 5.7–52%. During non-epidemic periods, this proportion attributable can, not surprisingly, be as low as 1% (range 1–17%) (Cherry, 2005; Ward et al., 2005). Part of the reason for the variable findings in different studies include whether or not the study was conducted during an epidemic cycle, differing levels of awareness of pertussis among doctors and differences in diagnostic tools.

> 'But I haven't been "whooping"—so how can I have "whooping cough"?'

The clinical features of pertussis can range from the classical illness to a minimally symptomatic disease. Unimmunised children are more likely to experience the classical illness, which has three phases following a 7–10 day incubation period (Mattoo and Cherry, 2005)

During the catarrhal phase, the individual usually complains of a runny nose, runny eyes and a mild cough for 7–10 days. In atypical presentations, the catarrhal phase may be shorter, with the only complaint being pharyngeal discomfort.

The paroxysmal phase lasts 2–8 weeks. There are fits of coughing throughout the day and night (often worse at night). Typically, 5–10 powerful coughs will occur in one expiration followed by a deep and noisy inspiration. This inspiratory breath gives rise to the 'whoop' of whooping cough. To an observer (particularly a parent), the paroxysm can be a terrifying spectacle. The individual may become cyanosed, with bulging neck veins and eyes, a protruding tongue, profuse salivation and lacrimation. The paroxysm may be followed by a post-tussive vomit. Although the individual may be normal between paroxysms, children, in particular, are prone to weight loss and are often subdued.

Reports of the mechanical consequences of the pressures generated by the paroxysms are staggering. They include carotid artery dissection, intracranial haemorrhage, cough syncope, fractured ribs, subconjunctival haemorrhage, incontinence, hernias, ruptured vertebral discs, ruptured diaphragm, epistaxis, melaena, ulcerated frenulum, rectal prolapse, pneumothoraces and severe alkalosis with seizures (Matto and Cherry, 2005; Skowronski et al., 2003).

Overall, about 5% of individuals with pertussis develop complications, most commonly neurological and respiratory. The proportion of complications is highest in infants <6 months. The respiratory complications include pneumonia and otitis media (due to pertussis itself or to secondary infection); neurological complications include encephalopathy and seizures, possibly secondary to paroxysm-induced hypoxia (although the cause is not fully understood). The incidence of encephalopathy is about 0.9/100000 cases (World Health Organization, 2005).

The convalescent phase occurs next. There is a gradual (rather than sudden) reduction in the frequency and severity of symptoms. It normally lasts 1–2 weeks. During this stage, an intercurrent viral respiratory tract infection can precipitate further paroxysms but these are not due to pertussis.

In addition to these classical symptoms, pertussis can present atypically, particularly in previously immunised children or partially immunised adolescents and adults. There may simply be a chronic cough without the whoop or post-tussive vomiting. The proportion of whooping amongst adults varies, but has been as low as 8% in some studies (8–82%) (Hewlett, 2005); therefore, Hilary could still have pertussis despite the absence of a whoop. Post-tussive vomiting of classical pertussis occurs in only 17–50% of adult cases (Hewlett and Edwards, 2005).

Asymptomatic infection can also occur. A randomised controlled trial examining the efficacy of the acellular vaccine found that seroconversion to pertussis among asymptomatic participants was 5–10 times more common than among symptomatic individuals (Ward et al., 2005).

Fever is not a major feature of this infection—do not dismiss a diagnosis of pertussis because of the absence of a history of fever.

> Lin examines Hilary; there are no abnormal findings. She thinks Tony's suggestion of pertussis is a good one. She is not sure if Hilary meets the case definition so she calls the local public health unit (PHU). Dr Kevin Minto at the unit is able to assist her.

CASE 16 PERTUSSIS

Public health notification and response

Pertussis is a notifiable disease in many parts of the world. GPs cannot be expected to remember or have records of case definitions for every notifiable disease, but most PHUs are happy to be called.

Although case definitions for pertussis might vary from region to region, the WHO (2003) case definition is probably fairly representative:
- case diagnosed as pertussis by a physician OR
- person with a cough lasting at least two weeks with at least one of the following symptoms: paroxysms (i.e. fits) of coughing, inspiratory whooping or post-tussive vomiting (i.e. vomiting immediately after coughing) without other apparent cause OR
- case confirmed by a laboratory by isolating *B. pertussis*, detecting genomic sequences by means of polymerase chain reaction (PCR) or positive paired serology

Cases may be clinically confirmed (a case that meets the clinical case definition but is not laboratory confirmed) or laboratory confirmed (a case that meets the clinical case definition and is laboratory confirmed).

Patients with pertussis may have only a chronic cough without an accompanying whoop, paroxysm or post-tussive vomit; such patients would not meet the case definition and therefore would not be notified as a case of pertussis. This is one reason that cases of pertussis in the community are likely to be underestimated. The other factor is the limitation of diagnostic tests.

Lin's local definition is almost identical to the WHO's but includes an extra criterion for laboratory detection: a single high IgA.

Lin asks Hilary specifically about accompanying whoops, paroxysms or post-tussive vomiting. She does admit to having vomited once after a paroxysm of coughing, so she meets the case definition for clinically-confirmed pertussis.

Lin says to Kevin, 'Should I have waited for microbiological confirmation before calling you?'

In most areas, clinically confirmed pertussis, even in the absence of microbiological confirmation, is still notifiable as soon as possible. This is because pertussis is highly infectious through droplet transmission or contact with contaminated surfaces: it has an attack rate of up to 80% in susceptible contacts (Tiwari et al., 2005). It is vital to provide treatment for the index case and susceptible contacts as soon as possible, and waiting days for test results to come back will only increase the risk of infecting more contacts. Also, negative test results do not exclude pertussis.

Lin gives Hilary's details to Kevin. He will contact her later that day to start contact tracing.

Lin now wants to test Hilary for pertussis. However, she can't recall with certainty the timing of tests. She calls the microbiologist at the local hospital for advice.

Investigations

Testing for *B. pertussis* is directed towards identifying either the bacterium (through culture or PCR) or an antibody response to the bacterium (serology).

But all tests for pertussis have limited or uncertain sensitivity for various reasons which are outlined in Table 16.1: the positive predictive value of most of these tests is good but the negative predictive value is limited. This means that a positive test in a patient with a prolonged cough illness is likely to be pertussis but a negative test does not exclude it. Part of the uncertainty regarding the efficacy of tests for pertussis is that there is no reliable gold standard against which to measure them. While culture of *B. pertussis* is used as the gold standard, the test is handicapped by its poor sensitivity.

Lin finds it difficult to absorb all this information quickly. 'So how should I proceed?' she asks the microbiologist.

Given the poor sensitivity and technical difficulties in getting cultures for *B. pertussis*, PCR is preferable to culture if testing is available. Therefore, a reasonable approach would be a combination of PCR and serology, as outlined in Table 16.2.

Table 16.1 Testing for pertussis

Test	Advantages	Disadvantages
Culture	This is the gold standard, with a 100% positive predictive value. It differentiates *B. pertussis* from *B. parapertussis*, an organism that causes a minority of pertussis cases and a milder form of the disease.	The disadvantages of culture far outweigh its advantages. *B. pertussis* is only isolated from areas with ciliated respiratory epithelium. A nasopharyngeal specimen is required and throat, anterior nose and sputum samples are of little value (Mattoo and Cherry, 2005). *B. pertussis* may not grow for up to seven days, delaying confirmation. The sensitivity is very poor, 0–67% (Hallander, 1999; von Konig et al., 2002). The yield from nasopharyngeal swabs is poorer than from aspirates but this is a more difficult procedure. The yield is almost 30% better with immediate inoculation of the nasopharyngeal specimen onto an appropriate culture medium, which is unlikely to happen in general practice or even hospitals (Hallander et al., 1993).† There is only a small window of opportunity for culturing, up to 2–4 weeks after the onset of the catarrhal phase, up to 1–3 weeks after the onset of the paroxysmal phase or only for a few days after starting antibiotics (NSW Health, 2005). Cotton swabs cannot be used, only Dacron or calcium alginate swabs.‡
PCR	This can be performed on throat swabs. It has a higher sensitivity than culture, increasing identification rate 2.6–4 times (Schlapfer et al., 1995; Schmidt-Schlapfer et al., 1997). It cannot be as readily affected by prior antibiotic therapy. It remains positive for longer than cultures—up to six weeks after the onset of symptoms (Tozzi et al., 2005)—but sensitivity decreases with time. It can differentiate *B. pertussis* from *B. parapertussis* (depending on the primers used).	It is not 100% sensitive, so negative results do not exclude pertussis. It may not be available in many developing countries, which have the highest burden of disease. False-positives can occur (Mattoo and Cherry, 2005). It requires Dacron swabs; calcium alginate swabs cannot be used.‡

(Continued)

Table 16.1 Testing for pertussis (Continued)

Test	Advantages	Disadvantages
Serology	Enzyme-linked immunosorbent assays (ELISA) can be directed against a number of pertussis antigens or only a few, including pertussis toxin, pertactin, filamentous haemagglutinin and fimbria.[*] Only IgG and IgA are used to make a diagnosis of pertussis, based on a single high titre or a two-fold rise between baseline and convalescent titres.[§] IgA is specific for infection rather than immunisation; a raised IgG titre can occur with either but a single IgG titre against pertussis toxin above 100–125 IU/mL is consistent with acute infection (Tozzi et al., 2005).	It cannot make an early diagnosis. A single IgA test has poor sensitivity, 24–62% in one study, although this used a clinical case definition of pertussis as its gold standard (Poyntent et al., 2002). IgA can persist indefinitely after an infection. IgA testing is not very reliable in infants. Many clinicians will not consider pertussis as a diagnosis until the cough has been present for weeks, by which time it will be too late to take a baseline titre. Specificity can be a problem with ELISA kits using FHA and PRN, which can cross-react with other *Bordetella* spp.
Direct fluorescent antibody (DFA) testing	It uses nasopharyngeal secretions, which are easily obtainable.	It is relatively insensitive and non-specific.

[†]Regan-Lowe medium is a widely used medium for culturing pertussis. It consists of cephalexin (to inhibit the growth of oropharyngeal flora), charcoal (to absorb toxins) and horse blood (to promote growth of *B. pertussis*). The original culture medium developed by Bordet and Gengou (Bordet-Gengou medium) in the early 1900s is also still popular; however, the Regan-Lowe medium has the advantage that it can be stored in the refrigerator for one month (Hallander, 1999).

[‡]The disadvantage is compounded by the fact that swab containers often do not say whether they are cotton, calcium alginate or Dacron; therefore, clinicians may have difficulty identifying the swab they need, even if they remember which one to use.

[*]Although only pertussis toxin is specific for *B. pertussis* (the others are also expressed by other *Bordetella* spp), a rise in fimbrial haemagglutinin correlates with acute *B. pertussis* infection (Poyntent et al., 2002).

[§]Interestingly, data suggest that a fall in IgG titre against pertussis toxin and filamentous haemagglutinin can also represent acute infection (Simondon et al., 1998). This is somewhat akin to acute episodes of gout being precipitated by a rise or fall in serum uric acid levels.

CASE 16 PERTUSSIS

Table 16.2 Testing for pertussis with PCR and serology

	<2 weeks after symptoms onset	2–6 weeks after symptoms onset	>6 weeks after symptoms onset
PCR†	yes	yes	no
Baseline serology‡	yes	yes	no
Convalescent serology 2–4 weeks later	yes	yes	no
Single serology adequate	no	maybe	yes

†If PCR is not available, nasopharyngeal cultures can be taken in the first 2–4 weeks after the onset of symptoms.
‡Serology is not reliable in children <2 years.

> Given that Hilary has been unwell for almost four weeks, the microbiologist suggests a serology and PCR.
> 'Will blood tests be helpful in pointing towards pertussis?' Tony wants to know.

The classical finding in children with pertussis is leukocytosis with a predominant lymphocytosis and, to a lesser degree, neutrophilia. This is due to the action of a virulence factor, pertussis toxin, which causes more white cells to enter the blood from extravascular sites; these cells remain in the blood rather than leave the circulation. In fact, there appears to be an association between the death of children with pertussis and higher levels of lymphocytosis and leukocytosis, possibly related to the pooling of cells in the pulmonary vasculature (Pierce et al., 2000).

However, adults and other partially immunised groups may have a normal white cell count and differential (Mattoo and Cherry, 2005).

> Hilary asks, 'Should I wait for the blood tests to come back before I start treatment?'

Treatment

Lin needs to consider who should be treated and whether treatment should begin before or after laboratory confirmation.

Pertussis is a highly communicable disease that can cause severe disease or death, particularly in infants. Since it may take many days for the results of these tests to become available and be conveyed to the patient, empiric antibiotic therapy is the recommended approach in many parts of the world. Delaying treatment to wait for results may also result in increased secondary transmission to contacts, thereby increasing the workload of public health officers in contact tracing.

The aims of treating cases of pertussis are to reduce the severity and duration of illness and the period of communicability. However, in practice, the latter objective is more often achieved than the former. A systematic review of the role of antibiotics in whooping cough concluded that they did not alter the clinical course of the illness, although they did render the case non-infectious (Altunaiji et al., 2005).

Since the benefit of treatment with antibiotics is directed towards eradication of the organism from the nasopharynx, treatment is considered unnecessary once spontaneous clearing of the nasopharynx occurs. In 80–90% of cases, spontaneous clearing of pertussis occurs three weeks after the onset of the cough; however, it may take six weeks in infants (Tiwari et al., 2005).

Based on this, the recommendations are to commence treatment within 21 days of the onset of symptoms in Australia and the UK (National Health and Medical Research Council, 2003; South Yorkshire Health Protection Unit, 2005) or within 21 days of the onset of the cough in the US and Canada (Anonymous, 2003; Tiwari et al., 2005). In the US, infants can be treated up to six weeks after the onset of the cough (Tiwari et al., 2005). Nevertheless, one wonders how accurate data on the persistence of *B. pertussis* in the nasopharynx are, given the poor sensitivity of culture techniques.

'We follow the US and Canadian recommendations,' the microbiologist explains. 'Since Hilary has had a cough for three weeks, she should be commenced on antibiotics.'

'What should I use?' Lin asks.

Macrolide antibiotics are the standard antibiotic therapy for pertussis. Until recently, erythromycin was the only choice; however, randomised controlled trials have compared 14 days of erythromycin to two other macrolides, clarithromycin and azithromycin. The trials concluded that both these macrolides are as effective as erythromycin in eradicating *B. pertussis*, with the added benefits of fewer side effects than erythromycin and better compliance (Langley et al., 2004; Lebel and Mehra, 2001). The only disadvantage of clarithromycin and azithromycin is that they are more expensive than erythromycin.

Erythromycin resistance does occur but documented cases are rare (Lee, 2000); it is not currently an emerging problem.

In patients with an allergy to macrolides, the sulpha drug trimethoprim/sulfamethoxazole can be used. For those patients allergic to both macrolides and sulpha drugs, there are a number of antibiotics with in vitro activity against *B. pertussis* (e.g. fluoroquinolones, fusidic acid, amoxycillin, chloramphenicol). It is unclear whether this in vitro effect will translate to a clinical impact on the infection (Bourgeois et al., 2003; Collignon and Turnidge, 1999; Tiwari et al., 2005).

'What about roxithromycin?' Tony asks.

Roxithromycin is a macrolide antibiotic commonly used in Australia and New Zealand. Although one would assume that like other macrolides it would be effective against pertussis, this is by no means certain. While it does have an in vitro effect on *B. pertussis*, it is unclear whether this would translate to efficacy in the clinical setting (Brett et al., 1998).

'I hate taking pills,' Hilary says. 'How long will I be on this for?'

The typical duration of therapy is five days for azithromycin and seven for clarithromycin. US experts recommend 14 days for erythromycin (Tiwari et al., 2005) while Canadian, UK and Australian health authorities recommend seven days (Anonymous, 2003; National Health and Medical Research Council, 2003; South Yorkshire Health Protection Unit, 2005). A randomised controlled trial found that seven days of erythromycin was as effective as 14 days at microbiological eradication of pertussis from the nasopharynx (Halperin et al., 1997).

Lin prescribes clarithromycin for Hilary but lets her know that, although it will render her non-infectious, it may not improve her symptoms.
Hilary is naturally disappointed and asks if there is anything else that can improve her cough.

Pillay and Swingler (2003) performed a systematic review of the impact of the following interventions on the cough of pertussis: antihistamines, pertussis immunoglobulin, corticosteroids and inhaled salbutamol. They concluded that there was insufficient evidence to draw firm conclusions; the only benefit was a borderline impact for pertussis immunoglobulin.

There is insufficient evidence for Lin to make an evidence-based decision on what to offer Hilary for her cough; however, she prescribes her a corticosteroid puffer and some cough syrup and hopes for the best.
'Can I go to work, Doctor?'

Isolation measures

Patients with pertussis are considered non-infectious once they complete five days of antibiotic therapy; therefore, Hilary will have to stay home for five days.

Hilary thanks Lin and heads off home. As he promised earlier, Kevin calls Hilary about contact tracing. He explains about post-exposure prophylaxis (PEP).

For public health officers, difficulties responding to a pertussis notification highlight many of the obstacles encountered when dealing with a number of other communicable diseases (Anonymous, 2003):
- With an average of 10–12 secondary contacts for every index case, interviews can take around four hours in total, which is a lot of time when resources are limited.

- Maintaining the index case's confidentiality can be difficult when talking to contacts.
- Chemoprophylaxis may be refused because of cost.
- Chemoprophylaxis may be refused because of potential side effects, particularly since most contacts are asymptomatic at the time they are approached by public health teams. This is in contrast to a well-publicised fulminant infection such as meningococcal disease, where contacts may be terrified until they receive chemoprophylaxis.
- There is a lack of awareness among some clinicians that pertussis is a disease of adults and not just children.
- There may be poor documentation of immunisation status.

> Hilary is very interested in the process. 'How do you decide who will need treatment? And what exactly can you give people to protect them?'

Overall, there seems to be agreement between most countries on which high-risk (vulnerable) contacts should receive PEP. The differences lie with the lower-risk or non-vulnerable contacts.

'High-risk' does not necessarily refer to susceptibility to infection but to those people who are at risk of a severe infection or who could transmit the infection to others who would be at risk of severe infection. This typically includes household and institutional contacts (National Health and Medical Research Council, 2003), particularly:

- any infant <12 months, irrespective of immunisation status
- any child 12–24 months who has not received three doses of vaccine against pertussis
- any woman in the last trimester of pregnancy
- any adult or child who attends or works at a childcare facility

Lower-risk (non-vulnerable) contacts, for PEP purposes, typically include (Anonymous, 2003; Tiwari et al., 2005):

- household contacts who are only partially immunised against pertussis
- non-household contacts who are only partially immunised against pertussis and have had face-to-face contact and/or shared confined air for ≥1 hour

> Hilary's house is full because of a family reunion. Kevin's contact history reveals that Hilary has two vulnerable household contacts: a sister who is 37 weeks pregnant (Anne) and another sister who has a three-week-old baby (Sarah).
> Hilary is naturally worried. 'But Doctor, shouldn't Sarah's antibodies protect her baby? And she's breastfeeding—won't that help?'

Maternal antibodies do provide protection for the infant against many infections in the first few months of life. Unfortunately, pertussis is not one of them. Irrespective of the mother's immune status, the three-week-old must be protected against pertussis. Data from the US show that 90% of deaths from pertussis occur in infants <6 months of age (Mattoo and Cherry, 2005). Pertussis has even been implicated as a possible cause of sudden infant deaths (Heininger et al., 2004).

Erythromycin is the antibiotic traditionally given. However, it has been associated with infantile hypertrophic pyloric stenosis (IHPS) in the neonate (Cooper et al., 2002; Honein et al., 1999). For this reason, azithromycin is the preferred antimicrobial agent for infants <1 month (it has not been associated with IHPS to date). If azithromycin is not available, then erythromycin should be given: the risk to neonates of a life-threatening course of pertussis outweighs the risk of IHPS from erythromycin (Tiwari et al., 2005).

> 'I know Sarah won't want to take medicine when she's breastfeeding. Does she actually need an antibiotic? And is it safe for the baby?'

If Sarah is partially immunised against pertussis, then she needs PEP. Guidelines recommend erythromycin for the mother (National Health and Medical Research Council, 2003). However, there are conflicting studies over whether giving erythromycin to breastfeeding mothers will result in an increased risk of IHPS in the newborn. Since 50% of erythromycin in the maternal circulation will pass to breast milk, it is certainly a biologically plausible possibility (Louik et al., 2002; Sørensen et al., 2003).

Although it has not been officially recommended as yet, azithromycin could be an alternative to erythromycin because, as discussed above, it has not been associated with cases of IHPS.

CASE 16 PERTUSSIS

> 'What about Anne? Are you sure she needs anything? I mean, everyone always tells you not to take anything when you're pregnant.'

Erythromycin is recommended for pregnant women in the last trimester of pregnancy (National Health and Medical Research Council, 2003). The safety in pregnancy of the antibiotics used for pertussis is as follows (Anonymous, 2006):

- erythromycin—Category A (drugs that have been taken by a large number of pregnant women and women of childbearing age without any proven increase in the frequency of malformations or other direct or indirect harmful effects on the fetus having been observed)
- azithromycin—Category B1 (drugs that have been taken by only a limited number of pregnant women and women of childbearing age without an increase in the frequency of malformation or other direct or indirect harmful effects on the human fetus having been observed. Studies in animals have not shown evidence of an increased occurrence of fetal damage.)
- clarithromycin—Category B3 (drugs that have been taken by only a limited number of pregnant women and women of childbearing age without an increase in the frequency of malformation or other direct or indirect harmful effects on the human fetus having been observed. Studies in animals have shown evidence of an increased occurrence of fetal damage, the significance of which is considered uncertain in humans.)
- trimethoprim/sulfamethoxazole—Category C (drugs that, owing to their pharmacological effects, have caused or may be suspected of causing harmful effects on the human fetus or neonate without causing malformations. These effects may be reversible. Accompanying texts should be consulted for further details.)

> Hilary's husband, who is currently asymptomatic, is also given PEP. He is concerned about being an infection hazard at work and wonders if he should stay at home for five days like Hilary.

Contacts of pertussis cases are considered non-infectious if they are asymptomatic.

> Hilary asks, 'Can my dog get pertussis? He has been coughing quite a bit for the last few days.'

B. pertussis is a purely human pathogen but *B. bronchoseptica* can cause respiratory illness in animals, especially dogs (kennel cough) and pigs. It is also an uncommon cause of zoonotic infection (Mattoo and Cherry, 2005).

> Kevin successfully resolves the contact tracing and administration of PEP for Hilary's case. A few weeks later, he receives a call from a GP.
> 'Hi, I have a 24-year-old woman requesting immunisation with the acellular vaccine against pertussis. The only problem is that she had a pertussis-like illness last year, although we never took serology or cultures to confirm it. If she did have pertussis, is it dangerous to immunise her?'

People with previous pertussis infections can be safely immunised with the acellular vaccine (National Health and Medical Research Council, 2003).

According to approximate estimates, immunisation provides only about 6–12 years of immunity while infection provides longer protection of around 15 years (von Konig et al., 2002; WHO, 2005). Neither provides life-long immunity.

> Kevin's registrar, Dr Kathleen Bell, asks what types of vaccines are available for pertussis.

Broadly speaking, there are two types of pertussis vaccines: whole cell and acellular. They are compared in Table 16.3.

Table 16.3 A comparison of whole cell and acellular pertussis vaccines

	whole cell	acellular
Contents	inactivated *B. pertussis*	*B. pertussis* components[†]
Cost	cheaper	more expensive
Local side effects	more	less
Systemic side effects	more	less
Effectiveness	yes	yes

[†]The acellular vaccine consists of components of *B. pertussis*, including pertussis toxin +/− combinations of other adhesins, such as filamentous haemagglutinin, pertactin and fimbriae.

> Kathleen asks, 'I want to get a pertussis booster immunisation with dTpa but I had a tetanus-diphtheria (TD) booster just two years ago. Will it be a problem?'

dTpa is an acellular vaccine recommended for older children, adolescents and adults. The use of small and capital letters in vaccine names refers to the amount of antigen which they contain: dTpa contains a large amount of tetanus antigen (T) but smaller amounts of diphtheria and pertussis antigens (dp).

Kathleen is concerned that the immunity generated from her recent TD booster will lead to a vigorous local reaction if she is exposed to the large tetanus antigen component of dTpa. However, a Canadian study has recently shown that dTpa can be safely administered to children and adolescents as little as 18 months after a previous immunisation with tetanus toxoid such as TD or Td (Halperin et al., 2006).

> 'Is the acellular vaccine 100% effective?' she asks.

No vaccine is completely effective. Although the results of efficacy studies vary, it is thought that the best whole cell and acellular pertussis vaccines can achieve 85% efficacy (WHO, 2005).

One interesting phenomenon has been the observation of antigenic shift in pertussis strains during immunisation programs with the whole cell vaccines. This resulted in circulating strains of *B. pertussis* that may not have been effectively neutralised with the whole cell vaccines being used at the time, thereby contributing to the increase in pertussis in the community (Poynten et al., 2004).

References

Altunaiji, S., Kukuruzovic, R, Curtis, N. et al. (2005) Antibiotics for whooping cough (pertussis). Cochrane Database Of Systematic Reviews 1, CD004404.

Anonymous (2006) Drug use in pregnancy and breastfeeding (amended 2006 Apr). In: *eTG complete* (CD-ROM). Therapeutic Guidelines Limited; Melbourne.

Anonymous (2003) National consensus conference on pertussis. *Canada Communicable Disease Report* 29(S3), 1–33.

Bourgeois, N., Ghnassia, J.C., Doucet-Populaire, F. (2003) In vitro activity of fluoroquinolones against erythromycin-susceptible and -resistant *Bordetella pertussis*. *Journal of Antimicrobial Chemotherapy* 51(3), 742–43.

Brett M., Short P., Beatson S. (1998) The comparative in-vitro activity of roxithromycin and other antibiotics against *Bordetella pertussis*. *Journal of Antimicrobial Chemotherapy* 41(Suppl B), 23–27.

Cherry, J.D. (2005) The epidemiology of pertussis: a comparison of the epidemiology of the disease pertussis with the epidemiology of *Bordetella pertussis* infection. *Pediatrics* 115(5), 1422–27.

Collignon, P., Turnidge, J. (1999) Fusidic acid in vitro activity. *International Journal of Antimicrobial Agents* 12(Suppl 2), S45–48.

Cooper, W.O., Griffin, M.R., Arbogast, P. et al. (2002) Very early exposure to erythromycin and infantile hypertrophic pyloric stenosis. *Archives of Pediatrics & Adolescent Medicine* 156(7), 647–50.

Department of Health and Ageing (2006) *National Notifiable Diseases Surveillance System*. Available from www9.health.gov.au/cda/Source/Rpt_3_sel.cfm (Accessed 17 June, 2006)

Galanis, E., King, A.S., Varughese, P. et al. (2006) Changing epidemiology and emerging risk groups for pertussis. *Canadian Medical Association Journal* 174(4), 451–52.

Hallander, H.O. (1999) Microbiological and serological diagnosis of pertussis. *Clinical Infectious Diseases* 28(Suppl 2), S99–106.

Hallander, H.O., Reizenstein, E., Renemar, B. et al. (1993) Comparison of nasopharyngeal aspirates with swabs for culture of *Bordetella pertussis*. *Journal of Clinical Microbiology* 31(1), 50–52.

Halperin, S.A., Sweet, L., Baxendale, D. et al. (2006) How soon after a prior tetanus-diphtheria vaccination can one give adult formulation tetanus-diphtheria-acellular pertussis vaccine? *Pediatric Infectious Disease Journal* 25(3), 195–200.

Halperin, S.A., Bortolussi, R., Langley, J.M. et al. (1997) Seven days of erythromycin estolate is as effective as fourteen days for the treatment of *Bordetella pertussis* infections. *Pediatrics* 100(1), 65–71.

Heininger, U., Kleeman, W.J., Cherry, J.D. et al. (2004) A controlled study of the relationship between *Bordetella pertussis* infections and sudden unexpected deaths among German infants. *Pediatrics* 114(1), e9–15.

Hewlett, E.L. (2005) *Bordetella* species. In Mandell, G.L., Bennett, J.E., Dolin, R. (eds) *Principles and Practice of Infectious Diseases*. Churchill Livingstone; Philadelphia.

Hewlett, E.L., Edwards, K.M. (2005) Clinical practice. Pertussis—not just for kids. *New England Journal of Medicine* 352(12), 1215–22.

Honein, M.A., Paulozzi, L.J., Himelright, I.M. et al. (1999) Infantile hypertrophic pyloric stenosis after pertussis prophylaxis with erythromycin: a case review and cohort study. *Lancet* 354(9196), 2101–05.

Langley, J.M., Halperin, S.A., Boucher F.D. et al. (2004) Azithromycin is as effective as and better tolerated than erythromycin estolate for the treatment of pertussis. *Pediatrics* 114(1), e96–101.

Lebel, M.H., Mehra, S. (2001) Efficacy and safety of clarithromycin versus erythromycin for the treatment of pertussis: a prospective, randomized, single blind trial. *Pediatric Infectious Disease Journal* 20(12), 1149–51.

Lee, B. (2000) Progressive respiratory distress in an infant treated for presumed pertussis. *Pediatric Infectious Diseases Journal* 19(5), 475, 492–93.

Louik, C., Werler, M.M., Mitchell, A.A. (2002) Erythromycin use during pregnancy in relation to pyloric stenosis. *American Journal of Obstetrics and Gynecology* 186(2), 288–90.

Mattoo, S., Cherry, J.D. (2005) Molecular pathogenesis, epidemiology, and clinical manifestations of respiratory infections due to *Bordetella pertussis* and other *Bordetella* subspecies. *Clinical Microbiology Reviews* 18(2), 326–82.

National Health and Medical Research Council (2003) *Australian Immunisation Handbook. 8th Edition*. National Health and Medical Research Council; Canberra. Available from www9.health.gov.au/immhandbook (Accessed 9 January, 2006)

NSW Health. (2005) *Pertussis. Response Protocol for NSW Public Health Units*. Available from www.health.nsw.gov.au/infect/pdf/pertussis.pdf (Accessed 1 June, 2006)

Pierce, C., Klein, N., Peters, M. (2000) Is leukocytosis a predictor of mortality in severe pertussis infection? *Intensive Care Medicine* 26(10), 1512–14.

Pillay, V., Swingler, G. (2003) Symptomatic treatment of the cough in whooping cough. Cochrane Database of Systematic Reviews 4, CD003257.

Poynten, M., McIntyre, P.B., Mooi, F.R. et al. (2004) Temporal trends in circulating *Bordetella pertussis* strains in Australia. *Epidemiology and Infection* 132(2), 185–93.

Poynten, I.M., Hanlon, M., Irwig, L. et al. (2002) Serological diagnosis of pertussis: evaluation of IgA against whole cell and specific *Bordetella pertussis* antigens as markers of recent infection. *Epidemiology and Infection* 128(2), 161–67.

Schlapfer, G., Cherry, J.D., Heininger, U. et al. (1995) Polymerase chain reaction identification of *Bordetella pertussis* infections in vaccinees and family members in a pertussis vaccine efficacy trial in Germany. *Pediatric Infectious Diseases Journal* 14(3), 209–14.

Schmidt-Schlapfer, G., Liese, J.G., Porter, F. et al. (1997) Polymerase chain reaction (PCR) compared with conventional identification in culture for detection of

Bordetella pertussis in 7 153 children. *Clinical Microbiology and Infection* 3(4), 462–67.

Simondon, F., Iteman, I., Preziosi, M.P. et al. (1998) Evaluation of an immunoglobulin G enzyme-linked immunosorbent assay for pertussis toxin and filamentous hemagglutinin in diagnosis of pertussis in Senegal. *Clinical and Diagnostic Laboratory Immunology* 5(2), 130–34.

Skowronski, D.M., Buxton, J.A., Hestrin M. et al. (2003) Carotid artery dissection as a possible severe complication of pertussis in an adult: clinical case report review. *Clinical Infectious Diseases* 36(1), e1–4.

Sørensen, H.T., Skriver, M.V., Pedersen, L., et al. (2003) Risk of infantile hypertrophic pyloric stenosis after maternal postnatal use of macrolides. *Scandinavian Journal of Infectious Diseases* 35(2), 104–6.

South Yorkshire Health Protection Unit. (2005) *Guidelines for chemoprophylaxis and immunisation in persons exposed to pertussis.* Available from www.hpa.org.uk/infections/topics_az/whoopingcough/images/SYHPU_pertussis_guidelines.pdf (Accessed 10 July, 2006)

Tiwari, T., Murphy, T.V., Moran J. et al. (2005) Recommended antimicrobial agents for the treatment and postexposure prophylaxis of pertussis: 2005 CDC Guidelines. *Morbidity and Mortality Weekly Reports Recommendations and Reports* 54(RR-14), 1–16.

Tozzi, A.E., Celentano, L.P., Ciofi degli Atti, M.L. et al. (2005) Diagnosis and management of pertussis. *Canadian Medical Association Journal* 172(4), 509–15.

von Konig, C.H., Halperin, S., Riffelmann, M. et al. (2002). Pertussis of adults and infants. *Lancet Infectious Diseases* 2(12), 744–50.

Ward J.I., Cherry J.D., Chang S-J. et al. (2005) Efficacy of an acellular pertussis vaccine among adolescents and adults. *New England Journal Of Medicine* 353(15), 1555–63.

World Health Organization (WHO) (2005) Pertussis vaccines—WHO position paper. *Weekly Epidemiological Record* 80(4), 31–39.

World Health Organization (WHO) (2003) *WHO recommended standards for surveillance of selected vaccine-preventable diseases.* World Health Organization; Geneva. Available from www.who.int/vaccines-documents/DocsPDF06/843.pdf (Accessed June 27, 2006)

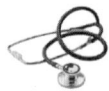

Case 17 Poliomyelitis
Roger feels weak ...

Poliomyelitis at a glance ...

- **Agent:** family Picornaviridae; genus *Enterovirus*; species poliovirus
- **Geographical distribution:** wild-type virus—Asia and Africa account for endemic regions and regions with re-established transmission of disease; vaccine-associated paralytic poliomyelitis—rare but can occur in any country using oral polio vaccine
- **Main modes of transmission:** close personal contact with faeco-oral transmission; houseflies and contaminated water have also been implicated
- **Person-to-person transmission:** yes
- **Animal-to-person transmission:** no (purely human reservoir)
- **Incubation period:** 7–10 days (2–35 days)
- **Infectious period:** usually up to 6 weeks after infection onset, while virus is being shed in the stool; can rarely be shed for many months in the stool of immunodeficient people
- **Clinical features:** four classical clinical syndromes—asymptomatic infection, abortive infection, aseptic meningitis with or without transient paralysis, paralytic disease (spinal, bulbospinal, bulbar)
- **Identification:** polymerase chain reaction (PCR) and culture of virus from stool, oropharynx (only early in the infection) and, rarely, cerebrospinal fluid (CSF)
- **Treatment:** supportive measures and rehabilitation
- **Post-exposure prophylaxis:** nil
- **Vaccine:** live oral polio vaccine (OPV) or a parenterally-administered inactivated polio vaccine (IPV)

Main characters

Dr Mercedes Jones	infectious diseases registrar
Dr Petra Smith	neurology intern
Roger Green	boy with fever and weakness
Dr Wanda Lam (PhD)	infection control nurse
Dr Glen Ford	public health physician

Dr Mercedes Jones, the infectious diseases registrar, receives a page from Dr Petra Smith, the neurology intern.

'Hi, we have just admitted a young patient in the emergency department (ED) with new-onset weakness. We would appreciate your advice regarding possible infective diagnoses and the appropriate investigations and treatment.'

Mercedes walks down to the ED and meets the patient. His name is Roger Green, a 12-year-old boy from Nigeria. He arrived in the country ten days ago with a school group celebrating a cultural festival. One week ago, he became unwell.

On Days 1 and 2 he had fevers and shivers, a mild bifrontal headache, sore throat and reduced appetite. He rested in bed. A general practitioner (GP) wondered about streptococcal pharyngitis and gave him an intramuscular (IM) injection of penicillin in the left leg.

From Days 3–5, he felt well, even going on a long run on Day 4. However on Day 6, after being well for three days, he developed a headache, neck stiffness and fevers.

Yesterday, Day 7, he noticed generalised muscle aches and painful cramps and spasms in his legs. Today, he awoke to find that his left leg was weak. He has had no difficulty passing urine or opening his bowels.

On examination, Roger doesn't look that unwell. He has a fever of 38.3°C and mild neck stiffness. However, the major examination finding is asymmetrical weakness of the lower limbs. He has 4/5 weakness of hip flexion of the right lower limb but 3/5 weakness of hip flexion, hip extension, knee flexion and dorsiflexion of the left lower limb. Both knee jerks are reduced and the left ankle jerk is absent. Babinski response is downgoing bilaterally. Sensory findings are intact, including saddle sensation.

'What neurological picture does that add up to?' Mercedes asks.

CASE 17 POLIOMYELITIS

Roger has an acute flaccid paralysis (AFP). His AFP is asymmetric and involves only the lower limbs.

> Mercedes believes that Roger's AFP may be caused by an infection. In particular, she is thinking of poliomyelitis.
> Petra says, 'I can understand why you're thinking infection, given the febrile prodrome. But how did you pinpoint poliomyelitis?'

What is poliomyelitis?

A febrile prodrome does point to an infective cause of AFP. The features that specifically support a diagnosis of poliomyelitis are:

Biphasic illness Poliomyelitis can cause a biphasic illness. Initially, there is an influenza-like illness—with fevers, myalgias, headache and sore throat—which spontaneously resolves. Then, after a 2–5 day asymptomatic period, a meningitic-type illness occurs followed soon by paralysis. However, a biphasic picture is uncommon in children over 15 years and adults; their illness is usually monophasic (Marx et al., 2000).

Physical activity and intramuscular injections during the early illness These might increase the risk of developing paralytic polio (Howard, 2005). Roger did exercise just after getting over the minor illness and received a penicillin injection during his early illness.

Absence of sensory symptoms

Asymmetric AFP

> 'I thought that polio was pretty much eradicated and that you only find a few cases in India. Are you sure they have polio in Nigeria?' asks Petra.
> Mercedes isn't sure but she knows how to find out. The website for the Global Polio Eradication Initiative (www.polio-eradication.org) has this information. It confirms that at that time (June 2007) Nigeria had endemic poliomyelitis. It also informs her that the other nations with endemic polio are India (as Petra suggested), Pakistan and Afghanistan.
> Roger became ill three days after leaving Nigeria. This would fit with the incubation period of poliomyelitis, typically 7–10 days (range 2–35 days).

> Petra says, 'I saw a kid during my paediatrics term with a similar picture. They turned out to have an enterovirus infection... Ummm, "EV 70-something". Is polio similar to these enteroviruses?'

Poliomyelitis itself is actually a member of the genus *Enterovirus* and the family Picornaviridae. Non-polio enteroviruses can cause AFP. In particular, enterovirus 71 (EV 71) can be associated with outbreaks of AFP (it also causes hand, foot and mouth disease [HFMD] in children).

> 'So it sounds like there are potentially lots of causes of AFP. How do we work out if it is polio or not?'

Differential diagnoses

The differential diagnosis of AFP is broad, with both infective and non-infective causes (Table 17.1).

In broad terms, the following will help lead to a diagnosis (polio or otherwise):

- history and examination
- MRI spine
- electromyography/nerve conduction studies (EMG/NCS)
- cerebrospinal fluid (CSF) examination (lumbar puncture)
- microbiologic tests of specimens
- serum creatine kinase (CK) (raised in primary muscular disorders)
- muscle biopsy if the above investigations suggest a muscular origin
- detection of high levels of heavy metals (e.g. blood lead level)

The history and examination may provide a number of supportive features:

Vaccination history Poliomyelitis is less likely if the patient has been fully immunised. Vaccine-associated paralytic poliomyelitis (VAPP) is a possibility if the patient or a household contact has recently been vaccinated against polio.

Recent consumption of canned food This raises the possibility of botulism, especially if the food was home canned. However botulism tends to be symmetric and usually commences with cranial nerve palsies, unlike Roger's illness.

Table 17.1 Causes of acute flaccid paralysis

Viral	poliovirus, enterovirus
	coxsackie virus
	Japanese encephalitis
	West Nile virus
	HIV
	Epstein-Barr virus (EBV)
	cytomegalovirus (CMV)
	varicella zoster virus (VZV)
	Murray Valley virus
Non-viral infective causes	*Mycoplasma*
	Borrelia
	diphtheria
	botulism
Disorders of the neuromuscular junction	myasthenia gravis
	Eaton-Lambert syndrome
Neuropathies	acute inflammatory demyelinating polyneuropathy
	acute motor axonal neuropathy
	critical illness neuropathy
	lead poisoning
	other heavy metal poisoning
Spinal cord diseases	trauma
	infarction
	cord compression
	transverse myelitis
Muscular conditions	polymyositis
	other myositis
	myopathy
Functional weakness	

SOURCE Adapted from Howard, 2005

History of an animal bite This should include asking about tick and snakes, even many years ago. It raises the possibility of tick paralysis, paralytic rabies (also known as dumb rabies), especially if post-exposure prophylaxis (PEP) was not used at the time. Patients often give a history of paraesthesia or disturbed sensation at the site of the bite.

Travel history If the patient has travelled to regions where other infective agents of AFP are found—e.g. polio or West Nile virus—these must be considered in the diagnosis provided the incubation period and time of travel fit.

Prodrome illness A febrile prodrome definitely supports an infective cause of AFP. Guillain-Barré syndrome (GBS) must also be considered when an infection-like illness occurs before onset of the AFP. Botulism is typically not associated with fevers.

History of head or back trauma

Interval between the febrile illness and onset of weakness
Two-thirds of patients with GBS experience an infection in the preceding month. However, the interval between the febrile illness and onset of symptoms is usually at least 10 days, rather than the three-day interval in Roger's case.

> Roger is unsure of his vaccination history. His mother would probably know but she is back in Nigeria. To his knowledge, neither he nor anyone in his household have been recently vaccinated against polio. He doesn't remember ever having an animal or tick bite or any trauma to his head or back. This is his first trip outside Nigeria.
>
> 'Does his examination support a diagnosis of polio?' Petra asks.

Polio tends to cause asymmetric AFP and the weakness most commonly involves the proximal musculature, with the lower limbs more frequently involved than the upper limbs (Modlin, 2005). GBS and botulism typically cause symmetric disease. In patients with tick paralysis, the tick can usually be found on the body at the time of examination.

> 'What tests should I order?' Petra wants to know.
> 'Let's start with an MRI,' Mercedes replies.
> 'What are you looking for?'

Investigations

Paralytic polio is due to inflammation of the grey matter of the spinal cord, specifically the anterior horn cells. The term poliomyelitis reflects this anatomical predilection: polios means grey, myelos means marrow (referring to the grey matter of the cord,) and -itis indicates inflammation.

Paralytic polio can cause changes in the anterior grey matter on MRI. However, the test is not very sensitive (people with paralytic polio may still have a normal MRI spine) and does not have a good positive predictive value either (other viruses can cause MRI changes in the anterior grey matter in AFP, e.g. EV 71) (Huang et al., 1999). Therefore the main advantage of MRI spine in this situation is to exclude other diagnoses, such as transverse myelitis, cord compression and demyelination.

The MRI spine is normal, which still means that paralytic polio is potentially the diagnosis.
'Okay, let's order an EMG.'

EMG/NCS can be helpful. It may provide diagnostic findings characteristic of paralytic polio and exclude motor axon or anterior horn disease (Solomon and Willison, 2003). Characteristic findings are:

- reduced compound muscle action potentials (CMAP)
- normal sensory nerve action potentials (SNAP)
- positive sharp waves and fibrillations

The presence of reduced velocities in both motor and sensory nerves as well as delayed distal latencies would support an acute demyelinating process such as GBS and make polio unlikely.

Roger undergoes EMG/NCS: it demonstrates reduced CMAP, normal SNAP, positive fibrillations and sharp waves. There is no evidence of demyelination. Polio is still a possibility.
'A lumbar puncture is the next step,' Mercedes says.
'What would you expect to find?'

As Melnick (1996) points out, as with most viral infections affecting the central nervous system, polio will produce CSF with a pleocytosis usually under 500 cells/μL (early on a polymorphonuclear response occurs, followed by a mononuclear response within a few days) and a raised protein count.

Preliminary CSF analysis may reveal albuminocytologic dissociation (raised protein in the absence of pleocytosis). This is associated with GBS and would make polio unlikely.

Roger's CSF is clear with normal pressure. Within half an hour, the lab calls with a pleocytosis of 200 white cells/μL (60% polymorphs, 40% mononuclears) and a raised protein of 60 mg/dL. The Gram stain is negative, which also supports a diagnosis of polio.
'So have we confirmed our diagnosis?'

The MRI, EMG/NCS and CSF findings do not confirm poliomyelitis but they do make a diagnosis of GBS unlikely. A confirmatory diagnosis requires identification of the poliovirus. In addition, microbiologic tests need to be performed to look for other infectious causes of AFP (Table 17.2).

The molecular laboratory receives the CSF, stool and throat specimens. They will start PCR testing tomorrow. Dr Wanda Lam (PhD), the infection control nurse, wants to know what precautions should be taken when nursing this patient with specific regard to poliovirus.

Isolation measures

People infected with poliovirus will shed virus in stool for around six weeks. This is irrespective of whether they have been naturally infected with wild-type poliovirus (whether symptomatic or asymptomatic) or are shedding a vaccine strain after being immunised with the oral vaccine. However, the concentration of virus in stool decreases with time: virus can be recovered from the stool of 80% of patients in the first two weeks of illness but only 25% in the third two-week period after illness. There is also a period of shedding in the oropharynx but only for 2–3 days, on average. Immunodeficient people can shed poliovirus in the stool for many months but this seems to be rare.

In other words, the main mode of spread is faeco-oral, usually from person-to-person. Occasionally, sewage-derived water can be a

Table 17.2 Microbiological tests for causes of AFP other than polio[†]

Sample	Test
Serum	Paired baseline and convalescent sera for poliovirus, enteroviruses, coxsackie viruses, *Mycoplasma*, rabies, Japanese encephalitis, HIV, EBV, CMV, VZV, West Nile virus, Murray Valley virus, *Borrelia*
Stool	Polymerase chain reaction (PCR) and culture for enterovirus and poliovirus
	Culture for *C. botulinum* and *botulinum* toxin
CSF	PCR and culture for CMV, VZV, EBV, enterovirus, rabies and poliovirus[‡]
	IgM for some of the infections listed above under 'Serum' (e.g. rabies, West Nile virus, *Borrelia*)—talk to the microbiology laboratory about which infections can be tested for in this manner
Throat	PCR and culture for poliovirus and enterovirus
	Culture for *C. diphtheriae* and test for *C. diphtheria* toxin

[†]This list covers the important infective causes of AFP. However, not all tests need to be ordered for every case. Investigations should be guided by the patient's exposure history and findings. For example, patients unlikely to have botulism should not be tested for this.
[‡]It is worth examining the CSF for poliovirus but rare to isolate it (Modlin, 2005). Other enteroviruses, on the other hand, are more likely to be isolated from CSF (Melnick, 1996). Isolation of poliovirus from the CSF is particularly useful in VAPP due to the oral (Sabin) vaccine—one would expect recently-vaccinated individuals to shed poliovirus in faeces, so without CSF confirmation clinicians can only guess that vaccination is the culprit.
SOURCE: Adapted from Modlin, 2005 and Melnick, 1996

vehicle of infection through drinking, bathing or irrigation. Even houseflies have been implicated as transmitting the virus (Halsey et al., 2004; Melnick, 1996).

Therefore, for suspect or confirmed polio patients, the following precautions would be reasonable in the hospital setting:

- single room and bathroom/toilet
- gloving and gowning before entering the room
- good hand hygiene before and after entering the room (good hand hygiene should apply to all patient contact anyway!)

> The lab performs the enterovirus PCR the next day. The stool culture comes back positive for enterovirus.

> Petra is excited. 'So his AFP is due to an enterovirus and not to poliovirus.'

Enterovirus PCR testing will detect any enterovirus, including poliovirus—it cannot discriminate between types of enterovirus. However, the type of enterovirus can be determined once the virus has been cultured. Enterovirus cultures take only about 48 hours.

Nevertheless, the fact that the enterovirus PCR was positive in stool and not in CSF is typical of poliovirus.

> 'So let's start treatment for poliovirus or enterovirus. Can't we use pleconaril?'

Treatment

Pleconaril is a drug that prevents enteroviruses uncoating their viral capsid, stopping them from replicating their RNA. Research findings have been favourable (Rotbart et al., 2001) but the pharmaceutical company has abandoned production of the oral formulation; it is collaborating with another pharmaceutical company to trial a pleconaril nasal spray for rhinovirus infections (Webster, 2005).

> 'So how can paralytic polio be treated?'

Treatment is predominantly supportive. The paralysis extends for about three days and then stops as the fever subsides (Modlin, 2005). Supportive measures include (Howard, 2005):

Strict bed rest to prevent extension of the paralysis
Adequate analgesia and frequent passive movements to prevent joint ankylosis and contractures
Assisted ventilation (invasive or non-invasive) if acute respiratory failure occurs
Splinting, stretching, good physiotherapy and appropriate orthoses as soon as the infection has resolved and the patient starts to mobilise; this reduces the risk of limb deformity and improves strength and function

CASE 17 POLIOMYELITIS

> Two days later, the stool cultures become positive. On the following day, molecular studies on the cultured virus reveals that it is poliovirus.
> Mercedes asks the lab, 'Now that you've isolated poliovirus, will you analyse it further?'

Actually, the laboratory will be able to discern whether the poliovirus is:

- wild-type (three serotypes exist)
- a vaccine strain of polio
- circulating vaccine-derived poliovirus (cVDPV)

> The lab determines that Roger has a cVDPV. Petra is puzzled: 'What is cVDPV?'

The oral (Sabin) polio vaccine is a live vaccine. Like wild-type poliovirus, the vaccine strain is shed in the faeces for some weeks after vaccination. This led to concerns that, in the setting of reduced community immunity to poliovirus, person-to-person transmission of vaccine strains could cause outbreaks of paralytic disease, hence the term circulating vaccine-derived polioviruses (cVDPV).

This has occurred, with outbreaks of cVDPV reported in different parts of the globe. Those infected by cVDPV have usually been incompletely immunised. A vaccine-derived strain of poliovirus is regarded as a cVDPV if it has diverged by >1% of VPI (major capsid surface protein) nucleotides from the original vaccine strain (Kew et al., 2004).

According to World Health Organization (2005) estimates, less than half of infants in Nigeria had had the third dose of polio vaccine. While this may not reflect the levels of immunisation when Roger was an infant, it shows that there have been problems with achieving high levels of complete polio immunisation in Nigeria. Incomplete immunisation would have left Roger susceptible to cVDPV.

> Petra asks whether she should call the public health unit.

Public health notification and response

Irrespective of whether a case involves wild-type or a vaccine strain, it should be reported. In fact, in many countries in the world where polio is endemic a clinical presentation with AFP alone is notifiable, even if a microbiologic diagnosis has not yet been made.

> Roger is left with negligible weakness on the right leg but moderately severe weakness on the left. He is naturally upset but is determined to commence rehabilitation. His teacher asks, 'Will he get any more problems from the polio in the future or is this it?'

Prognosis

There is a condition known as post-polio syndrome (PPS), which occurs in a high proportion of individuals with previous paralytic polio. There is typically a median interval of 36 years (range 8–71 years) between the acute attack of paralytic polio and the onset of PPS. There are a variety of symptoms associated with PPS but the most common features are fatigue (both general and muscular), new weakness (usually of the areas affected by the original episode of polio) and pain. This can result in functional deterioration.

The cause is not clear, but is thought to be a combination of age-related wear-and-tear along with degeneration of the enlarged motor units that were affected by polio (Trojan and Cashman, 2005).

> Mercedes sighs. 'Poor Roger. What bad luck to get paralytic polio.'
> Petra asks, 'Why do you keep saying paralytic polio? Polio always causes paralysis, doesn't it?'

Polio can present with the following clinical syndromes (Melnick, 1996):

- asymptomatic infection
- abortive infection (influenza-like illness that resolves)
- aseptic meningitis with or without transient paralysis
- paralytic polio: spinal 79%, bulbospinal 19% or bulbar 2%

Asymptomatic disease accounts for over 90% of polio infections and abortive infections for 4–8%. Paralytic polio occurs in only 1% of infections but causes serious problems with morbidity and mortality.

The overall mortality for paralytic disease ranges from 2–5% in children to 30% in adults. Bulbar paralytic polio is particularly dangerous because of its association with autonomic disease, haemodynamic instability, respiratory failure and dysphagia; therefore, bulbar paralytic polio can be associated with mortality rates up to 75% (Howard, 2005; National Health and Medical Research Council, 2003).

> Mercedes speaks to one of the public health physicians, Dr Glen Ford, because she is not clear on one point. 'Dr Ford, my patient got polio from a virus that ultimately was derived from a vaccine strain. Why use a dangerous live vaccine at all? It doesn't make any sense.'

There are two vaccines for poliovirus: oral polio vaccine (OPV), which contains live attenuated virus, and the inactivated polio vaccine (IPV), which contains inactivated virus. Both IPV and OPV contain types 1, 2, 3 of poliovirus.

The advantages of OPV over IPV have been:

- ease of administration
- far better induction of intestinal immunity through IgA secretion (Melnick, 1996)
- passage to unimmunised contacts through faeco-oral transmission while the vaccine strain of virus is shed in stool
- cheaper cost

The main risks of OPV are VAPP and cVDPV.

The risk of VAPP is low. The US has recorded rates of around five cases per million children vaccinated and Australia has one-tenth the US rate. In times of epidemic polio, the rate of wild-type polio infection was much higher than the rate of VAPP and the benefits of OPV far outweighed the risk.

However, because of the success of the global eradication program, many countries now have only extremely rare or no cases of wild-type polio. In this situation, the rates of VAPP have become unacceptable to heath departments. Therefore, countries like the US and Australia now recommend IPV instead of OPV for vaccination programs (National Health and Medical Research Council, 2003).

Recently, the monovalent oral type 1 poliovirus vaccine was developed. It is almost three times more effective against type 1 poliovirus than the trivalent vaccine. It will be useful in countries such as India where type 1 poliovirus still circulates because the trivalent vaccine led to preferential seroconversion to the other polioviruses, especially type 2 (Grassley et al., 2007).

References

Grassly, N.C., Wenger, J. Durrani, S., et al. (2007) Protective efficacy of a monovalent oral type 1 poliovirus vaccine: a case-control study. *Lancet* 369 (9570), 1356-62.

Halsey, N.A., Pinto. J., Espinosa-Rosales, F. et al. (2004) Search for poliovirus carriers among people with primary immune deficiency diseases in the United States, Mexico, Brazil, and the United Kingdom. *Bulletin of the World Health Organization* 82(1), 3–8.

Howard, R.S. (2005) Poliomyelitis and the postpolio syndrome. *British Medical Journal* 330(7503), 1314–18.

Huang, C.C., Liu, C.C., Chang, Y.C. et al. (1999) Neurologic complications in children with enterovirus 71 infection. *New England Journal of Medicine* 341(13), 936–42.

Kew, O.M., Wright, P.F., Agol, V.I. et al. (2004) Circulating vaccine-derived polioviruses: current state of knowledge. *Bulletin of the World Health Organization* 82(1), 16–23.

Marx, A., Glass, J.D., Sutter, R.W. (2000) Differential diagnosis of acute flaccid paralysis and its role in poliomyelitis surveillance. *Epidemiologic Reviews* 22(2), 298–316.

Melnick, J.L. (1996) Current status of poliovirus infections *Clinical Microbiology Reviews* 9(3), 293–300.

Modlin, J.F. (2005). Poliovirus. In Mandell, G.L., Bennett, J.E., Dolin, R. (eds) *Principles and Practice of Infectious Diseases*. Churchill Livingstone; Philadelphia.

National Health and Medical Research Council (2003) *Australian Immunisation Handbook. 8th Edition*. National Health and Medical Research Council; Canberra. Available from www9.health.gov.au/immhandbook (Accessed 2 December, 2005)

Rotbart, H.A., Webster, A.D., Pleconaril Treatment Registry Group (2001) Treatment of potentially life-threatening enteroviral infections with pleconaril. *Clinical Infectious Diseases* 32(2), 228–35.

Solomon, T., Willison, H. (2003) Infectious causes of acute flaccid paralysis. *Current Opinion in Infectious Diseases* 16(5), 375–81.

Trojan, D.A., Cashman, N.R. (2005) Post-poliomyelitis syndrome. *Muscle & Nerve* 31(1), 6–19.

Webster, A.D. (2005) Pleconaril—an advance in the treatment of enteroviral infection in immuno-compromised patients. *Journal of Clinical Virology* 32(1), 1–6.

World Health Organization (2005) *Immunisation coverage with 3rd dose of polio vaccine in infants, 2005*. World Health Organization; Geneva. Available from www.who.int/immunization_monitoring/diseases/ Polio_coverage_map.jpg (Accessed 5 December, 2005)

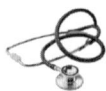

Case 18 Q fever
Ben aches and has a dry cough …

> **Q fever at a glance …**
>
> - **Agent:** family Coxiellaceae; genus *Coxiella*; species *Coxiella burnetii*
> - **Geographical distribution:** worldwide (except New Zealand)
> - **Main mode of transmission:** aerosol usually through direct or indirect animal contact
> - **Person-to-person transmission:** yes (extremely rare)
> - **Animal-to-person transmission:** yes
> - **Incubation period:** 2–3 weeks (4 days–6 weeks)
> - **Clinical features:** acute Q fever—most commonly, asymptomatic disease, febrile illness with or without pneumonia, or hepatitis; chronic Q fever—most commonly endocarditis but a wide variety of syndromes is possible
> - **Identification:** serology is the mainstay; nested polymerase chain reaction (PCR) has good positive predictive value; cultures are technically difficult
> - **Treatment:** tetracyclines are treatment of choice for acute Q fever; combination therapy may be the ideal treatment for chronic Q fever
> - **Post-exposure prophylaxis:** nil
> - **Vaccine:** inactivated vaccine exists but is not used widely

Main characters

Dr Rex Bader	general practitioner
Dr Renata Rupart	general practice registrar
Mr Ben Danstretch	young man with fevers
Ms Val Danstretch	Ben's sister
Dr Samisoni Pillay	public health official
Mr Matheus Olivetti	farmer
Ms Carla Sloan	health official from the bioprotection unit

Dr Rex Bader is a busy city general practitioner (GP). He works with his registrar, Dr Renata Rupart. The next patient is Mr Ben Danstretch, who is in town visiting his sister, Val (a regular patient of Rex's). Val accompanies Ben today.

Ben has been unwell for the last 48 hours with fevers up to 38.5°C, a headache, dry cough and myalgias. He arrived in the city two weeks ago from a nearby rural town to help Val and her cat—the cat having just given birth—move to a new apartment.

Ben is an abattoir worker and was working up until he came to visit Val. He is an otherwise healthy young man on no regular medications and with no known allergies.

Rex is concerned about the possibility of Q fever.

'Why?' asks Renata.

What is Q fever?

Q fever is a bacterial infection transmitted from animals and can present in this manner. In some parts of the world, abattoir workers must be vaccinated against Q fever before they can work, if they have not already been infected previously. The incubation period of Q fever is 2–3 weeks (4 days–6 weeks) (Parker et al., 2006), which would fit with Ben's history.

Ben tells Rex he has never heard of Q fever and, to his knowledge, has never been immunised against it.

Rex asks Renata to examine Ben and describe her findings. 'He looks moderately unwell. He doesn't have any signs of meningism; the only positive signs are a tachycardia of

CASE 18 Q FEVER

> 100 beats/minute, tachypnoea of 20 breaths/minute and some crackles in the lung bases.
> 'That suggests community-acquired pneumonia. Wouldn't that make Q fever less likely? After all, Q fever is extremely rare, isn't it?

One of the most common presentations of Q fever is community-acquired pneumonia. It accounts for 1% of cases of community-acquired pneumonia requiring hospitalisation in the UK and Europe. Unlike other patients with community-acquired pneumonia, Q fever patients are more likely to have a headache, which is more likely to be severe (Marrie, 2004). Myalgias, arthralgias and pleuritic chest pain are other common features (Parker et al., 2006).

Ben has a dry cough. Only 28% of patients with radiologically-confirmed pneumonia due to Q fever have a cough (Marrie and Raoult, 2005) and half of these have a dry cough. If Ben does have Q fever pneumonia, then Renata was lucky to hear crackles—they are normally found in only about a third of patients (Marrie, 2004).

> Rex tells Ben that he has pneumonia, possibly due to Q fever. Ben asks how it got the name.

In 1935 in Brisbane, Australia, Derrick investigated an outbreak of illness among abattoir workers. He suspected a new infectious disease, which he called Q fever, Q for 'query' because the cause was unknown. Later, the organism responsible, *Coxiella burnetii*, was identified. *C. burnetii* is phylogenetically related to *Legionella* (Coleman et al., 2004).

> Rex asks Renata for other causes of community-acquired pneumonia.

Differential diagnoses

Some causes of community-acquired pneumonia, especially in abattoir workers, include:

- *Streptococcus pneumoniae* (pneumococcus)
- *Haemophilus influenzae*

- *Mycoplasma pneumoniae*
- *Chlamydia psittaci*
- *Chlamydia pneumoniae*
- legionellosis
- influenza
- Q fever
- leptospirosis
- tularaemia
- brucellosis (uncommonly)

Rex now asks Renata how she would like to investigate Ben. She suggests baseline serology for Q fever and blood cultures. 'Cultures will easily identify Q fever as the cause, won't they?'

Investigations

This is an appropriate set of tests but Q fever is not easily identified on blood cultures without special techniques such as the shell vial cell culture system. Even these will identify only up to 15% of cases (Marrie, 2004). Because *C. burnetii* is highly infectious, cultures must occur in labs with biosafety level 3 conditions so most laboratories do not attempt them.

Serology is the mainstay of diagnosis. A number of different serologic techniques can be used including microimmunofluorescence, microagglutination, complement fixation titres and enzyme immunoassay (EIA). The sensitivity and specificity of each technique vary. Unfortunately, they often do not give a diagnosis in the acute setting: diagnostic confirmation must wait till the patient has recovered and convalescent serology returns a positive result.

Polymerase chain reaction (PCR) is not available in many laboratories. One laboratory's nested PCR had a specificity of 100%; however, the sensitivity was only 26% and was higher in the first two weeks of the illness (Fournier and Raoult, 2003). This means that the positive predictive value of the test is very good but it has a poor negative predictive value.

Rex sends Ben to the radiology practice and pathology laboratory next door. He returns two hours later with a chest X-ray and blood results. The chest X-ray is normal. 'Is that what you were expecting?' Renata asks, surprised.

Around 50% of people with Q fever pneumonia will have a normal chest X-ray. Abnormalities, when present, vary from interstitial infiltrates to rounded opacities, lobar infiltrates, hilar lymphadenopathy and pleural effusions (Martin and Marty, 2001).

Results for the acute Q fever serology won't be available for 48 hours but other blood results are shown in Table 18.1. A urinalysis is also positive for blood. Rex asks Renata whether the results are consistent with Q fever.

Ben has thrombocytopenia, leukocytosis, raised liver function tests and microscopic haematuria. Leukocytosis is seen in 25% of cases of Q fever and nearly 100% will have abnormal liver function tests. Generally, the transaminases are elevated 2–3 times normal. Bilirubin is usually normal. Thrombocytopenia occurs in 10% but thrombocytosis can also occur. Fifty percent of cases will have microscopic haematuria.

An autoimmune screen was not performed but Q fever can generate autoantibodies such as anti-smooth muscle antibodies, anticardiolipin and antimitochondrial antibodies (Marrie, 2004; Marrie and Raoult, 2005).

Renata is especially fascinated with the abnormal liver function tests: 'Don't people with Q fever hepatitis get a characteristic histological appearance?'

People with acute Q fever develop granulomas in their liver. The granulomas consist of a central lipid vacuole surrounded by a dense fibrin ring. Under the microscope, they look like round doughnuts and are therefore known as 'doughnut granulomas'. When the hepatitis is due to chronic rather than acute Q fever, doughnut granulomas tend not to be present. Instead, there is a lymphocytic infiltrate with foci of spotty necrosis (Fournier et al., 1998).

Table 18.1 Early blood results for Ben

Test	Normal range
Haemoglobin 140	130–180 g/L
Mean cell volume 82	80–100 Fl
White cell count 12[†]	3.5–11 × 10^9/L
Platelet count 120[†]	150–450 × 10^9/L
Sodium 137	135–145 mmol/L
Potassium 4.0	3.6–5.1 mmol/L
Chloride 98	95–107 mmol/L
Bicarbonate 25	22–32 mmol/L
Urea 6.2	2.9–7.1 mmol/L
Creatinine 100	60–100 μmol/L
Calcium 2.15	2.25–2.58 mmol/L
Troponin <0.1	0–0.1 μg/L
Albumin 35	33–48 g/L
Bilirubin 20	0–25 μmol/L
ALP 110	38–126 U/L
GGT 30	0–30 U/L
AST 40	<45 U/L
ALT 180[†]	<45 U/L

[†]denotes an abnormal result

'Are doughnut granulomas specific for Q fever?'

Fibrin-ring granulomas are not specific for Q fever and are associated with a number of other conditions. The following list is adapted from Marazuela et al., 1991; Ponz et al., 1991; and Tjwa et al., 2001:

Infective causes   Q fever, Epstein-Barr virus, cytomegalovirus, hepatitis A virus, visceral leishmaniasis, toxoplasmosis, Boutonneuse fever (Mediterranean spotted fever)

Non-infective causes   Hodgkin's lymphoma, allopurinol

CASE 18 Q FEVER

Ben is naturally concerned. 'Am I going to die?'

Prognosis

The mortality rate from Q fever is 1–2.4%. Most untreated patients recover, with the fever disappearing after a median of 10 days (5–57) (Marrie and Raoult, 2005; Parker et al., 2006).

'Which antibiotics do you suggest?' Renata asks Ben.

Treatment

The treatment of choice for Q fever pneumonia is oral doxycycline for 10 days. Alternatives include a fluoroquinolone (such as ciprofloxacin) or a macrolide plus rifampicin (Marrie, 2004).

Rex commences Ben on 10 days of doxycycline. He reviews him 48 hours later and is pleased to find that he is feeling better.

Ben has some questions. 'Doctor, I wash my hands thoroughly at the abattoir. I don't understand how I could have contracted this infection.'

Ben is unlikely to have contracted Q fever through poor hand washing (although his good hand washing habits should not be discouraged!). Parker et al. (2006) divide the routes of transmission of Q fever into three categories:

Person-to-person spread
Direct animal exposure   Aerosolisation of infected particles from slaughtered or parturient animals is a well-recognised risk factor. As an abattoir worker, Ben would have been exposed through direct contact with animal carcasses. Farm workers and veterinarians are two other groups likely to be directly exposed to Q fever.
Indirect animal exposure   People who do not have direct contact with animals can still be exposed to aerosols, for instance via a truck

transporting livestock or contaminated hay through a town. The aerosols consist of contaminated dust particles from desiccated reproductive fluids and, less often, from animal urine and faeces (Martin and Marty, 2001). Wind can spread Q fever aerosols for kilometres (Hawker et al., 1998). Other indirect modes of transmission include ingestion of contaminated food or milk and fomite transmission via shoes and wool contaminated with animal excreta (Woldehiwet, 2004).

> Val also has a question: 'Doctor, a friend in Southern Spain called us yesterday. When I told him that Ben had pneumonia and that it was due to Q fever, he was very surprised. He said that there is a lot of Q fever in Southern Spain but that it only affects the liver, not the lungs. I'm confused—has Ben got Q fever pneumonia?'

One of the remarkable features of Q fever is the geographical variation in clinical manifestations. Val's friend is quite right—in Southern Spain, Q fever manifests predominantly as hepatitis; however, the same organism will mainly cause pneumonia in eastern Canada and both pneumonia and hepatitis in southern France. The route of transmission may play an important role in the geographical variation of clinical manifestations (Marrie et al., 1996; Raoult et al, 2005).

> Rex explains that pneumonia is the predominant local clinical manifestation of Q fever. Val then asks, 'So people with acute Q fever infection either get pneumonia or hepatitis?'

Acute Q fever most commonly causes asymptomatic infection (60% of cases). Of the remaining 40% with symptomatic acute infection, the majority have a self-limiting febrile illness with or without pneumonia or hepatitis. However, Q fever can cause many clinical syndromes. Some patients present without fever, which makes the diagnosis more difficult (Parker et al., 2006).

Chronic Q fever most typically manifests as endocarditis, usually in the immunocompromised and those with previously abnormal valves. The risk of developing endocarditis from acute Q fever can be as high as 40%. For this reason, it is recommended that all patients with acute Q fever should undergo a transthoracic echocardiogram to detect valve lesions and have follow-up phase I serology at three and six months (see below for an explanation of phases). If the IgG titre is ≥800 in phase I, then PCR and a transoesophageal echocardiogram should be performed (Landais et al., 2007).

It can also manifest as osteomyelitis, prosthetic vascular infection, pulmonary fibrosis, skin eruptions and chronic fever, among other things (Marrie and Raoult, 2005).

> Rex tells Dr Samisoni Pillay, a local public health official, about Ben. 'I saw this young abattoir worker with pneumonia two-and-a-half weeks ago. I have just received his convalescent serology for Q fever taken on Day 14 of illness. I must admit that I always have trouble interpreting Q fever serology. I wonder if you could help me please?'
>
> Samisoni is more than happy to help and soon receives the faxed results:
>
> Q fever immunofluorescence for Ben Danstretch (DOB 25-01-1980)
>
> anti-phase II IgG—1:400 (normal <200)
> anti-phase II IgM—1:100 (normal <50)
> anti-phase I IgG—not detected (normal <800)

C. burnetii can undergo structural variation of its lipopolysaccharide wall. This is known as phase variation and is important for the pathogenicity of the organism. Antibodies to phase II predominate in acute Q fever while antibodies to phase I predominate in chronic infection.

In Rex's laboratory, an anti-phase II IgG ≥200 and an anti-phase II IgM ≥50 reflect recent infection but an anti-phase I IgG ≥800 is diagnostic for chronic Q fever. The cut-off titre values for Q fever vary in different regions of the world depending on factors such as the background prevalence of the disease.

> Samisoni goes over the concept of phase variation and confirms that Ben's serology is indeed consistent with acute Q fever. 'Thanks for that. Q fever is notifiable, isn't it?

Public health notification and response

In many countries, Q fever is notifiable to health departments or public health units. This is presumably because it is recognised both as a zoonosis and an occupational hazard for certain groups working in close proximity to animals and animal products. Furthermore, it is a vaccine-preventable disease. Public health surveillance data on Q fever notifications can identify trends and susceptible groups, resulting in positive public health actions to reduce the rate of the disease.

Since Q fever is a notifiable disease, Samisoni obtains the details of the case and speaks to Ben about his risk factors for Q fever. Like Rex, Samisoni concludes Ben must have been infected at the abattoir. Ben now wants to know whether he should be vaccinated against Q fever.

A vaccine exists but only a few countries in the world use it, for example, Australia. The vaccine has 100% efficacy and trials have demonstrated good long-term cell-mediated immunity in concert with relatively low seroconversion rates of 50–80% (National Health and Medical Research Council, 2003). It should be used for individuals at risk of contracting Q fever, such as abattoir workers, veterinarians, farmers, zoo workers, those who transport animals and stockyard workers (National Health and Medical Research Council, 2003). In Australia it is mandatory for employers of these groups to ensure their workers are vaccinated. Samisoni must inform the abattoir manager of the need to vaccinate the remaining workers or face prosecution.

However, people who have had Q fever before must not have the vaccine because of the risk of a serious hypersensitivity reaction. Individuals should have serologic testing and skin testing before being vaccinated (National Health and Medical Research Council, 2003). For two reasons, Ben does not need to be vaccinated: first, his infection means he has now developed natural immunity to Q fever; second, previous Q fever is a contraindication.

Samisoni informs Ben's local public health unit about the notification and the need to contact Ben's employer about vaccinating his co-workers.

Three weeks pass. Samisoni is on call for the weekend. His pager beeps: it's Rex. 'Samisoni, you won't believe it, but Ben's

> sister, with whom he has been staying for the past month, also developed pneumonia about two weeks ago. Could she have Q fever too, and could she have caught it from Ben?'

Q fever is highly infectious—inhaling only one organism is sufficient to cause disease (Martin and Marty, 2001). However, human-to-human transmission is extremely rare, with cases documented in the setting of autopsies, sexual intercourse and during the delivery of a baby (Parker et al., 2006).

> Samisoni wonders if there is any other common exposure that Ben and his sister may have shared. Rex recalls that Ben arrived to stay with his sister just prior to Val's pet cat giving birth. Domestic cats are an important source of Q fever infection in the urban setting (Fournier et al., 1998) and it is the reproductive fluids and tissues of these animals that are likely to have the highest amount of *C. burnetii*.
>
> Rex is surprised. 'I thought that only cows, sheep and goats were the animal reservoirs of Q fever.'

Although cows, sheep and goats are the animals most commonly recognised as reservoirs for *C. burnetii*, a wide variety of animals can be infected including dogs, rodents, small mammals, fish, amphibians, swine, birds and ticks (Parker et al., 2006).

Despite ticks being infected with *C. burnetii*, transmission to humans through tick bites is rare and may not even occur. However, inhalation of tick faeces, which are found in animal hides and clothing, can be a source of human infection (Parker et al., 2006).

> 'The other issue is that Val might be pregnant,' Rex says. 'We are performing an urgent test today. If it is Q fever, could it affect the pregnancy?'

Q fever during pregnancy has been associated with spontaneous abortion, low birth weight and premature birth (Raoult et al., 2005). The pathogenesis is unknown but may relate to immune complex deposition and subsequent vascular thromboses and vasculitis (Raoult et al., 2000).

> 'If the cat was infected with Q fever, would it have been sick?'

Although Q fever can cause problems such as abortions, many animals will be asymptomatic.

> Samisoni says it would be unlikely for Val to have Q fever, although it a remote possibility. There is more likely to be another cause for her community-acquired pneumonia.
> 'How can we confirm whether the cat was responsible for any infection?' Rex asks.

It is unlikely that a standard laboratory would be able to assist in the diagnosis but a specialised veterinary laboratory may be able to test reproductive fluids and tissue with PCR and culture as well as perform serologic assays on the cat. Because the cat delivered many weeks ago, it is likely that bedding soiled with reproductive tissues and fluids would have been thrown out, so they will have to rely on serology.

> Although Q fever from her cat seems unlikely, Samisoni asks Val's permission to test her cat for Q fever serology. Val agrees and a specimen is sent from the cat to the major veterinary laboratory in the country's capital city.
> The lab calls a few days later to confirm that the cat's serology is negative. Meanwhile, Val's *Legionella* urinary antigen has returned positive.
> Later in the week, Samisoni receives another enquiry about Q fever. Mr Matheus Olivetti asks, 'I want to buy a farm and have livestock. Apart from vaccinating the farm workers against Q fever, how else can I protect my workers and livestock?'

Protective measures include (Woldehiwet, 2004):

- sterilising and pasteurising milk
- ensuring all vehicles that transport animals are thoroughly washed and disinfected (this should happen routinely anyway)
- cleaning or destroying bedding that animals use when giving birth (this is more an issue in countries where animals give birth indoors)

- if Q fever is a big problem with animals, using the animal vaccine available in some countries
- routine hand washing after contact with animals or bedding material

> By this stage, Samisoni is hoping that he gets no more calls about Q fever. However, Ms Carla Sloan, from the bioprotection unit, calls to ask whether bioterrorism could be a factor in Ben's case.
> 'I don't think so, but I admit I didn't realise Q fever was a potential bioterrorism agent.'

Q fever produces a spore-like form that is resistant to adverse environmental conditions. In fact, the organism can remain infectious for over a month on fresh meat in cold storage, 7–10 months on surfaces at 15–20°C, over three years in skim milk at room temperature and for 4–5 months in formalin fixed tissues. It can even survive in paraffinised tissue blocks, so its durability would make it a good biological agent.

Additionally, it is a highly infectious bacterium—one organism is sufficient to cause infection The World Health Organization estimated that an aerosol of weaponised Q fever would result in a similar number of casualties to comparable amounts of aerosolised tularaemia or anthrax. Consequently, the Centers for Disease Control and Prevention (CDC) classify *C. burnetii* as a Type B biologic agent (Cutler et al., 2006). The only disadvantage of Q fever, from a bioterrorism viewpoint, is that it would have a lower mortality than the other two agents (Martin and Marty, 2001).

C. burnetii is so durable because it can exist in two forms, a small cell variant (SCV) and a large cell variant (LCV). The SCV is like a spore and allows the organism to persist in difficult external environmental conditions. The LCV form allows the organism to persist within the acidic environment of monocytes and macrophage phagolysosomes (Cutler et al., 2006).

> A few months pass Samisoni calls Rex to enquire about Ben and Val. Rex tells him that, unfortunately, Ben developed Q fever endocarditis. His echocardiogram showed a pre-existing heart valve lesion and 30–50% of patients with acute Q fever and underlying heart valve disease will go on to develop Q fever endocarditis (this is why all patients with acute Q fever should undergo echocardiography).

> 'I know most forms of bacterial endocarditis need 4–6 weeks of antibiotics. Is that also the case with Q fever?' Samisoni asks.

Q fever endocarditis is not easy to treat. Patients often require more than the minimum of 18 months of antibiotic therapy (with or without valve replacement) before clinicians are prepared to cease treatment.

> Rex explains that Ben is on a combination of doxycycline and hydroxychloroquine. Samisoni is surprised by this: 'I thought hydroxychloroquine wasn't an antibiotic. Why do you use it to treat an infection like Q fever?'

Hydroxychloroquine is not an antibiotic but is used to treat Q fever. The pH within the phagolysosomes of the host cells in which *C. burnetii* live is too low for the bactericidal activity of doxycycline. Adding hydroxychloroquine increases the pH of the phagolysosome, enhancing doxycycline's bactericidal activity (Raoult et al., 1999).

References

Coleman, S.A., Fischer, E.R., Howe, D. et al. (2004) Temporal analysis of *Coxiella burnetii* morphological differentiation. *Journal of Bacteriology* 186(21), 7344–52.

Cutler, S.J., Bouzid, M., Cutler, R.R. (2006) Q fever. *Journal of Infection* 54(4), 313–18.

Fournier, P.E., Raoult, D. (2003) Comparison of PCR and serology assays for early diagnosis of acute Q fever. *Journal of Clinical Microbiology* 41(11), 5094–98.

Fournier, P.E., Marrie, T.J., Raoult, D. (1998) Diagnosis of Q fever. *Journal of Clinical Microbiology* 36(7), 1823–24.

Hawker, A.I., Ayres, J.G., Blair, I. et al. (1998) A large outbreak of Q fever in the West Midlands: windborne spread into a metropolitan area? *Communicable Disease and Public Health* 1(3), 180–87.

Landais, C., Fenollar, F., Thuny, F. et al. (2007) From acute Q fever to endocarditis: serological follow-up strategy. *Clinical Infectious Diseases* 44(10), 1337–40.

Marazuela, M. Moreno, A., Yebra, M. et al. (1991) Hepatic fibrin-ring granulomas: a clinicopathologic study of 23 patients. *Human Pathology* 22(6), 607–13.

Marrie, T.J., Raoult, D. (2005) *Coxiella burnetii* (Q fever). In Mandell, G.L., Bennett, J.E., Dolin, R. (eds) *Principles and Practice of Infectious Diseases*. Churchill Livingstone; Philadelphia.

Marrie, T.J. (2004) Q fever pneumonia. *Current Opinion in Infectious Diseases* 17(2), 137–42.

Marrie, T.J., Stein, A., Janigan, D. et al. (1996) Route of infection determines the clinical manifestations of acute Q fever. *Journal of Infectious Diseases* 173(2), 484–87.
Martin, G.J., Marty, A.M. (2001) Clinicopathologic aspects of bacterial agents. *Clinics in Laboratory Medicine* 21(3), 513–48.
National Health and Medical Research Council (2003) *Australian Immunisation Handbook. 8th Edition.* National Health and Medical Research Council; Canberra. Available from http://www9.health.gov.au/immhandbook (Accessed 25 June, 2005)
Parker, N.R., Barralet, J.H., Bell, A.M. (2006) Q fever. *Lancet* 367(9511), 679–88.
Ponz, E., Garcia-Pagan, J.C., Bruguera, M. et al. (1991) Hepatic fibrin-ring granulomas in a patient with hepatitis A. *Gastroenterology* 100(1), 268–70.
Raoult, D., Marrie, T.J., Mege, J.L. (2005) Natural history and pathophysiology of Q fever. *Lancet Infectious Diseases* 5(4), 219–226.
Raoult, D., Tissot-Dupont, H., Foucault, C. et al. (2000) Q Fever 1985–1998: clinical and epidemiologic features of 1,383 infections. *Medicine* 79(2), 109–23.
Raoult, D., Houpikian, P., Tissot Dupont, H. et al. (1999) Treatment of Q fever endocarditis: comparison of two regimens containing doxycycline and ofloxacin or hydroxychloroquine. *Archives of Internal Medicine* 159(2), 167–73.
Tjwa, M., De Hertogh, G., Neuville, B. et al. (2001) Hepatic fibrin-ring granulomas in granulomatous hepatitis: report of four cases and review of the literature. *Acta Clinica Belgica* 56(6), 341–48.
Woldehiwet, Z. (2004) Q fever (coxiellosis): epidemiology and pathogenesis. *Research in Veterinary Science* 77(2), 93–100.

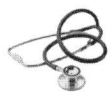

Case 19 Rabies
Desta is acting strangely …

Rabies at a glance …

- **Agent:** family Rhabdoviridae; genus *Lyssavirus*; species rabies virus
- **Geographical distribution:** worldwide (New Zealand, Papua New Guinea, Australia is rabies-free)
- **Animal-to-human transmission:** yes
- **Human-to-human transmission:** theoretically possible but never reliably documented in modern medical literature
- **Incubation period:** 1–2 months (under 7 days–over 6 years)
- **Clinical features:** typically, an acute encephalitis associated with hydrophobia and autonomic neuropathy; less commonly, acute flaccid paralysis (paralytic rabies)
- **Identification:** various techniques (antibody testing, reverse transcriptase polymerase chain reaction, culture) can be applied to various tissues (cerebrospinal fluid, skin from the nape of neck, serum, saliva, tears)
- **Treatment:** almost universally fatal (unproven treatment protocol with a combination of ribavirin, interferon-alpha, ketamine, human rabies immunoglobulin and rabies vaccine)
- **Post-exposure prophylaxis:** combination of wound cleaning, human rabies immunoglobulin and rabies vaccine
- **Vaccine:** inactivated vaccine (neurological adverse effects more likely with nerve tissue vaccines than cell culture vaccines)

CASE 19 RABIES

Main characters

Dr Mayu Akiyama	infectious diseases registrar
Ms Desta Sahle	young woman with acute confusion
Ms Jaakkina Barck	medical student doing an infectious diseases rotation
Dr Niamh O'Hare	public health physician
Ms Susan Smith	young woman bitten by a bat
Mr Peter Black	veterinarian

Dr Mayu Akiyama is an infectious diseases registrar in a regional hospital. He is asked to see a 20-year-old woman who was admitted to the high dependency unit two days earlier with an acute confusional state. Her name is Desta Sahle.

Desta is lying in bed, awake but restless and wriggling about and not capable of supplying a good history. Her mother and father are there and tell Mayu all that they know.

'She has always been a healthy girl. She is studying hospitality at the technical college and gets good grades. Then, four days ago, she started to act strangely: her attention span dropped. She would be confused for hours and then become normal again. She was sweating a lot, but we couldn't get her to keep up her fluids. Every time we gave her water, she would take a few sips and look really uncomfortable. Then she refused to drink at all. We got worried and brought her to hospital two days ago. She just seems to have become more and more confused and agitated and has developed some diarrhoea.'

The neurology resident has little to add to the history. 'The patient is becoming more and more unwell. She has been sweating profusely and salivating, been intermittently febrile and is completely confused. Today, she has had two episodes of supraventricular tachycardia, for which we have just commenced an amiodarone infusion.

'We managed to perform a lumbar puncture (LP) on the day of admission. She had a mild lymphocytic pleocytosis but the cerebrospinal fluid (CSF) was otherwise normal. Her MRI showed a few hyper-intense spots in the hypothalamus on T2-weighted images. She hasn't improved with intravenous

> (IV) acyclovir or broad-spectrum antibiotics. Her herpes simplex virus polymerase chain reaction (PCR) is pending.
> 'Could this be rabies?'

What is rabies?

Desta's discomfort with drinking water is likely to be hydrophobia, a symptom classically associated with rabies and found in 50–80% of cases. The reason for hydrophobia is presumably to reduce the amount of phobic spasms. These spasms occur because rabies causes exaggerated contractions of pharyngeal and inspiratory muscles, resulting in uncomfortable pharyngeal spasms. Precipitants for the pharyngeal spasm can be drinking or even simply being offered a drink (hydrophobia) or having air blown on the face or chest (aerophobia). Rarely, violent phobic spasms can cause pneumomediastinum (Kietdumrongwong and Hemachudha, 2005); therefore, one can understand the reluctance of people with rabies to drink.

The arrhythmias, diarrhoea, profound sweating and salivation are autonomic features that would also support a diagnosis of rabies.

The MRI and LP results, while non-specific, would also be consistent with rabies. In rabies, the MRI (usually on T2 imaging) may show high intensity areas in the hypothalamus, hippocampus and brain stem (Bleck and Rupprecht, 2005).

The death in 1849 of the famous American author Edgar Allan Poe during an acute confusional illness was only recently attributed to rabies when a physician reviewed his case notes. Poe's notes appear to describe hydrophobia as part of his acute confusional state, so rabies could well have been responsible for his demise (Benitez, 1996).

The confusion and agitation is consistent with an encephalitic picture. In summary, encephalitic or furious rabies is the likely diagnosis (there is another form of rabies known as paralytic or dumb, which will be discussed later).

> Mayu voices her concerns about rabies to Desta's parents. They look surprised. 'Doctor, isn't rabies transmitted by dogs? Desta hasn't been bitten by a dog—she'd have told us about that surely.'

CASE 19 RABIES

Rabies is a zoonosis that can be transmitted to humans by a variety of animals. Dogs are the major reservoirs of the virus worldwide but all mammals are susceptible to the rabies virus, including bats, dogs, mongooses, domestic cats, rabbits, hamsters, skunks, racoons, hyenas and jackals (Bleck and Rupprecht, 2005; Warrell and Warrell, 2004).

> As Mayu explains this to Desta's parents, her mother gasps.
> 'Oh doctor, I remember Desta mentioning that she woke up in her apartment to find a dead bat in her bedroom. It would have flown in through the open window at night. But she didn't have any signs of a bite and she didn't touch it. In fact, she picked it up with a shovel and threw it into the rubbish bin. Also, this happened 12 months ago, so this in no way could be related to her current illness, could it?'

It is possible to contract rabies from bats without even being aware of any contact. Messenger et al. (2002) found that 14/32 people with rabies due to insectivorous bats in the US could not recall any bites or contact with bats whatsoever. In fact, in some countries the discovery of a dead bat in one's bedroom would be sufficient to warrant immediate rabies post-exposure prophylaxis (PEP), irrespective of whether or not there was a bite.

Although the incubation period in the majority of cases is 1–2 months, incubation periods can be as short as seven days (especially if the virus is directly inoculated into neural tissue) or as long as over six years (Hemachudha et al., 2002). The cause of the long incubation period is not clear but may relate to local replication of the virus in striated muscle at the site of inoculation prior to its entry into peripheral nervous tissue. Other factors may be the site and severity of the bite and the amount of inoculum received. Also, once the virus enters the peripheral nerves it travels retrogradely to the central nervous system using axoplasmic transport at a rate of 50–100 mm/day, which also adds time to the incubation period (Warrell and Warrell, 2004).

> Mayu realises she hasn't asked the parents about any prodromal symptoms that would further support a diagnosis of rabies. She runs through a mental list.

Patients may complain of itching or paraesthesias at the site of the healed animal bite prior to the onset of the encephalitis and this sensation can extend up the affected limb or side of the face. The pruritus can be so intense as to result in excoriations. This progressive reaction, starting at the bite site, is typical of rabies. Fevers and flu-like symptoms may also be present (Hemachudha et al., 2002). The prodrome, if present, will not last for more than a week.

> Desta's father thinks that she may have had an itchy forehead a few days before coming to hospital but isn't too sure. Her parents are still not willing to accept that their daughter may have rabies.
> 'Shouldn't people with rabies have fits and be paralysed?'

Seizures, cranial nerve defects and hemitract signs such as hemiparesis are not typical of encephalitic rabies (Hemachudha et al, 2002).

> 'Doctor, could this be anything else?'

Differential diagnosis

The presence of the phobic spasms and hydrophobia makes all other diagnoses unlikely (Bleck and Rupprecht, 2005). In the absence of phobic spasms and hydrophobia, however, a list of differential diagnoses must be considered for encephalitic rabies and paralytic rabies (the differences between these two types of rabies are discussed below), including:

For encephalitic rabies other causes of viral encephalitis, acute hepatic porphyria, tetanus, strychnine poisoning, drug abuse/withdrawal, serotonin syndrome
For paralytic rabies Guillain-Barré syndrome, other causes of acute flaccid paralysis (see Case 17), transverse myelitis

> 'How can you confirm whether my daughter has rabies, Doctor?'

Investigations

There are a number of tests for rabies. It is recommended that they *all* be performed in order to increase the sensitivity of testing. Often, multiple specimens may be needed (Bleck and Rupprecht, 2005; Centers for Disease Control and Prevention, 2003; Warrell and Warrell, 2004). Tests include:

Skin biopsy This has long been regarded as the gold standard in diagnosing rabies. The biopsy is taken from the nape of the neck above the hairline to detect rabies antigen by an immunofluorescent antibody (IFA) test and/or rabies RNA by reverse transcriptase polymerase chain reaction (RT-PCR). The rationale behind using skin from this site is that the virus migrates to and settles in hair follicles. Typically, a specimen should have at least 10 hair follicles, including the cutaneous nerves that are associated with the follicles (Centers for Disease Control and Prevention, 1998). It is 50% sensitive in the first week of illness and sensitivity rises from the second week.

Lumbar puncture to detect virus by culture, RNA by RT-PCR and antibodies. The preliminary examination of CSF (e.g. cell count, protein) may be normal or only mildly abnormal with a slight mononuclear pleocytosis and minor elevation in protein, which are unhelpful in differentiating rabies from other illnesses.

Samples of saliva and tears for RT-PCR

Serum and CSF for antibody testing

It is difficult to interpret the presence of antibodies in patients who have been previously vaccinated for rabies. Nevertheless, a high antibody concentration in the CSF, even in vaccinated individuals, has been regarded as diagnostic of rabies. In vaccinated patients, one should collect a second CSF sample to look for rising titres. In unvaccinated patients, antibodies are often only seen in the second week of clinical illness (50% by Day 8 of illness, 100% by Day 15) but their presence is diagnostic. Antibodies, both in serum and CSF, are likely to be negative in Desta's early illness and not of much assistance, although they could serve as baseline levels.

Mayu organises all the above tests for Desta. Luckily, the rabies reference laboratory is 300 km away and they are able to perform the tests and provide results within 48 hours.

While waiting for the tests, Ms Jaakkina Barck, one of the infectious diseases medical students, has some questions. 'About two years ago, I saw a rabies patient in the emergency department.

> I am pretty sure that he had paralysis of the lower limbs and wasn't confused like this patient. Could the doctors there have been wrong about the diagnosis?'

Although rabies can have various clinical manifestations, nearly all cases present as furious rabies or paralytic rabies. Furious rabies, also known as classical or encephalitic rabies, accounts for almost 80% of clinical presentations. Paralytic rabies, also known as dumb rabies accounts for about 20% (Bleck and Rupprecht, 2005). Desta's presentation with the hyperactivity and hydrophobia is consistent with furious rabies.

Paralytic rabies presents with a flaccid paralysis with sphincteric involvement, and may easily be confused with Guillain-Barré syndrome. It is only later that the cerebral involvement becomes apparent. It is also worth noting that only 50% of patients with paralytic rabies develop phobic spasms, compared to all patients with furious rabies (Hemachudha et al., 2002). Non-classical signs include myoclonus, choreiform movements of the bitten limb, brainstem signs, ataxia and Horner's syndrome, to name but a few (Hemachudha et al., 2002).

> 'I know that one of the emergency physicians thought rabies was unlikely because the patient didn't have percussion myoedema. Is that right?'

Percussion myoedema is a clinical sign best elicited by percussing the muscle over the deltoid, thigh and chest. This results in mounding of the muscle, which spontaneously resolves over a few seconds.

It supposedly is found only in paralytic rabies, not in the furious form which Desta has, and can occur also in other conditions, such as hyponatraemia, renal failure and hypothyroidism (Hemachudha et al., 2002). With regard to stage of illness, percussion myoedema can occur in the prodrome and persists thereafter (Bleck and Rupprecht, 2005).

> The reference laboratory calls back: Mayu is right and Desta has rabies. The IFA and RT-PCR of her skin biopsy were positive, as was the RT-PCR of saliva. As suspected, antibodies weren't detectable at such an early stage of the illness.

Mayu conveys these findings to Desta's parents. They are understandably upset. 'What will happen to her?'

Prognosis

The mortality rate of rabies in the absence of pre-exposure or post-exposure immunisation is almost 100%. No medications have been shown to be effective. Desta has experienced three of the fives stages of rabies—an incubation period, prodrome and acute neurological syndrome—and she will almost certainly progress to the next two stages, namely, coma followed 10–14 days later by death from a cardiac or respiratory cause (Hemachudha et al., 2002).

Treatment

A working group has suggested that combination therapy may be of benefit in certain cases. This, however, has not been proven or guaranteed to work (Jackson et al., 2003). Five possible agents which may be used are:

1. Rabies vaccine intradermally in multiple sites
2. Human rabies immunoglobulin intramuscularly
3. Ribavirin intravenously and intraventricularly
4. Interferon-alpha intravenously and intraventricularly
5. Ketamine, a non-competitive antagonist of the N-methyl-D-aspartate

In the only reported case of survival from rabies without any pre- or post-exposure prophylaxis, the treatment included inducing a coma and using ketamine, phenobarbital, benzodiazepines, ribavirin and amantadine (Willoughby et al., 2005). The 15-year-old girl had residual neurological defects five months later (Centers for Disease Control and Prevention, 2004a).

The intensivist working in the high dependency unit wonders about the role of corticosteroids in reducing the inflammation.

Corticosteroids worsened the outcome in experiments on mice with rabies 35 years ago (Enright et al., 1970).

The intensive care team, in consultation with experts in neurology and infectious diseases, institute combination therapy. However, Desta falls into a coma and dies five days later.

Rabies is a notifiable disease, so Mayu contacts the public health unit. She speaks to Dr Niamh O'Hare. 'Hi, I believe that you have already been notified of a case of rabies in a girl who died yesterday?'

'That's right.'

'A very sad business indeed. However, three nurses who looked after this girl have been asking me about whether they need post-exposure prophylaxis for rabies (POPR).

'One of them got splashed in the eye with respiratory secretions while suctioning the patient's airway. The other nurse's exposed arm got splashed with urine when she changed the catheter bag; she had no cuts or tears on the skin where the urine hit her. The third nurse got splashed with saliva on his hand; again the skin was intact.

'I have no idea how to advise them. Can you help me out please?'

Public health notification and response

Except in the setting of solid organ and corneal transplants (Centers for Disease Control and Prevention, 2004b), there have been no well-documented cases of human-to-human transmission of rabies, although Helmick et al. (1987) list some anecdotal reports going back hundreds of years. Certainly it is a theoretical possibility. As with any occupational exposure, the risk of infection is related to the nature of the injury and the type of body fluid involved.

With regard to the type of body fluid involved, rabies virus has been isolated in saliva, tears, CSF, nerve tissue, corneal tissue and solid organs. It has not been found in blood, urine or faeces. As for the type of injury, it is believed that the infectious fluids can only infect the healthcare worker through contact with mucous membranes or broken skin. Intact skin is a barrier to infected fluids.

Knowing this, Niamh should advise Mayu as follows. The first nurse was exposed to infectious fluids (airway secretions probably mixed with saliva) on mucous membranes (the eye) and should receive POPR. The second nurse was hit by a non-infectious fluid (urine) on intact skin and so does not need POPR. The third nurse was hit by an infectious fluid (saliva) but on intact skin and therefore does not need POPR.

Mayu thanks Niamh for his advice. 'Now I also had a call from the patient's boyfriend about whether he needs to do anything. He tells me that they have been sexually active, even on the day that she first became sick. I guess he needs POPR?'

Contacts of index cases with rabies should receive POPR if they have had contact with the saliva or neurological tissue of an infectious case, for example, kissing on the mouth, sexual activity, bites, or sharing food, cups or cutlery (NSW Health, 2004). Desta's boyfriend definitely needs POPR because his mucous membranes would have come in contact with her infectious saliva.

Mayu thanks Niamh for his advice and says goodbye. A few minutes later, Niamh receives a call from a general practitioner (GP) about an elderly female patient. The patient was walking in the park and saw a dog acting very strangely, yelping and frothing at the mouth. It came up to her and licked her on the hand, then ran off. She has never seen the dog before.
'Could she get rabies?'

US experts recommend quarantining domestic animals that have bitten humans and observing them for a 10-day period. If the animal develops signs of a rabies-like illness during that time, it is put down immediately and sent within 24–48 hours for a post-mortem to exclude rabies. This provides adequate time for the human who was bitten by the animal to receive adequate protection from POPR (National Association of State Public Health Veterinarians, 2005). In fact, in some regions with a high prevalence of rabies or in individuals with a high-risk injury, it may be worth commencing POPR and discontinuing it if the animal is well after 10 days or the test results are negative for rabies. Stray or wild animals are put down immediately and sent for a post-mortem. Unfortunately, in this case the dog's whereabouts are unknown.

Where rabies is endemic—which is most of the world—some countries (e.g. the US) have policies of the mandatory or recommended vaccination of domestic animals and livestock against rabies (National Association of State Public Health Veterinarians, 2005). Niamh's country is one where rabies vaccination of all domestic dogs and cats is mandatory. After the initial vaccination, boosters must be given every 12 months. Pet owners have to provide certification that the immunisation is up to date. It would be very uncommon for a vaccinated animal to develop rabies but it is still worth erring on the side of caution and quarantining the animal for 10 days.

Although rabies vaccination of domestic animals is a good idea, it requires a lot of time and resources to implement and monitor and this is simply not possible for some countries. In this case, however, the identity of the dog and therefore its vaccination status are unknown.

The other issue is the type of exposure. The patient was licked on the skin by the dog. The World Health Organization (2002) has protocols for dealing with the different types of animal exposures. It divides exposures into categories I to III, with III being the most serious. Being licked on intact skin by a potentially rabid animal is the lowest risk group, category I. The recommendation is for no action provided the history is reliable. However, if there is any uncertainty about whether the licked skin was intact or not, then vaccination alone (without using immunoglobulin) is recommended.

> The GP says the patient is 100% certain her skin was intact when the dog licked her. Niamh explains that this is a category I exposure and requires no action.
>
> Two weeks later, Niamh receives a call from Ms Susan Smith, who returned from a trip to Australia yesterday. 'I was bitten by a bat on the east coast of Australia three days ago. But my travelling companion told me that there is no rabies in Australia. So I didn't do anything. I just wanted to double check with the experts, such as yourself. I hope I'm not wasting your time.'

Rabies is only one of seven different genotypes of lyssavirus. Rabies was the first lyssavirus to be identified and is probably the best known. Six of the seven genotypes of lyssavirus, including rabies, can be transmitted by bats. The five other genotypes of lyssavirus are Lagos bat virus, Mokola, Duvenhage, European bat lyssavirus type 1 and European bat lyssavirus type 2 (Warrell and Warrell, 2004).

The most recently discovered lyssavirus is the Australian bat lyssavirus (ABL, genotype 7). As the name suggests, ABL is transmitted only by insectivorous or frugivorous bats and has been linked to two deaths in Australia. From these two cases, it appears that ABL has the same terrible clinical course as rabies. Therefore, while Susan is not at risk of rabies itself, the bat bite could have exposed her to ABL. This is a serious injury indeed.

> 'There must be something I can do to protect myself—is there a vaccine or something?'

There are no specific vaccines for ABL. However, POPR appears to be effective (Hooper et al., 1997).

> Niamh conveys this to Susan. She is naturally alarmed and keen to commence immunisation. However, Niamh first wants to know whether she cleaned the wound when she was bitten. Susan is slightly annoyed by the question:
> 'Why are you wasting time asking me if I cleaned the wound? That's not going to stop me getting this bat virus infection. Give me the needles—they are the priority!'

Although immunisation is definitely a necessary part of POPR, the importance of cleaning the wound cannot be emphasised enough. Warrell and Warrell (2004) note that simply washing the wound thoroughly with soap and water can increase survival by 50%! Also it is advisable to follow this up by applying a virucidal agent such as povidone-iodine to the wound (National Health And Medical Research Council, 2003). Another principle of wound management in rabies is to avoid using primary sutures in the wound (i.e. leaving the wound open) until it has been infiltrated with immunoglobulin.

> Susan apologises to Niamh once she hears why he wanted to know whether she had cleaned the wound. Apparently, Susan was so revolted at the thought of being bitten by a bat that she immediately cleaned the wound thoroughly with soap, water and a number of antiseptic agents.
> 'So what shots will I need?'

POPR involves five doses of rabies vaccine and one dose of human rabies immunoglobulin (HRIG). One mL of vaccine should be given at Days 0, 3, 7, 14 and 30, intramuscularly or subcutaneously. As much HRIG as possible must be infiltrated in and around the wound. The remaining HRIG should be given intramuscularly. This can be particularly uncomfortable for the patient but failing to administer HRIG in and around the wound, even if all five doses of vaccine have been given, can still result in rabies (Wilde et al., 1996). HRIG must be administered within seven days of the first dose of vaccine or not given at all.

Availability of both HRIG and equine immunoglobulin is a big problem in many countries, especially developing ones, but there are alternatives to standard POPR.

Multi-site intradermal (rather than intramuscular) injections of vaccine is one strategy for hastening the neutralising antibody response. However, HRIG is still the preferred treatment. There has recently been one death from rabies in a child who received multi-site intradermal vaccinations without immunoglobulin (Sriaroon et al., 2003). Also, chloroquine (an antimalarial) may interfere with the neutralising antibody response from the multi-site intradermal method. Individuals taking chloroquine should have intramuscular injections (Van den Enden, 2005).

> Susan hears this and says, 'Five doses of vaccine . . . sounds painful. I guess they better be given in my bottom where there's more flesh and less pain!'

The antibody response to rabies vaccine is best when the vaccine is administered in the deltoid area.

> 'Are there any side effects I should know about?'

There are two kinds of rabies vaccines: cell culture vaccines and nerve tissue vaccines. The nerve tissue vaccines are more likely to be associated with serious neurological complications, such as Guillain-Barré syndrome and encephalomyelitis. Consequently, the cell culture vaccines are preferred but they are associated with higher production costs which may make them inaccessible to some developing nations (Jackson, 2002). The most common adverse events are a sore arm at the site of injection, headaches, malaise and nausea. Serious allergic reactions are rare (National Health And Medical Research Council, 2003).

HRIG is also safe (Rupprecht and Gibbons, 2004). However, some countries use the cheaper equine rabies immunoglobulin (from horses) and this tends to be associated with more adverse events (Jackson, 2002).

> 'By the way, I take prednisone for rheumatoid arthritis. Does that mean the immunisations won't work?'

Immunosuppressive diseases or medications can reduce the antibody response to the immunisation course. Immunosuppressed individuals should have their antibody titres checked 2–4 weeks after completing the immunisation course (National Health and Medical Research Council, 2003).

> 'Is there anything else I should do?'

Tetanus and other bacterial infections could complicate this wound. Susan should show the wound to a doctor and get a tetanus immunisation and/or antibiotics if necessary.

> Niamh soon gets a call from Mr Peter Black, a veterinarian.
> 'I'm about to spend 12 months working in Sri Lanka before returning to work in the zoo, where I'll be handling a variety of animals. I have never been vaccinated for rabies. Do I need rabies vaccination?'

Two common indications for pre-exposure prophylaxis for rabies (PEPR) are spending prolonged periods of time in a country where rabies is endemic and ongoing contact with animals that could develop rabies, as happens with veterinarians, animal handlers, park rangers and people working in labs with live lyssaviruses (National Health and Medical Research Council, 2003). Peter meets the criteria for PEPR on both counts. PEPR normally consists of three injections of vaccine intramuscularly or subcutaneously given at Days 0, 7 and 28.

> Peter says, 'I thought I'd need it. But I have two questions. First, do I need to check the antibody levels after these shots? And second, if I do get bitten in Sri Lanka, will I have to have the full POPR?'

In the absence of an immunosuppressive illness, routine testing of antibody levels is not necessary. One advantage of receiving PEPR is that Peter will need only three rather than the usual five immunisations of POPR if he is ever bitten (National Health and Medical Research Council, 2003).

> 'Will I need boosters, especially if I continue working at the zoo for many years?'

Peter can have a booster every two years or have his antibody titres checked, getting a booster if the levels are low. Individuals working in labs with live lyssaviruses should have antibody levels measured every six months (National Health and Medical Research Council, 2003).

> 'Out of curiosity, do you know why it's called rabies?'

Rabies is the Latin word for madness. The word lyssa (as in lyssavirus) is derived from the Greek word for madness. Who can criticise anyone from ancient times for creating these names after they encountered a crazed, vicious dog, foaming at the mouth?

References

Benitez, R.M. (1996) A 39-year-old man with mental status change. *Maryland Medical Journal* 45(9), 765–66.

Bleck, T.P., Rupprecht, C.E. (2005) Rabies virus. In Mandell, G.L., Bennett, J.E., Dolin, R. (eds) *Principles and Practice of Infectious Diseases*. Churchill Livingstone; Philadelphia.

Centers for Disease Control and Prevention (2004a) Recovery of a patient from clinical rabies—Wisconsin, 2004. *Morbidity and Mortality Weekly Report* 53(50), 1171–73.

Centers for Disease Control and Prevention (2004b) Investigation of rabies infections in organ donor and transplant recipients—Alabama, Arkansas, Oklahoma, and Texas, 2004. *Morbidity and Mortality Weekly Report* 53(26), 586–89.

Centers for Disease Control and Prevention (2003) *Rabies diagnosis*. Available from www.cdc.gov/ncidod/dvrd/rabies/Diagnosis/diagnosi.htm (Accessed 19 June, 2007)

Centers for Disease Control and Prevention (1998) *Collection of samples for diagnosis of rabies in humans*. Available from www.cdc.gov/ncidod/dvrd/rabies/professional/Prof.forms/antem.htm (Accessed 18 July, 2005)

Enright, J.B., Franti, C.E., Frye, F.L. et al. (1970) The effects of corticosteroids on rabies in mice. *Canadian Journal of Microbiology* 16(8), 667–75.

Helmick, C.G., Tauxe, R.V., Vernon, A.A. (1987) Is there a risk to contacts of patients with rabies? *Reviews of Infectious Diseases* 9(3), 511–18.

Hemachudha, T., Laothamatas, N., Rupprecht, C.E. (2002) Human rabies: a disease of complex pathogenetic mechanisms and diagnostic challenges. *Lancet Neurology* 1(2), 101–09.

Hooper, P., Lunt, R., Gould, A. et al. (1997). A new lyssavirus—the first endemic rabies-related virus recognized in Australia. *Bulletin de l'Institut Pasteur* 95(4), 209–18.

Jackson, A.C., Warrell, M.J., Rupprecht, C.E. et al. (2003) Management of rabies in humans. *Clinical Infectious Diseases* 36(1), 603.

Jackson, A.C. (2002) Update on rabies. *Current Opinion in Neurology* 15(3), 327–31.

Kietdumrongwong, P., Hemachudha, T. (2005) Pneumomediastinum as initial presentation of paralytic rabies: a case report. *BMC Infectious Diseases* 5, 92.

Messenger, S.L., Smith, J.S., Rupprecht, C.E. (2002) Emerging epidemiology of bat-associated cryptic cases of rabies in humans in the United States. *Clinical Infectious Diseases* 35(6), 738–47.

National Association of State Public Health Veterinarians, Inc. (NASPHV) (2005) Compendium of animal rabies prevention and control, 2005. *Morbidity and Mortality Weekly Report Recommendations and Reports* 54(RR-3), 1–8.

National Health and Medical Research Council (2003) *Australian Immunisation Handbook. 8th Edition*. National Health and Medical Research Council; Canberra. Available from www9.health.gov.au/immhandbook (Accessed 19 May, 2006)

NSW Health (2004) *Rabies and other lyssavirus infections. Response protocol for NSW Public Health Units*. Available from www.health.nsw.gov.au/infect/pdf/rabies.pdf (Accessed 20 June, 2007)

Rupprecht, C.E., Gibbons, R.V. (2005) Prophylaxis against rabies. *New England Journal of Medicine* 352(15), 1608–10.

Rupprecht, C.E., Gibbons, R.V. (2004) Prophylaxis against rabies. *New England Journal of Medicine* 351(25), 2626–35.

Sriaroon, C., Daviratanasilpa, S., Sansomranjai, P. et al. (2003) Rabies in a Thai child treated with the eight-site post-exposure regimen without rabies immune globulin. *Vaccine* 21(25–26), 3525–26.

Van den Enden, E. (2005) Prophylaxis against rabies. *New England Journal of Medicine* 352(15), 1608–10.

Warrell, M.J., Warrell, D.A. (2004) Rabies and other lyssaviruses. *Lancet* 363(9413), 959–69.

Wilde, H., Sirikawin, S., Sabcharoen, A. et al. (1996) Failure of postexposure treatment of rabies in children. *Clinical Infectious Diseases* 22(2), 228–32.

Willoughby, R.E., Tieves, K.S., Hoffman, G.M. et al. (2005) Survival after treatment of rabies with induction of coma. *New England Journal of Medicine* 352(24), 2508–14.

World Health Organization (2002) *Current WHO guide for rabies pre and post-exposure treatment in humans.* World Health Organization; Geneva. Available from www.who.int/rabies/en/WHO_guide_rabies_pre_post_exp_treat_humans.pdf (Accessed 15 December, 2005)

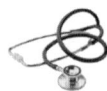

Case 20 Severe Acute Respiratory Syndrome (SARS)
Tommy has a cough and shortness of breath …

SARS at a glance …

- **Agent:** family Coronaviridae; genus *Coronavirus*; species SARS coronavirus
- **Geographical distribution:** Southern China is the major primary source but global spread from areas of local transmission may occur via travellers
- **Mode of transmission:** predominantly droplet; aerosolisation and contaminated surfaces are other potential modes
- **Person-to-person transmission:** yes
- **Incubation period:** 6 days (2–10 days)
- **Infectious period:** while symptomatic, maximally so during the second week of illness
- **Clinical features:** a fever-myalgia syndrome followed by gastrointestinal and respiratory symptoms which can proceed to severe pneumonia; young children have a milder illness than adults
- **Identification:** virus can usually be detected through reverse transcriptase polymerase chain reaction (RT-PCR) or culture of respiratory, faecal and urine specimens but the timing of the peak excretion of virus varies between the different anatomical sites; seroconversion can be detected, ideally with baseline and convalescent sera
- **Prophylaxis:** personal protective equipment and other infection control measures
- **Treatment:** no clear guidelines exist but promising agents include corticosteroids, ribavirin, protease inhibitors, niclosamide, nitric oxide, interferons, glycyrrhizin and RNA interference treatment
- **Post-exposure prophylaxis:** nil
- **Vaccine:** still at the research stage

Main characters

Dr Mary Timbu	general practitioner
Mr Tommy Anand	man with a cough and shortness of breath
Mr Cyrus Verreault	infectious diseases nurse at a public health unit
Dr Roy Powers	infectious diseases specialist
Ms Gillian Smead	head infection control nurse at a hospital

> The international medical community is on alert following an outbreak of severe acute respiratory syndrome (SARS) in Asia. Dr Mary Timbu is a general practitioner (GP) in a large city in a developed country that has had four suspect cases so far. Her receptionist puts through a call from a patient, Mr Tommy Anand, requesting an urgent appointment. Tommy has been to an affected area and is feeling unwell. 'What should I do?' he asks.

What is SARS?

Severe acute respiratory syndrome (SARS) is caused by a positive-sense, single-stranded RNA coronavirus: SARS-coV.

SARS coV causes pulmonary damage directly, via viral destruction of epithelium and macrophages in the bronchi and alveoli, and indirectly, via the production of immune system mediators (Perlman and Dandekar, 2005). It can be fatal.

It could be disastrous to allow a SARS patient into a waiting room, so GPs should determine whether a patient is a suspect SARS case *before* they arrive at the practice. One way is by triaging patients over the phone to see whether they meet the case definition for SARS.

Case definitions are readily available from a number of sources, such as online from the World Health Organization (WHO) and health departments. It is simply a matter of printing them out or writing them down and keeping them close at hand when required. Cases are classified into three groups: suspect, probable and confirmed.

> Mary has a copy of the case definition for suspected SARS patients:
> - fever >38°C AND

CASE 20 SEVERE ACUTE RESPIRATORY SYNDROME (SARS)

> - cough or difficulty breathing AND
> - one or more of the following exposures during the 10 days prior to onset of symptoms
>
>   - close contact with a person who is a suspect or probable case of SARS
>   - history of travel to an area with recent local transmission of SARS
>   - residence in an area with recent local transmission of SARS
>
> Tommy has a cough and shortness of breath. He was in a country of local SARS transmission three days prior to the onset of symptoms. He hasn't measured his temperature but he has been hot and sweaty.
>
> He could well be a suspect case of SARS. Mary runs through the options with him.

Three options are available for GPs confronted by suspected SARS patients:

- refer them to hospital
- assess them during a home visit
- assess them in the practice, taking appropriate measures to prevent cross-infection

The final two options depend on GPs being appropriately equipped with personal protective equipment (PPE) and confident about using it correctly. The PPE for SARS includes (Department of Health and Ageing, 2004):

- N95 (or P2) masks
- disposable, sterile gloves
- disposable, long-sleeved gowns
- protective eyewear
- alcohol hand rub
- surgical masks
- disposable garbage bags
- disposable thermometers or thermometer covers for once-only use
- hospital-grade disinfectant
- a single stethoscope, which is disinfected after use

A N95 mask has an efficiency ≥95% against particulate aerosols free of oil and reduces the risk of exposure to particles 0.1–>10 microns. It is equivalent to a P2 mask, often worn in Europe.

Mary decides to go to Tommy's house. She dons her PPE and goes inside, immediately giving him a surgical mask to wear. He looks slightly unwell, as if he has the flu. He tells her went overseas for two weeks on business. His business colleague was hospitalised for acute appendicitis and he visited her in hospital on a number of occasions. Four days ago, during his flight home, he began to feel hot and cold with generalised muscle aches. On arrival, airport authorities checked his temperature but found him to be afebrile and sent him home. Today, he became slightly short of breath with a non-productive cough.

Physical examination shows he is febrile to 38.7°C, tachycardic and tachypnoeic but his lungs are unremarkable. Clearly, Tommy meets the case definition for a suspect case of SARS.

Mary phones Mr Cyrus Verreault, an infectious diseases nurse at the nearest public health unit, who alerts the emergency medicine physician at the local teaching hospital and arranges an ambulance to transfer Tommy. The ambulance service has a protocol for picking up suspect SARS patients, involving wearing PPE and disinfecting the ambulance before it is used again. The emergency department has also prepared for such an occasion: a dedicated assessment area has been closed off.

Tommy has blood taken and a chest X-ray performed. The X-ray shows patchy bilateral opacities consistent with an infective process. He now meets the case criteria for probable SARS.

'What abnormalities would we expect to see on the blood tests of patients with SARS?' an emergency department intern asks.

SARS can cause laboratory abnormalities (Liu et al, 2004). However, these are non-specific and should not be used to confirm or exclude a diagnosis. They include the following (bracketed figures represent the percentage of patients with the abnormal finding on admission and later on in their hospitalisation, respectively):

- lymphopaenia due to direct invasion of T cells (70%, 95%)
- neutropaenia

- thrombocytopaenia (28%, 40%)
- coagulopathy
- haemophagocytosis
- hypoxaemia on arterial blood gas testing
- raised liver AST (27%, 49%)
- raised liver ALT (16%, 43%)
- raised lactate dehydrogenase (58%, 88%)
- raised creatine kinase (18%, 32%)

Tommy's blood tests show a mild lymphopaenia, hypoxaemia of 73 mm Hg and a raised ALT.

Dr Roy Powers, an infectious diseases specialist, is called. He agrees to the admission and reviews Tommy once he has been transferred to a negative-pressure room on the infectious diseases ward.

Naturally, Tommy is worried. His anxiety is heightened by not being able to see people's faces, since everyone who enters the room must wear PPE.

'Could this be anything other than SARS?'

Differential diagnoses

The case definition for probable SARS consists of fevers, respiratory symptoms and chest X-ray changes but these could be due to a number of infections. The differential diagnosis includes bacterial illnesses and other viral causes of pneumonia such as parainfluenza, adenoviruses, coronaviruses, rhinoviruses and respiratory syncytial virus.

'What tests do you want me to order to confirm the diagnosis of SARS?' Roy's resident asks.

Investigations

Identifying the virus is the key to confirming the diagnosis. This is usually achieved through reverse transcriptase polymerase chain reaction (RT-PCR), virus isolation or serology.

Most respiratory viruses are maximally shed from the respiratory tract within the first few days of illness and usually not beyond 10 days. However, with SARS-coV respiratory shedding increases over the first week, remains high over the second week (Chan et al., 2004) and often continues for over two weeks.

SARS-coV is also shed from stool, peaking just a few days after the peak in respiratory tract shedding. The ability to detect virus in stool is highest at the beginning of the second week, remains high for a further two weeks and continues for more than six weeks after symptom onset. Consequently, stool analysis can sometimes be used to confirm a late diagnosis of SARS. SARS-coV is also shed in urine, with peak shedding occurring at Weeks 3 or 4.

For this reason, cases of SARS are considered to be infectious while symptomatic but maximally so during the second week of illness (Centers for Disease Control and Prevention, 2005).

Based on these shedding properties, diagnostic protocols have been developed for the types of specimens used and the timing of their collection (Department of Health and Ageing, 2003a):

- Collect combined nose and throat swabs and, if possible, sputum on Day 4 when the SARS-coV first appears in the respiratory tract. Bronchoalveolar lavage, tracheal or nasopharyngeal aspirates, if undertaken, should be performed with maximum precautions in a negative-pressure area.
- On Day 7 collect further respiratory specimens and the first faecal specimen.
- Collect further faecal specimens at Days 10 and 14 and every 3–4 days while patient is under investigation.
- Collect serology on presentation and on Days 7, 14, 28 and 90.
- Test for other respiratory pathogens such as *Streptococcus pneumoniae, Haemophilus influenzae, Legionella, Chlamydia psittaci,* Q fever, *Mycoplasma pneumoniae,* influenza and respiratory syncytial virus.

All biological specimens from suspect or probably SARS patients must be delivered *by hand*—not sent through pneumatic or chute systems where spillage could unnecessarily put laboratory staff at risk—and the laboratory notified that specimens for SARS-coV testing are being sent.

CASE 20 SEVERE ACUTE RESPIRATORY SYNDROME (SARS)

> Since it is only the fourth day of Tommy's illness, no faecal specimens are collected. Nasopharyngeal and throat swabs are collected without incident. The reference laboratory is expecting the specimen and will have a result early tomorrow.
>
> Tommy is concerned about his family. 'My wife and my five-year-old son, what will happen to them? Will they get SARS? Can they visit me?'
>
> Roy doesn't know and phones Cyrus for advice.

Household members of potential SARS patients are usually regarded as close contacts, that is, someone 'who has lived, worked or had other dealings where they have been within 1 metre of a case or had direct contact with respiratory secretions without PPE' (Department of Health and Ageing, 2003b).

Different countries treat close contacts differently. In developed countries a typical approach is for close contacts to:

- continue with their daily routine but for 10 days measure their temperature daily and make daily contact with public health officers to discuss their clinical status
- remain in quarantine at home
- return to their normal routine once tests suggest that the index case does not have SARS

> Cyrus lets Tommy know the family are now aware that they must remain in quarantine for 10 days if he is confirmed as having SARS. Tommy is upset but understands the necessity for such measures. Cyrus explains that he needs to find out who his other close contacts have been.
>
> On the following day, Tommy is clinically unchanged apart from the onset of diarrhoea.
>
> 'Is that a surprise?' Roy's resident asks.

SARS-coV is excreted in faeces, so gastrointestinal manifestations are unsurprising. Diarrhoea is extremely common. Liu et al. (2004) found that 66% of SARS patients had diarrhoea at some stage in their clinical course, usually 6 +/−3.3 days from the onset of fevers.

The pathogenesis for the diarrhoea relates to ACE2, which is the host cell surface receptor for SARS. ACE2 is found in the lungs and gastrointestinal tracts, hence the respiratory and gastrointestinal manifestations (Perlman and Dandekar, 2005).

Roy receives a call from the chief microbiologist at the reference laboratory. It seems that both the nasopharyngeal and throat swabs are RT-PCR-positive for SARS-coV—Tommy is the country's first confirmed case of SARS.

Roy gives the news to Tommy, who is clearly shaken. 'Be honest, Doctor. What's going to happen to me. When will I get the terrible pneumonia? Am I going to die?'

Prognosis

The clinical progression of SARS can be divided into three phases (Liu et al., 2004; Peiris et al., 2003):

Phase 1 (week 1) a systemic process, characterised early on by fever and myalgias with more organ-specific involvement later in the week. This phase is probably related to viral replication and cytolysis, with improvement after a few days.

Phase 2 (week 2) fever, desaturation and, sometimes, diarrhoea. The presence of transient lung infiltrates in 50% of cases suggests something more than a purely viral effect, such as an immunological process. The latter half of this phase (Days 10–15) is characterised by severe clinical worsening associated with a fall in viral load and seroconversion to IgG.

Phase three respiratory complications Twenty percent of Peiris et al.'s cohort went on to develop ARDS. Other studies found 15% of patients required mechanical ventilation.

The overall mortality is around 10% but increases to over 50% in people over 60 years old (Groneberg et al,. 2005).

Tommy listens soberly to this information. 'So I have a nine in 10 chance of pulling through. Is there any treatment for this virus?'

Treatment

The treatment of SARS with various agents has been extensively studied during and since the original outbreaks. Groneberg et al. (2005) reviewed the literature and drew the following conclusions:

Ribavirin This provides some benefit. However, since it was given in combination with steroids, uncertainty exists as to which agent was responsible for the benefit. In vitro studies showed ribavirin did inhibit replication of the virus at clinically achievable levels (Stroher et al., 2004). Ribavirin is a toxic agent, causing haemolytic anaemia, hypocalcaemia and hypomagnesaemia in about half of patients (Knowles et al., 2003).

Corticosteroids These may play a role because the clinical deterioration in the second week could be due to an immunological process. As with ribavirin, the effect of steroids is uncertain because it is usually used in combination with other agents. Ho et al. (2003) showed that patients who received early high doses of pulsed steroids required less oxygen, had earlier radiographic improvement and required much less rescue pulsed steroids. Corticosteroid therapy is not without risk: 28/67 (42%) of SARS patients with large joint pain who had all received ribavirin and corticosteroids had avascular necrosis identified about four months after steroid therapy (Hong and Du, 2004).

Anti-HIV protease inhibitors The addition of both lopinavir and ritonavir to SARS patients who had received a standard treatment protocol significantly reduced the death rate, need for intubation, need for emergency pulsed steroids for sudden respiratory deterioration and rate of nosocomial superinfections (Chan et al., 2003). In vitro, nelfinavir or calpain inhibitor VI or III have shown promise (Barnard et al., 2004).

RNA interference treatment Administering small interfering RNAs (siRNAs) can result in mRNA degradation of identical sequence specificity. In vitro studies have shown inhibition of infection, replication and cytopathic changes of SARS (Zhang et al., 2004, He et al., 2003).

Glycyrrhizin (a constituent of liquorice roots) This inhibited SARS-coV replication in vitro (Cinatl et al, 2003).

Nitric oxide (NO) Inhaled NO gas led to an immediate improvement in oxygenation that continued after NO treatment was stopped (Keyaerts et al., 2004).

Niclosamide This anthelminthic inhibits SARS-coV replication (Wu et al., 2004).

Interferons Interferons are likely to have some benefits as prophylaxis or treatment.

'Is there a vaccine yet?'

Research is ongoing into both passive and active immunisation. With regard to passive immunisation, use of monoclonal antibodies from SARS patients both neutralised infection in vitro and prevented viral replication. Viral-vector and DNA vaccines appear to be the most promising options for active immunisation (Groneberg et al., 2005).

There are no clear guidelines for the pharmacological treatment of SARS. However, on the basis of the available data, Roy commences Tommy on a combination of ribavirin, methylprednisolone, lopinavir and ritonavir. The intensive care unit agrees to accept him into a single negative-pressure room, more for electrolyte monitoring while on ribavirin than for his respiratory status.

Roy calls Cyrus, voicing his concerns about border entry screening not detecting Tommy as a suspect SARS patient on arrival at the airport. The country does border screening for SARS for all passengers entering the country from areas of local transmission and all those exiting the country. However, this relies on passengers reading information sheets and answering questions about whether they have fever or respiratory symptoms; if they do, they are taken across to a quarantine officer for further screening.

'Cyrus, how did this guy get through the border screening?'

It turns out that Tommy did not have respiratory symptoms or feel like he had a fever when he arrived in the country, so he was not picked out by the airport authorities as a potential SARS case.

'So, Cyrus, what good is border screening for SARS?'

Isolation measures

Data from several countries with border screening programs and from mathematical models highlight the limitations of this strategy. In Australia, of 29 suspect SARS patients who were symptomatic at the airport, only four were detected by border screening (14%); reasons for failure included passengers not hearing or understanding verbal messages or lying about symptoms (Samaan et al., 2004).

According to St John et al. (2005), five SARS patients entered Canada over a three-month period but none were ill on arrival. They concluded that the prevalence of SARS would be 1.1 cases per 1 million incoming passengers, giving border entry screening a positive predictive value of 0%, and that the C$7.55 million spent on border screening would be better spent on acute care facilities (the areas most likely to first be sought by suspect SARS patients).

A UK model from Pitman et al. (2005) also found that entry screening was unlikely to be effective in preventing the importation of SARS patients. They calculated that only 1–21% of infected individuals would progress from being asymptomatic to symptomatic disease during a 10-hour flight and therefore be detectable, and this figure does not allow for symptomatic passengers not disclosing their illness to airport authorities.

Even if passengers become ill during the flight, they may only have fever and myalgia without respiratory symptoms. Liu et al. (2004) found that SARS patients developed respiratory symptoms 4.5 +/−1.9 days after the onset of fevers and therefore might not be picked up at border screening.

Roy asks, 'But why didn't those thermal scanners pick up his fever?'

The definition for a suspect case of SARS includes a fever >38°C. However, this does not take into account the natural features of a fever. Body temperature varies according to time of day, so a one-off temperature reading, such as during border screening, may occur when a passenger is afebrile. Also, temperature varies with anatomical site: a temperature of 38°C orally is different to 38°C measured at the tympanic membrane. Furthermore, passengers may have taken an antipyretic to rid themselves of fever (Senanayake, 2006).

Roy receives a call from Ms Gillian Smead, the head infection control nurse. 'The company selling N95 masks has just tripled the price because of a worldwide shortage. The hospital CEO wants to know if we can safely use surgical masks. What do you think?'

Derrick and Gomersall (2005) examined the filtration effectiveness of multiple surgical masks compared to a single surgical mask or to an N95 mask. They determined that people needed to wear five surgical masks to double the filtration factor achieved from wearing a single surgical mask. However, even this was far below the fit factor of 100 required for a respirator, so they concluded that N95 masks are always preferable. However, they noted that this did not necessarily mean that surgical masks would be ineffective against SARS. If SARS was spread by droplet transmission and fomites, a surgical mask would likely be effective. Even with airborne transmission, wearing surgical masks, particularly multiple surgical masks, might have some effect depending on the infective dose of the virus.

Gamage et al. (2005) examined the literature on infection control measures used during the SARS outbreak. Many studies had limitations but it appeared that both surgical and N95 masks were more effective than no mask if no aerosol-generating procedures were used. Not surprisingly, the risk of SARS increased in those who did not wear masks constantly during times of exposure. Ha et al. (2004) examined a hospital where N95 masks were not available till the third week of the SARS outbreak: not one healthcare worker using only surgical masks during this period developed SARS.

Roy admits data are lacking but, although surgical masks may be effective against droplet transmission, N95 masks clearly are more effective filters. Therefore, his recommendation is for the CEO to buy N95 masks if possible.

'Roy, I presume that you are still happy to continue isolation measures, avoid nebulisers and have terminal cleaning of rooms occupied by SARS patients?'

CASE 20 SEVERE ACUTE RESPIRATORY SYNDROME (SARS)

Varia et al. (2003) found that the risk of contracting SARS is greatest if exposures <1 m from the patient occurred. This makes sense, given that droplets travel up to 1 m. There was a sequential decrease in risk of SARS transmission with an exposure <3 m or >3 m. Aerosol-generating procedures such as the use of nebulisers increase the risk of transmission of SARS and should be avoided where possible.

SARS-coV can survive on plastic surfaces for up to 48 hours, for two days in normal stool and up to four days in diarrhoea. Therefore, environmental routes of infection are highly plausible and provide the rationale for environmental cleaning/decontamination of surfaces that have been in contact with SARS patients (World Health Organization, 2003).

> Gillian asks, 'I didn't realise that the virus could survive in stool for so long. Was that the route of transmission in Amoy Gardens?'

The SARS-coV that was responsible for the outbreak at the Amoy Gardens apartment complex probably originated from stool. However, the outbreak was principally remarkable for the wide ranging airborne spread of the virus. The vehicle for this was probably the toilet system, which had poor seals around the floor drains, allowing the virus to spread through the building's ventilation system (Yu et al., 2004).

> Initially, Tommy's respiratory function deteriorates but he does not require mechanical ventilation and soon improves. Within 10 days he is better and treatment is stopped.
> Unfortunately, Cyrus from the public health unit has to tell him that his son has developed probable SARS. Tommy is extremely upset. 'He's only five years old. He must be more vulnerable than an adult.'

Although SARS is an extremely serious condition, the best outcomes have been in children ≤12 years old. Not one child has died from SARS and very few have needed intensive care unit (5%) or mechanical ventilation (1%). There may be some chronic sequelae in children who have had SARS, namely ongoing radiologic abnormalities on high-resolution chest CT scans and reduced exercise capacity (Li and Ng, 2005).

> Everyone is pleased to hear that, although Tommy's son's respiratory swabs are also RT-PCR-positive for SARS-coV, the boy recovers quickly over the next four days without intensive care. In fact, he is more interested in whether his beloved pet cat will get SARS. 'Is he safe, Doctor?'

SARS probably evolved from a coronavirus in animals somewhere in China's Guangdong province. The palm civet, which is a local delicacy there, had been the chief suspect but more recently bats have been found to carry the virus, and they may be the primary source (Normile, 2005). In particular, horseshoe bats have been identified as a reservoir for a virus that is genetically very similar to SARS-coV (Wang et al., 2006). In the laboratory setting, scientists have been able to infect a wide range of animals including monkeys, ferrets and domestic cats (Groneberg et al., 2005).

> Roy calls Cyrus with the result of the boy's RT-PCR.
> 'Cyrus, SARS is extremely infectious. I presume you had to trace the passengers on Tommy's flight home?'

Public health notification and response

SARS is moderately infectious compared to other communicable diseases, with an estimated reproductive number (R_0) of 2.7, excluding 'super shedding' situations (R_0 refers to the number of secondary cases generated by a single case in a susceptible population) (Riley et al., 2003). In comparison, measles can have an R_0 >15 in unvaccinated populations (Trottier and Philippe, 2003).

CASE 20 SEVERE ACUTE RESPIRATORY SYNDROME (SARS)

> Presumed transmission of SARS during flights has occurred. However, the risk is likely to be low because the main route of infection is through droplets (Leder and Newman, 2005). One study found that the risk of infection was highest in those sitting in the three rows in front of the index case, although infection was still possible in those seated elsewhere in the plane (Olsen et al., 2003). The fact that those in front of the index case were at highest risk makes sense if droplet spread through coughing is the main mode of transmission.

> Cyrus follows the local guidelines for SARS and air travel. This recommends contact tracing of all passengers sitting four rows in front and behind Tommy. He and the other infectious diseases officers contact all the passengers; none of them have developed symptoms.
> An officer asks Cyrus, 'Do you think that any of the passengers could have had asymptomatic infection?'

Many infections can have protean manifestations, from asymptomatic infection detected only through seroconversion to severe life-threatening disease requiring hospitalisation. However, a meta-analysis demonstrated that the seroprevalence of SARS in asymptomatic or subclinical populations is only 0.10% (and this does not discount the possibility of false-positive results) (Leung et al., 2005).

References

Barnard, D.L., Hubbard, V.D., Burton, J. et al. (2004) Inhibition of severe acute respiratory syndrome-associated coronavirus (SARSCoV) by calpain inhibitors and beta-D-N4-hydroxycytidine. *Antiviral Chemistry & Chemotherapy* 15(1), 15–22.

Centers for Disease Control and Prevention (2005) *Frequently asked questions about SARS.* Available from www.cdc.gov/ncidod/sars/faq.htm (Accessed 20 June, 2007)

Chan, P.K., To, W.K., Ng, K.C. et al. (2004) Laboratory diagnosis of SARS. *Emerging Infectious Diseases* 10(5), 825–31.

Chan, K.S., Lai, S.T., Chu, C.M. et al. (2003) Treatment of severe acute respiratory syndrome with lopinavir/ritonavir: a multicentre retrospective matched cohort study. *Hong Kong Medical Journal* 9(6), 399–406.

Cinatl, J., Morgenstern, B., Bauer, G. et al. (2003) Glycyrrhizin, an active component of liquorice roots, and replication of SARS-associated coronavirus. *Lancet* 361(9374), 2045–46.

Department of Health and Ageing (2004) *Interim Australian Infection Control Guidelines For Severe Acute Respiratory Syndrome (SARS)*. Available from www.health.gov.au/internet/wcms/publishing.nsf/content/health-sars-guidelines-index.htm/$file/3_icg.pdf (Accessed 30 March, 2006)

Department of Health and Ageing (2003a) *Specimen Collection Protocol For SARS*. Available from www.health.gov.au/internet/wcms/publishing.nsf/content/health-sars-guidelines-index.htm/$FILE/specimen.pdf (Accessed 30 March, 2006)

Department of Health and Ageing (2003b) *Recommendations For Tracing And Managing Contacts Of SARS Patients*. Available from www.health.gov.au/internet/wcms/publishing.nsf/content/health-sars-guidelines-index.htm/$FILE/tracing.pdf (Accessed 30 March, 2006)

Derrick, J.L., Gomersall, C.D. (2005) Protecting healthcare staff from severe acute respiratory syndrome: filtration capacity of multiple surgical masks. *Journal of Hospital Infection* 59(4), 365–68.

Gamage, B., Moore, D., Copes, R. et al. (2005) Protecting health care workers from SARS and other respiratory pathogens: a review of the infection control literature. *American Journal of Infection Control* 33(2), 114–21.

Groneberg, D.A., Poutanen, S.M., Low, D.E. et al. (2005) Treatment and vaccines for severe acute respiratory syndrome. *Lancet Infectious Diseases* 5(3), 147–55.

Ha, L.D., Bloom, S.A., Nguyen, Q.H. et al. (2004) Lack of SARS transmission among public hospital workers, Vietnam. *Emerging Infectious Diseases* 10(2), 265–68.

He, M.L., Zheng, B., Peng, Y. et al. (2003) Inhibition of SARS-associated coronavirus infection and replication by RNA interference. *Journal of the American Medical Association* 290(20), 2665–66.

Ho, J.C., Ooi, G.C., Mok, T.Y. et al. (2003) High-dose pulse versus nonpulse corticosteroid regimens in severe acute respiratory syndrome. *American Journal of Respiratory and Critical Care Medicine* 168(12), 1449–56.

Hong, N., Du, X.K. (2004) Avascular necrosis of bone in severe acute respiratory syndrome. *Clinical Radiology* 59(7), 602–08.

Keyaerts, E., Vijgen, L., Maes, P. et al. (2004) Inhibition of SARS co-V infection in vitro by S-nitroso-N-acetylpenicillamine, a nitric oxide donor compound. 11th International Congress on Infectious Diseases; Cancun, Mexico, March 4–7.

Knowles, S.R, Phillips, E.J., Dresser, L. et al. (2003) Common adverse events associated with the use of ribavirin for severe acute respiratory syndrome in Canada. *Clinical Infectious Diseases* 37(8), 1139–42.

Leder, K., Newman, D. (2005) Respiratory infections during air travel. *Internal Medicine Journal* 35(1), 50–55.

Leung, G.M., Lim, W.W., Ho, L.M. et al. (2005) Seroprevalence of IgG antibodies to SARS-coronavirus in asymptomatic or subclinical population groups. *Epidemiology and Infection* 134(2), 211–21.

Li, A.M., Ng, P.C. (2005) Severe acute respiratory syndrome (SARS) in neonates and children. *Archives of Disease in Childhood. Fetal and Neonatal Edition* 90(6), F461–65.

Liu, C.L., Lu, Y.T., Peng, M.J. et al. (2004) Clinical and laboratory features of severe acute respiratory syndrome vis-a-vis onset of fever. *Chest* 126(2), 509–17.

Normile, D. (2005) Virology. Researchers tie deadly SARS virus to bats. *Science* 309(5744), 2154–55.

Olsen, S.J., Chang, H.L., Cheung, T.Y., et al. (2003) Transmission of the severe acute respiratory syndrome on aircraft. *New England Journal of Medicine* 349(25), 2416–22.

Peiris, J.S., Chu, C.M., Cheng, V.C. et al. (2003) Clinical progression and viral load in a community outbreak of coronavirus-associated SARS pneumonia: a prospective study. *Lancet* 361(9371), 1767–72.

Perlman, S., Dandekar, A.A. (2005) Immunopathogenesis of coronavirus infections: implications for SARS. *Nature Reviews. Immunology* 5(12), 917–27.

Pitman, R.J., Cooper, B.S., Trotter, C.L. et al. (2005) Entry screening for severe acute respiratory syndrome (SARS) or influenza: policy evaluation. *British Medical Journal* 331(7527), 1242–43.

Riley, S., Fraser, C., Donnelly, C.A. et al. (2003) Transmission dynamics of the etiological agent of SARS in Hong Kong: impact of public health interventions. *Science* 300(5627), 1961–66.

Samaan, G., Patel, M., Spencer, J. et al. (2004) Border screening for SARS in Australia: what has been learnt? *Medical Journal of Australia* 180(5), 220–23.

Senanayake, S.N. (2006) The limitation of fever in case definitions for avian influenza and SARS. *Communicable Diseases Intelligence* 30(2), 250.

St John, R.K., King, A., de Jong, D. et al. (2005) Border screening for SARS. *Emerging Infectious Diseases* 11(1), 6–10.

Stroher, U., DiCaro, A., Strong, J.E. et al. (2004) Severe acute respiratory syndrome-related coronavirus is inhibited by interferon-alpha. *Journal of Infectious Diseases* 189(7), 1164–67.

Trottier, H., Philippe, P. (2003) Deterministic modeling of infectious diseases: measles cycles and the role of births and vaccination. *The Internet Journal of Infectious Diseases* 1(2). Available from http://www.ispub.com/ostia/index.php?xmlFilePath=journals/ijid/vol2n2/model3.xml (Accessed 2 July, 2007)

Varia, M., Wilson, S., Sarwal, S. et al. (2003) Investigation of a nosocomial outbreak of severe acute respiratory syndrome (SARS) in Toronto, Canada. *Canadian Medical Association Journal* 169(4), 285–92.

Wang, L.F., Shi, Z., Zhang, S. et al. (2006) Review of bats and SARS. *Emerging Infectious Diseases* 12(12), 1834–40.

World Health Organization (2003) *Consensus Document On The Epidemiology Of Severe Acute Respiratory Syndrome.* World Health Organization; Geneva. Available from www.who.int/csr/sars/en/WHOconsensus.pdf (Accessed 30 March, 2006)

Wu, C.J., Jan, J.T., Chen. C.M. et al. (2004) Inhibition of severe acute respiratory syndrome coronavirus replication by niclosamide. *Antimicrobial Agents and Chemotherapy* 48(7), 2693–96.

Yu, I.T., Li, Y., Wong, T.W. et al. (2004) Evidence of airborne transmission of the severe acute respiratory syndrome virus. *New England Journal of Medicine* 350(17), 1731–39.

Zhang, Y., Li, T., Fu, L. et al. (2004) Silencing SARS Co-V Spike protein expression in cultured cells by RNA interference. *FEBS Letters* 560(1-3): 141–46.

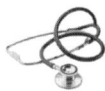

Case 21 Tetanus
George has a stiff jaw …

Tetanus at a glance …

- **Agent:** family Clostridiaceae; genus *Clostridium*; species *Clostridium tetani*
- **Geographical distribution:** worldwide
- **Main mode of transmission:** trauma
- **Person-to-person transmission:** no
- **Animal-to-person transmission:** no
- **Incubation period:** 7–14 days (1 day–many months)
- **Clinical features:** four patterns—generalised (most common), neonatal, localised and cephalic; typically associated with spasms, rigidity and autonomic disturbances
- **Identification:** very difficult to make a microbiologic or molecular diagnosis; occasional isolation of the organism from the wound; experimental real-time polymerase chain reaction (PCR) has been used to isolate the toxin from wounds but this is not freely available
- **Treatment:** a combination of antibiotics (metronidazole ideally), neutralisation of unbound toxin, supportive care and strategies directed towards control of spasms and autonomic disturbances
- **Post-exposure prophylaxis:** this can vary from no intervention required to combinations of vaccine and immunoglobulin, depending on wound type and individual immune status
- **Vaccine:** toxoid vaccine available, usually in combination with other vaccines

Main characters

Dr Ben Lister	infectious diseases physician
Dr Penny Catt	general practitioner
Mr George Trimble	patient with a stiff jaw
Dr Kris Mekano	infectious diseases registrar
Dr Kirk Holly	intensive care specialist
Mrs Trimble	his wife

> It is the middle of a long weekend. The on-call infectious diseases physician, Dr Ben Lister, receives a call from a peripheral hospital, about two hours drive away.
>
> 'Dr Lister, this is Penny Catt—I'm the GP (general practitioner) looking after the emergency department down here today. I need some advice. We have a 55-year-old man, Mr George Trimble, who injured his right hand with a pair of hedge clippers when he was gardening two weeks ago. He has turned up today complaining of a stiff jaw for the last 48 hours.
>
> 'I am worried he might have tetanus. He involuntarily bit on the spatula when I was trying to assess the gag reflex, but the examination was otherwise normal and the injury to his right hand has completely healed.'

What is tetanus?

Tetanus is a toxin-mediated infection characterised by rigidity, severe muscle spasms and autonomic disturbances. It is caused by an obligate anaerobic, spore-forming, Gram positive bacillus, *Clostridium tetani*. The word tetanus is derived from the Greek word for rigidity or stretching.

When the *C. tetani* spores germinate under anaerobic conditions, two toxins are produced, tetanolysin and tetanospasmin, with tetanospasmin being responsible for most of the clinical features of the illness. The toxin enters the peripheral nerves near the site of inoculation and uses trans-synaptic spread and retrograde axonal transport to reach the central nervous system. This occurs at a rate of 75–250 mm/day, taking 2–14 days (Attygalle and Rodrigo, 2004).

The toxin has a light and a heavy chain linked by disulfide bonds and causes sustained excitatory activity of alpha motor neurons and muscle spasms. This is achieved by cleaving synaptobrevin, a chemical that prevents pre-synaptic release of the two inhibitory neurotransmitters glycine and gamma-aminobutyric acid (GABA) (Bhatia et al., 2002).

> Penny says, 'He is fairly certain that he was vaccinated against tetanus as a child in the 1950s. That's why he didn't bother seeing a doctor at the time of injury. Do you know whether they were immunising against tetanus back in the 1950s?'

Tetanus vaccination has been part of the routine childhood immunisation schedules in many countries since the late 1940s.

> 'So, if he is right about being fully immunised in childhood, then he should still be protected against tetanus?'

Immunity to tetanus may wane in the ageing population, regardless of whether they received the full five doses of vaccine during childhood. There certainly is an increase in tetanus incidence as one gets older, with one analysis demonstrating that 60% of reported cases were in people >40 years (Rhee et al, 2005). McQuillan et al. (2002) also demonstrated a dramatic reduction in the proportion of people with protective antibody levels to tetanus with increasing age (31% of 70-year-olds compared to 91% of 6–11 year-olds). Older people may also increase their risk of exposure to tetanus because they spend more time gardening than younger people.

For these reasons, some countries recommend booster doses after receiving the five doses of vaccine in childhood, for example, a booster dose every 10 years, a single booster at age 50 years, or boosters at 45 and 65 years (Immunisation Advisory Centre, 2004; National Health and Medical Research Council, 2003; Public Health Agency of Canada, 2002).

Rare case reports describe tetanus in fully immunised individuals. While the reasons for this are uncertain, Vinson (2000) notes that the level of antibody usually regarded as protective (0.01 IU/mL) was the threshold to differentiate non-fatal cases of tetanus from fatal cases in guinea pigs, rather than the threshold to determine whether or not the guinea pigs developed tetanus at all. In other words, adequate antibody levels (0.01 IU/mL) may be a better predictor of survival from tetanus rather than a predictor of developing tetanus.

Penny confirms that the patient never received a tetanus booster and, moreover, is uncertain about how many immunisations he received in childhood.

'Is there any way to confirm the diagnosis?' Penny asks.

Investigations

Despite the advances in molecular microbiology, the diagnosis of tetanus is still a clinical one in most cases, with recognition of the typical clinical syndrome following a tetanus-prone injury. However, 15–30% of patients are unable to recall a preceding injury, making it just that bit more difficult to make a diagnosis (Attygalle and Rodrigo, 2004). Also, patients can have less well-recognised portals of entry that may delay the diagnosis, such as dental caries (Burgess et al., 1992) or otitis media (Mahoney, 1980).

Sometimes the toxin can be isolated, for instance, from the wound itself, using mouse bioassays or experimental real-time polymerase chain reactions (Akbulut et al., 2005). However, the toxin assays may not be readily available in developing nations, which account for the bulk of tetanus cases worldwide.

Isolation of the organism, *C. tetani*, from a wound, is possible but is technically difficult and does not distinguish toxin-producing strains of *C. tetani* from non-toxin-producing strains (Farrar et al., 2000).

Blood profiles are not helpful in diagnosis and the cerebrospinal fluid is usually normal. Once spasms have developed, electromyography may demonstrate loss of the silent period that occurs 50–100 ms after reflex contraction. Electrophysiological studies may show evidence of a predominantly sensory neuropathy (Bhatia et al., 2002)

George presents with trismus two weeks after a gardening injury, with a history of uncertain tetanus immunity and no post-exposure prophylaxis (PEP); therefore, tetanus must be regarded as the likely diagnosis. Since his wound has healed, microbiologic confirmation of the diagnosis is unlikely.

His physical examination findings also support the diagnosis. The spatula test involves touching the pharynx with a spatula. If the patient gags and the spatula is expelled, tetanus is considered unlikely. However, if the patient bites down on the spatula (due to a reflex contraction of the masseters), the test is positive provided no alternative cause is found (e.g. drug-induced dystonia). Apte and Karnad (1995) found the spatula test to be 94% sensitive and 100% specific for tetanus.

'As you know, Ben, our peripheral hospital is very small, with just a small emergency department and a single ward. Should we send our patient to your hospital?' asks Penny.

Prognosis

The mortality rate from tetanus varies according to the severity score and type of tetanus, being highest for neonatal tetanus at 70% and lowest for localised tetanus at 1–16% (Bhatia et al., 2002). Interestingly, tetanus associated with intramuscular injections of quinine has a very high mortality, even when compared to tetanus acquired from other intramuscular injections (Yen et al., 1994).

One study showed that tetanus patients who received intensive care management had a much lower mortality rate than those tetanus patients who did not (15% versus 43.58%) (Trujillo et al., 1987). The majority of deaths occurs in developing nations in Africa and Asia (Farrar et al., 2000). Nevertheless, good general medical and nursing care by staff experienced in the management of tetanus halves the mortality (Bhatia et al, 2002).

Ben's teaching hospital has an excellent intensive care unit which is happy to accept the transfer.

Penny calls again. 'The nurse has just told me that he is starting to get marked aching in the muscles of his neck and shoulders but no spasms yet. Is this what you would expect?'

In generalised tetanus, the clinical features typically develop in the following sequence (Bhatia et al., 2002; Farrar et al., 2000):

- increased tone and rigidity throughout the body
- generalised spasms
- autonomic disturbances

Trismus (lockjaw) is usually the first symptom of increased tone. Headaches, neck and backaches, and dysphagia can follow. Another well-recognised feature of increased tone in generalised tetanus is risus sardonicus (ironic smile) caused by contraction of the facial muscles.

Generalised spasms are extremely painful and can be so severe as to result in fractures, rhabdomyolysis, respiratory compromise and muscle rupture. They can occur spontaneously or be triggered by seemingly trivial stimuli, such as injections, sounds or touch. Although they can persist for a long time, the spasms are usually maximal in the first two weeks after their onset.

Autonomic disturbances usually begin a few days after the onset of spasms. They are characterised by arrhythmias, fluctuations in heart rate and blood pressure, increased salivation, ileus, high-output renal failure and bronchorrhoea. They are usually maximal during the second week of the illness.

Ongoing rigidity and spasms are usually responsible for the prolonged hospitalisation.

George is transferred to Ben's hospital about 12 hours later. The paramedics report that he began to develop painful spasms during the last hour of the journey. He now has risus sardonicus and is tachycardic at 125/minute, tachypnoeic, febrile to 39.4°C and experiencing painful spasms.

Ben asks his registrar, Dr Kris Mekano, to grade the severity of the patient's tetanus. Kris looks puzzled and says, 'I don't know how to do that.'

A number of scales have been developed to assess the severity of tetanus: the worse the severity, the worse the prognosis. These include the Dakar score, the Phillips score and the Ablett classification (Attygalle and Rodrigo, 2004; Bhatia et al., 2002; Farrar et al., 2000).

Ben uses the Dakar score, which is calculated at 48 hours of illness and uses the following variables (Farrar et al., 2000):

- incubation period (1 point if <7 days)
- period of onset (1 point if <2 days)
- site of injury (1 point for umbilicus, burns, open fracture, uterine, surgical wound, intramuscular injection)
- spasms, if present (1 point)
- fever above 38.4°C (1 point)
- tachycardia above 120 beats/minute in an adult (150 beats/minute in a neonate) (1 point)

Kris asks, 'What's the period of onset? Isn't that the same as the incubation period?'

The incubation period refers to the interval between inoculation with the organism and the onset of symptoms (12 days in this patient). In tetanus, the period of onset specifically refers to the interval between the onset of symptoms (e.g. trismus) and the onset of spasms. In this case, the period of onset for this patient is around 60 hours; he therefore would not get a point on the Dakar scale for this variable.

Kris calculates a score of 3/6 for George, which indicates mild-to-moderately severe disease.
    The intensivist, Dr Kirk Holly, assesses the patient.
    'How will you manage him?' Ben inquires.

Treatment

According to Bhatia et al. (2002), the principles of managing tetanus are:

- halting production of toxin from the wound (with antibiotics and debridement)
- neutralising unbound toxin
- managing muscle spasm
- controlling dysautonomia
- supportive measures (e.g. good airway management, nutritional support, bedsore prevention)

Kirk asks Ben, 'I would normally use penicillin or metronidazole for tetanus patients. Do you have a preference?'

The two antibiotics of choice for tetanus are penicillin and metronidazole. However, metronidazole is probably the preferred agent for the following reasons:

- Intravenous and intramuscular injections can precipitate spasms. One advantage of metronidazole over penicillin is that it can be administered rectally with good bioavailability (400 mg every six hours per rectum).
- Penicillin is more likely to cause central nervous system hyperexcit-ability. This may be because penicillin acts as a competitive antagonist of the inhibitory neurotransmitter GABA, the action of which has already been reduced by the tetanus toxin.

'And to deal with the toxin?'

Unbound toxin is neutralised through passive immunisation with equine, bovine or human immunoglobulin (antitoxin). The immunoglobulin binds unbound or circulating toxin. This shortens the course of the disease and may limit severity (Farrar et al., 2000). It is best to administer it as soon as possible because more toxin becomes bound with time and immunoglobulin is ineffective against bound toxin.

Not surprisingly, equine or bovine immunoglobulin has a higher rate of allergic reactions (20%, with 1% extremely serious reactions) than human antitoxin. Also, human immunoglobulin has a much longer half-life than the animal form. Therefore, human antitoxin is preferable. Unfortunately, much of the developing world has access only to equine antitoxin (Farrar et al., 2000).

'How will you treat the muscle spasm?' Ben asks.

Muscle spasm can be controlled with a combination of sedation and muscular blockade. Well-recognised sedatives used in tetanus include benzodiazepines (e.g. midazolam, diazepam) and propofol. Muscular blockade can be achieved with neuromuscular blocking agents (e.g. vecuronium, pancuronium, rocuronium), baclofen and dantrolene. Magnesium sulfate seems to have a promising role in controlling muscle spasm in tetanus (Bhatia et al., 2002).

'And the dysautonomia—how do you handle that?'

As with muscle spasm, sedatives (e.g. benzodiazepines, phenothiazines) and possibly magnesium sulfate have a role in controlling dysautonomia. Intrathecal baclofen and adrenergic blockers (e.g. labetalol, esmolol, clonidine) can also be used (Bhatia et al., 2002).

George's muscle spasms are immensely painful and compromise his airway, so he is sedated and mechanical ventilated.

His distraught wife asks, 'Could my husband have prevented this if he'd gone to the doctor earlier?'

Tetanus is preventable through PEP. The type of PEP varies according to the patient's immunisation status, the nature of the injury and local guidelines. The algorithm is complex and examples of the Australian and Canadian guidelines can be found at www.health.gov.au/immhandbook/ and http://www.phac-aspc.gc.ca/im/vpd-mev/tetanus_e.html.

Of course, such algorithms depend on the patient being able to recall their immunisation status correctly. Burton and Crane (2005) found that almost 35% of patients presenting to an emergency department with a wound were given unnecessary tetanus boosters on the basis of inaccurate or uncertain immunisation histories. They felt that this could be avoided by better communication with GPs and creating a more accessible database with immunisation details, for example, a centralised electronic system.

A future solution could involve measuring serum tetanus antibody levels in the emergency department. Researchers are examining the role of pinprick blood tests that can detect tetanus antibody levels within an hour (Colombet et al., 2005).

'Could it be anything other than tetanus, Doctor?'

Differential diagnoses

In this case, tetanus is the most likely diagnosis. However, Bhatia et al. (2002) list a number of conditions that can have similar features to tetanus:

Stiff man syndrome   This is a progressive muscular disease with fluctuating spasm and rigidity associated in a large proportion of cases with anti-glutamic acid decarboxylase (GAD) (Meinck and Thompson, 2002).

Drug-induced dystonias/dyskinesias   Due to drugs such as metoclopramide and prochlorperazine.

Strychnine poisoning   Although convulsions are one of the major feature of this condition, it can also cause muscle spasms as well as stiffness of the facial and neck muscles (Santhosh et al., 2003).

Bell's palsy
Painful conditions of the lower mandible
Globus hystericus
Tetany
Rabies
Acute abdomen

> Kris assures her that generalised tetanus is likely to be the diagnosis. But Mrs Trimble says, 'I thought that tetanus was a third-world disease. How can we have it here?'

C. tetani is found worldwide and widely in the environment. It can even be found in the intestinal flora of chickens, horses, domestic animals and humans. It is the success of immunisation programs and PEP in developed nations that has shifted the burden of disease to the developing world.

> 'Doctor, you keep saying my husband has generalised tetanus. Is that a type of tetanus? Are there other types?' asks Mrs Trimble.

Classically there are four patterns of tetanus (Bhatia et al., 2002):

Neonatal tetanus This accounts for 40% of deaths from tetanus worldwide. It is typically a disease of babies aged 5–15 days old and can be prevented by ensuring all pregnant women are adequately immunised against tetanus, using good hygiene during labour and keeping the umbilical cord stump clean. Although all forms of tetanus are terrible, neonatal disease is especially unpleasant: the spasms are worse than in adults and the mortality is very high (70%).

Localised tetanus As the name implies, the spasms are usually limited to the part of the body that was the site of inoculation. This tends to be a mild form of the disease with a low mortality; however, secondary generalisation can occur, with a higher mortality.

Cephalic tetanus This form often follows head injuries and middle ear infections. As the name implies, it tends to involve the cranial nerves, with the facial nerve being most commonly involved.

Generalised tetanus This is the most common form of the disease and is the type affecting George.

> Mrs Trimble has a worried look. 'My cat got pricked by the same pair of hedge clippers as my husband. She's not going to get tetanus too, I hope?'

Tetanus can occur in most mammals, although the susceptibility to infection varies. Horses and humans are highly susceptible. Cats have innate resistance to the organism but can still develop the disease (De Risio and Gelati, 2003). Mrs Trimble should take the cat to the vet.

Kris informs the local public health unit about this case.

Public health notification and response

Due to its seriousness and the fact that it is a vaccine-preventable disease, tetanus is a notifiable disease in most parts of the world. Health department surveillance to monitor trends in tetanus is therefore very important in identifying issues such as declining immunisation coverage and secondary vaccine failure.

George remains in intensive care for six weeks but is then discharged to the ward on the road to recovery.

References

Akbulut, D., Grant, K.A., McLauchlin, J. (2005) Improvement in laboratory diagnosis of wound botulism and tetanus among injecting illicit-drug users by use of real-time PCR assays for neurotoxin gene fragments. *Journal of Clinical Microbiology* 43(9), 4342–48.

Apte, N.M., Karnad, D.R. (1995) Short report: the spatula test: a simple bedside test to diagnose tetanus. *American Journal of Tropical Medicine and Hygiene* 53(4), 386–87.

Attygalle, D., Rodrigo, N. (2004) New trends in the management of tetanus. *Expert Review of Anti-Infective Therapy* 2(1), 73–84.

Bhatia, R., Prabhakar, S., Grover, V.K. (2002) Tetanus. *Neurology India* 50(4), 398–407.

Burgess, J.A., Wambaugh, G.W., Koczarski, M.J. (1992) Report of case: reviewing cephalic tetanus. *Journal of the American Dental Association* 23(7), 67–70.

Burton, T., Crane, S. (2005) Unnecessary tetanus boosters in the ED. *Emergency Medicine Journal* 22(8), 609–10.

Colombet, I., Saguez, C., Sanson-Le Pors, M.J. et al. (2005) Diagnosis of tetanus immunization status: multicenter assessment of a rapid biological test. *Clinical and Diagnostic Laboratory Immunology* 12(9), 1057–62.

De Risio, L., Gelati, A. (2003) Tetanus in a cat—an unusual presentation. *Journal of Feline Medicine and Surgery* 5(4), 237–40.

Farrar, J.J., Yen, L.M., Cook, T. et al. (2000) Tetanus. *Journal of Neurology, Neurosurgery, and Psychiatry* 69(3), 292–301.

Immunisation Advisory Centre (2004) *New Zealand Immunisation Schedule*. Available from www.immune.org.nz/site_resources/Professionals/Immunisation%20Schedule/Immunisation_Schedule_July_1_2004.pdf (Accessed 9 January, 2006)

Mahoney, J.L. (1980) Otogenic tetanus in Zaire. *The Laryngoscope* 90(7 Pt1), 1196–99.

McQuillan, G.M., Kruszon-Moran, D., Deforest, A. et al. (2002) Serologic immunity to diphtheria and tetanus in the United States. *Annals of Internal Medicine* 136(9), 660–66.

Meinck, H.M., Thompson, P.D. (2002) Stiff man syndrome and related conditions. *Movement Disorders* 17(5), 853–66.

National Health and Medical Research Council (2003) *Australian Immunisation Handbook. 8th Edition*. National Health and Medical Research Council: Canberra. Available from www9.health.gov.au/immhandbook (Accessed 9 January, 2006)

Public Health Agency of Canada (2002) *Tetanus—vaccine preventable diseases*. Available from www.phac-aspc.gc.ca/im/vpd-mev/tetanus_e.html (Accessed 9 January, 2006)

Rhee, P., Nunley, M.K., Demetriades, D. et al. (2005) Tetanus and trauma: a review and recommendations. *Journal of Trauma* 58(5), 1082–88.

Santhosh, G.J., Joseph, W., Thomas, M. (2003) Strychnine poisoning. *Journal of the Association of Physicians of India* 51, 739–40.

Trujillo, M.H., Castillo, A., Espana, J. et al. (1987) Impact of intensive care management on the prognosis of tetanus. Analysis of 641 cases. *Chest* 92(1), 63–65.

Vinson, D.R. (2000) Immunisation does not rule out tetanus. *British Medical Journal* 320(7231), 383.

Yen, L.M., Dao, L.M., Day, L.P. et al. (1994) Role of quinine in the high mortality of intramuscular injection tetanus. *Lancet* 344(8925), 786–87.

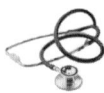

Case 22 Tuberculosis
John has a headache ...

Tuberculosis at a glance ...

- **Agent**: family Mycobacteriaceae; genus *Mycobacterium*; species *Mycobacterium tuberculosis* (other mycobacteria from the MTB complex can cause TB including *M. bovis, M. bovis* BCG, *M. africanum, M. canetti, M. microti, M. caprae*)
- **Geographical distribution**: worldwide
- **Main modes of transmission**: droplet spread; uncommonly, direct contact
- **Incubation period**: exposure to development of a positive tuberculin skin test takes 8–10 weeks; exposure to development of active TB infection takes months to decades
- **Infectious period**: infectious only with laryngeal and pulmonary TB, there are variable definitions for the end of the infectious period—the presence of three consecutive negative sputum smears collected more than eight hours apart and including one early morning sample OR appropriate anti-TB therapy for two weeks or more PLUS reduction in symptoms PLUS a reduction in the level of mycobacteria in sputum smears (e.g. going from 3+ AFBs in sputum to 1+ AFBs)
- **Clinical features**: most commonly pulmonary infection but TB can affect almost any organ system
- **Identification**: latent TB infection—tuberculin skin test or gamma-interferon-based blood test; active TB infection—microscopy, polymerase chain reaction (PCR), culture of tissue from the involved area
- **Treatment**: active TB infection—antimicrobial treatment with multiple antibiotics for a minimum of six months, depending on the primary site of infection; latent TB infection—6–9 months of isoniazid, although combination therapy can be used
- **Vaccines**: BCG vaccine, although it has limited efficacy

Main characters

Dr Julius Rathbone	infectious diseases physician
Dr Alex Degrassi	internal medicine registrar
Mr John Suller	diplomat with fevers, cough and a headache
Mrs Claudia Suller	Mr Suller's wife
Ms Stella Poulos	TB nurse

It's late on a Saturday night. Dr Julius Rathbone, the infectious diseases physician, receives a call from the emergency department.

'Hi, it's Dr Alex Degrassi, one of the registrars in emergency. I've just seen a man with probable meningitis. I've got the results of the lumbar puncture (LP), but I better give you the background of this case as it is probably relevant.

'Mr John Suller is a 40-year-old diplomat from one of the Sub-Saharan African embassies. He told me that he has had a persistent dry cough for three weeks, accompanied by fevers and night sweats. About four days ago, he developed a headache, which is gradually worsening. He has no focal neurological symptoms and an unremarkable physical examination apart from tachycardia and fever. His chest X-ray shows some left upper lobe scarring and possibly some mediastinal lymphadenopathy but there is no upper lobe consolidation or cavitating pneumonia.'

Alexander gives Julius the results of the LP (normal values are given in brackets):

- opening pressure: 32 cm H_2O (<30 cm H_2O)
- appearance: clear
- white cell count: $500 \times 10^6/L$ ($<5 \times 10^6/L$)
- red cell count: $2 \times 10^6/L$ ($4.5-6.5 \times 10^6/L$)
- white cell differential: 80% polymorphonuclear, 20% mononuclear
- protein count: 2 g/L (<0.45 g/L)
- glucose: 1.5 mmol/L (2.8–4.4. mmol/L)
- cerebrospinal fluid/serum glucose ratio: 25% (>60%)
- Gram staining: negative

He adds, 'I'm worried about bacterial meningitis, so I am going to commence empiric antibiotics to cover him for

Streptococcus pneumoniae, Neisseria meningitidis, Haemophilus influenzae and *Listeria monocytogenes*.

'I thought about tuberculosis (TB) but was put off by all those polymorphonuclear cells.'

What is tuberculosis?

TB is one of the best-known infections throughout history. It is caused by organisms from the *Mycobacterium tuberculosis* complex. While pulmonary TB is probably the best recognised manifestation, in fact almost any organ system can be involved. Its versatility in causing such a range of clinical manifestations is remarkable.

TB is a well-recognised cause of meningitis. Because John is from Sub-Saharan Africa, where the prevalence of TB is high, tuberculous meningitis (TM) should be a differential diagnosis even before the LP findings are known. Furthermore, John has left upper lobe findings on the chest X-ray consistent with pulmonary TB.

The findings of this LP could fit with a bacterial cause of meningitis but they also fit perfectly well with TM. Alex thinks TM unlikely because of the white cell differential in the cerebrospinal fluid (CSF). Characteristically, TM is associated with a marked predominance of mononuclear cells in the CSF; however, in the first 10 days or so there may be a predominance of neutrophils (Jeren and Beus, 1982) before a transition to the characteristic mononuclear pleocytosis.

Otherwise, according to Thwaites and Tran (2005) the results of the LP are consistent with TM, specifically:

- clear CSF (80–90% of cases)
- high protein (0.45–2.5 g/L, higher if there is spinal block)
- low CSF/blood glucose ratio (<0.5 in 95% of cases)

'I see,' Alex says. 'Does that mean I need to isolate the patient?'

Isolation measures

While TM is not communicable, pulmonary TB certainly is. John has a cough and chest X-ray changes; therefore, he should be placed in a single, negative-pressure room and no one should be allowed to enter without wearing a N95 respirator mask.

Alex asks, 'How do we confirm a diagnosis of TM?'

Investigations

TM is not easy to confirm and cases are often treated on a combination of clinical and laboratory suspicion. In fact, many studies break cases down into confirmed cases and suspect cases, with suspect cases often outweighing confirmed cases.

The three ways to confirm a diagnosis of TM are to:

- **Identify acid-fast bacilli (AFBs) on CSF microscopy**   To maximise the chance of identifying MTB on microscopy or culture, more than 5 mL of CSF is required (Thwaites et al., 2004a).
- **Grow *M. tuberculosis* (MTB) in a CSF culture**   This may take up to six weeks.
- **Identify MTB via a polymerase chain reaction (PCR)**   A meta-analysis confirmed that commercial TB PCR assays are very specific (98%) but have a poor sensitivity (56%) (Pai et al., 2003). In practical terms, this means that a positive test is very suggestive of a diagnosis of TM but a negative result is unreliable in excluding TM. One advantage of a positive TB PCR result over culture is that PCR rapidly increases the speed of the diagnosis.

'Would adenosine deaminase levels be useful?' Alex asks.

Adenosine deaminase (ADA) is an enzyme whose major role relates to lymphocyte proliferation and differentiation. The activity of ADA is increased in diseases with cell-mediated immunity, such as TB. For tuberculous pleural effusions, measuring ADA levels is useful. A meta-analysis concluded that raised levels have a sensitivity and specificity of 92% (Goto et al., 2003). The sensitivity and specificity of ADA levels in CSF are not as good as in pleural fluid (82% and 83%, respectively, in a recent study using a cut-off value of >11.39 U/L/min) but a positive result in the presence of other compelling clinical and laboratory evidence adds support to the diagnosis (Kashyap et al., 2006).

CASE 22 TUBERCULOSIS

> 'It appears that tuberculous meningitis is a difficult diagnosis to make even with all the lab investigations available!'

One study tried to predict a diagnosis of TM based on a combination of clinical and basic laboratory markers (Thwaites et al., 2002). This combination had probably a better efficacy than MTB-specific laboratory tests (i.e. 86% sensitivity and 79% specificity with prospective data). Co-infection with HIV, however, affects specificity because it introduces other differential diagnoses (e.g. cryptococcal meningitis). The predictors were:

- age
- duration of illness
- peripheral blood white cell count
- total CSF white cell count
- proportion of CSF white cells which are neutrophils

> 'Is there anyway to confirm the diagnosis in this particular case?'

Pulmonary TB is a possibility, so John's sputum should be examined.

There are more organisms in pulmonary TB than extrapulmonary TB, so the rate of smear positivity from sputum from people with pulmonary TB is much higher than from tissue or fluids from people with extrapulmonary TB. For example, the smear positivity in CSF and pleural fluid is only 5–10% (Tuberculosis Coalition for Technical Assistance, 2006).

> 'Does pulmonary TB preferentially affect one part of the lungs more than the others?'

TB can affect any part of the lungs or pleural cavity but the upper lobes are preferentially involved.

> 'Mainly the upper lobes—that's odd. What's the reason for that?'

The upper lobes have the highest oxygen tension of the lungs and MTB thrives in an oxygen-rich environment. It used to be thought that MTB was an obligate aerobe but it appears to have the biochemical and genomic capability to survive in an anaerobic setting (Wilson et al., 1999).

The laboratory confirms that staining of the CSF was negative for organisms, in particular, AFBs. Julius is keen to have John's sputum examined for AFBs. Given that John has a non-productive cough, he orders sputum induction.

Sputum induction is a non-invasive method of acquiring sputum from someone with a dry cough. One common method of inducing cough is to get the patient to inhale hypertonic saline through a nebuliser. The procedure carries a high risk of exposing others to infection, so it should be performed in a negative-pressure room (if available) with the healthcare worker wearing personal protective equipment, including at the very least, a N95 mask (Jensen et al., 2005).

'Wouldn't a bronchoscopy be more sensitive at picking up AFBs?'

The rate of smear and culture-positivity from bronchoscopy is similar to that from sputum induction (Conde et al., 2000) but carries more risks for the patient.

'How many sputum samples do you need?'

On average, the first sample is smear-positive in 85% of cases of pulmonary TB. The second sample adds a further 10% sensitivity and the third about 5%. Therefore, two samples are a minimum and more than three is unhelpful (Tuberculosis Coalition for Technical Assistance, 2006). At least one of the specimens should be early morning sputum because sputum from this time has the highest yield of organisms (Van Deun et al., 2002).

'So how sensitive is smear examination of sputum compared to culture?'

Smear examination is only 50–60% as sensitive as culture, although a positive test provides an immediate diagnosis while cultures can take up to six weeks to become positive (Tuberculosis Coalition for Technical Assistance, 2006). However, sputum culture can detect as few as 100 organisms/mL but sputum samples need to contain over 10 000 organisms/mL for smears to be positive—there is less than a 10% chance of smear positivity if there are <1000 organisms/mL (Van Deun et al., 2002). Interestingly, in some parts of the world women with suspected TB are less likely to be smear-positive than men (Khan et al., 2007). There are potentially many reasons for this (Alisjahban and van Creval, 2007).

There are ways to improve the yield of positive results from smears and culture, although they are dependent on the expertise of the technician and the availability of resources. Concentration by centrifugation or sedimentation is associated with a 20% higher sensitivity and smear-positive rate than direct smears. Fluorescence-based microscopy (using auramine) is 10% more sensitive than conventional light microscopy. Time for cultures to become positive can be improved by using liquid media (MGIT fluorescence and BACTEC radioactive media) instead of solid media (such as Lowenstein-Jensen and Ogawa media) (Tuberculosis Coalition for Technical Assistance, 2006). Even simple measures such as verbal instructions on how to produce a good sputam sample have proven effective in increasing rates of smear positivity (Khan et al., 2007).

Pulmonary TB is very infectious. The ID_{50} (the dose which would infect 50% of exposed individuals) is <10 bacilli (Public Health Agency of Canada, 1996). In fact, one droplet nucleus can be enough to infect an individual and coughing can generate 3000 droplet nuclei (each droplet containing 1–3 bacilli) (World Health Organization, 2004a).

> 'His CSF is smear-negative for AFBs. If his sputum is also smear negative, should we withhold anti-TB treatment until the cultures become positive?'

Treatment

Delaying treatment can result in the patient rapidly deteriorating and a poor outcome; therefore, if clinical suspicion is strong for TM, treatment should be commenced promptly (Kennedy and Fallon, 1979).

> Julius wants to commence anti-TB therapy within the next 24 hours. Sputum induction is performed and the first sample is smear-positive for AFBs.
> 'Should we order a TB PCR on the specimen?' Alex asks.

While culturing the mycobacterium will allow it to be formally identified, this may still take some weeks, even with a smear-positive specimen. Consequently, without TB PCR at this early stage there will be no microbiological confirmation that the AFB is indeed TB. It is generally recommended that all specimens positive for AFBs on staining should undergo TB PCR testing. The rationale is to confirm whether or not the AFB is *M. tuberculosis* or a non-tuberculous *Mycobacterium* (e.g. *M. avium* complex).

A positive TB PCR gives further weight to the argument for commencing empiric therapy against TB and initiating a contact investigation. In certain settings, a negative TB PCR in smear-positive sputum would be sufficient to withhold anti-TB therapy and to not initiate a contact investigation (National Tuberculosis Controllers Association and Centers for Disease Control and Prevention, 2005).

> The PCR is positive for TB complex. Alex asks, 'What is TB complex?'

TB in humans is predominantly caused by MTB but there are other mycobacteria that can also cause clinical TB in humans and together they form the TB complex, consisting of MTB, *M. africanum*, *M. bovis* (usually associated with cows and unpasteurised milk), *M. bovis* BCG strain, *M. caprae* (typically from goats), *M. canetti* and *M. microti* (typically from small rodents) (Huard et al., 2003). Although the introduction of pasteurisation has led to a dramatic reduction in *M. bovis* cases in humans, recent clusters of human cases have demonstrated that outbreaks still occur in developed nations and that person-to-person transmission of this infection (thought very rare for *M. bovis*) can occur (Evans et al., 2007).

> 'And are there any other infections he should be evaluated for?'

John should be counselled about testing for HIV. 25 countries have a prevalence of HIV over 5%, of which 24 are found in Sub-Saharan Africa—nine of these countries have a prevalence of HIV >15% (World Health Organization, 2004a). John comes from Sub-Saharan Africa.

Even if John is from a country with a low prevalence of HIV, the implications of co-infection are such that some countries screen all new TB patients for HIV.

> John agrees to an HIV test after receiving pre-test counselling. Alex asks, 'How serious is the problem of co-infection?'

More than 11 million people were co-infected with HIV and TB by the end of 2000, of whom 70% were in Sub-Saharan Africa. But HIV/TB co-infection is not a problem limited to the developing world. In the US, 26% of TB cases are attributable to HIV (Corbett et al., 2003). Co-infection has a number of implications:

- a higher risk of being infected by a contact with pulmonary TB (National Tuberculosis Controllers Association and Centers for Disease Control and Prevention, 2005)
- a much higher lifetime risk of latent TB infection (LTBI) becoming active disease. If John, aged 40 years old, has HIV, he would have had a 24–40% lifetime risk of reactivation TB compared to 3–7% in a non-HIV-immunocompetent individual (Horsburgh, 2004). Broadly, non-HIV people will have around a 10% lifetime risk of reactivation TB while HIV-positive people will have a 10% risk annually (Corbett et al., 2003)
- higher numbers of active TB infection in areas of high prevalence of HIV. In Sub-Saharan Africa, notifications of TB have increased by up to five times in the last 10 years (World Health Organization, 2004a). In consequence, health services are being overwhelmed, resulting in less people being treated adequately for TB. This, in turn, leads to a higher mortality from TB and higher rates of secondary infection and promotes the rise of multi-drug resistant strains of TB (MDR-TB)
- extrapulmonary and disseminated TB are more common in HIV-positive patients (World Health Organization, 2004a)
- patients with advanced HIV (CD4 counts <200 mm^3) may have atypical features of pulmonary TB, resulting in a delayed diagnosis. This includes higher rates of smear-negative sputum and chest X-rays less likely to demonstrate upper lobe cavities and infiltrates

and more likely to show mediastinal lymphadenopathy and miliary disease
- mortality rates over 50% in people with HIV-related TB (Corbett et al., 2003), which is much higher than would be expected in non-HIV patients

> The enzyme-linked immunosorbent assay (ELISA) for HIV is positive; within 24 hours, the diagnosis of HIV is confirmed by a Western Blot assay. John has HIV. Julius gently breaks the news to him.
>
> John asks, 'I know that you want to start the anti-TB treatment, but shouldn't I start on antiretroviral therapy against HIV as well?'

John must start therapy for tuberculosis. However, the issue of whether or not to start antiretroviral agents (ARVs) against HIV is more complex. Ultimately it comes down to whether the risks of delaying ARV outweigh the benefits of starting it.

The potential problems with combined ARVs and anti-TB therapy include:

Drug interactions Rifampicin decreases plasma levels of two major groups of ARV drugs: protease inhibitors (PIs) and non-nucleoside reverse transcriptase inhibitors (NNRTIs). Conversely, NNRTIs and PIs can both affect rifampicin levels. Another drug from the rifamycin class, rifabutin, has similar efficacy to rifampicin in the treatment of pulmonary tuberculosis (McGregor et al., 1996) but is less prone to interactions with ARVs. Certain ARVs and isoniazid can cause peripheral neuropathy but the toxicity can be worse if they are both used together (World Health Organization, 2004a).

Immune reconstitution disease (IRD) ARV can 'reinvigorate' the immune system and response, previously depleted by HIV. While this is a good thing in the long-term, it can result in transient clinical deterioration in the short-term as the reinvigorated immune system responds to the current infection. With pulmonary TB and ARV, this can result in clinical manifestations such as fever, worsening lung infiltrates, lymphadenopathy, hypercalcaemia and acute renal failure (Lipman and Breen, 2006). Interestingly, this paradoxical reaction can also occur early in the treatment course of TB in the absence of ARVs in non-HIV patients and may call for treatment with non-steroidal anti-inflammatory drugs or corticosteroids.

The general recommendation would therefore be to commence anti-TB therapy but defer ARV till at least the continuation phase of anti-TB therapy, that is, after two months. A situation that may warrant commencing anti-TB therapy and ARVs simultaneously is a case of advanced HIV, that is, a CD4 cell count of $<100 \times 10^6$/L (Dean et al., 2002).

> 'So what do I need to treat my TB?' John asks.

In situations where the organism is known or suspected to be sensitive to standard anti-TB drugs, the regimen would consist of 9–12 months of the following antibiotics (American Thoracic Society et al., 2003; National Collaborating Centre for Chronic Conditions, 2006):

- isoniazid (for the duration of therapy)
- rifampicin (for the duration of therapy)
- ethambutol (only for the first two months)
- pyrazinamide (only for the first two months)

The first two months, where all four drugs are used together, is commonly known as the intensive phase and the remainder of treatment on only two drugs is known as the continuation phase.

Corticosteroids have been demonstrated to reduce mortality in TM. This may be due to a combination of reduced CSF inflammation and a reduction in drug reactions from the anti-TB medications. Although it is unclear whether patients with TM co-infected with HIV benefit from the use of corticosteroids, it does not appear to do any harm and is probably worthwhile (Thwaites et al., 2004b). Both American Thoracic Society and UK guidelines recommend corticosteroids. It is usually ceased after about six weeks. Corticosteroids are also recommended in the treatment of tuberculous pericarditis (American Thoracic Society et al., 2003; National Collaborating Centre for Chronic Conditions, 2006).

> Alex asks, 'What about pyridoxine?'

Isoniazid can cause neurological disease (e.g. peripheral neuropathy) by impairing the effects of pyridoxine (vitamin B6). People especially susceptible to this adverse reaction from isoniazid include malnourished people, pregnant and lactating women, people who abuse alcohol and people with diabetes, HIV or renal failure (American Thoracic Society et al., 2003). While these groups definitely need pyridoxine supplementation during isoniazid therapy, some authors have recommended that all patients on isoniazid should have pyridoxine supplementation at a dose of <50 mg/day (Chan and Iseman, 2002).

Others dispute this on the basis that pyridoxine may antagonise the action of isoniazid. Even when pyridoxine is to be used, they argue that a much smaller dose can be used, given that 6 mg/day of pyridoxine is enough to prevent peripheral neuropathy (Ormerod et al., 2003).

Pyridoxine supplementation is recommended at higher doses if cycloserine, a second-line anti-TB agent, is being used to prevent neurotoxicity (American Thoracic Society et al., 2003).

> John is commenced on isoniazid, rifampicin, ethambutol, pyrazinamide, prednisone and pyridoxine (25 mg/day). 'How do these anti-tuberculous drugs work?' he asks.

In patients with a TB infection, there are four types of bacilli (World Health Organization, 2004a):

- metabolically active bacilli
- intracellular bacilli
- semi-dormant bacilli, which have intermittent episodes of metabolic activity
- dormant bacilli, which eventually die

It is the semi-dormant bacilli that are the hardest to eradicate, accounting for the long duration of therapy.

Isoniazid kills 90% of all the bacilli within the first few days of therapy, is most effective against the metabolically active bacilli and has little effect on the semi-dormant bacilli. Pyrazinamide is the most effective agent against intracellular bacilli and rifampicin kills the semi-dormant bacilli (World Health Organization, 2004a). Given the importance of isoniazid and rifampicin in killing bacilli, one can understand the problem presented by MDR-TB, where these agents cannot be used.

Isoniazid and pyrazinamide achieve excellent CSF levels. Rifampicin achieves only 10% of serum levels in the CSF and ethambutol has poor CSF penetration once the inflammation has subsided (Thwaites and Tran, 2005).

> 'So how long will I be infectious?'

National guidelines for determining infectivity vary but common recommendations include (National Tuberculosis Controllers Association and Centers for Disease Control and Prevention, 2005):

- three consecutive negative sputum smears collected more than eight hours apart and including one early morning sample OR
- appropriate anti-TB therapy for two weeks or more PLUS a reduction in symptoms PLUS a reduction in level of mycobacteria in sputum smears (e.g. going from 3+ AFBs in sputum to 1+ AFBs)

In general, it is also important to note that only pulmonary TB (including pleural disease) and laryngeal TB are considered infectious (National Tuberculosis Controllers Association and Centers for Disease Control and Prevention, 2005). If John had only TM and no pulmonary involvement, he would not have been considered infectious.

> Nursing staff are concerned about the risk of infection for staff, patients and visitors. The nurse unit manager asks how the risk of TB transmission can be minimised during John's hospital admission.

Isolation measures

Transmission of TB within healthcare settings can be reduced through administrative controls, environmental controls and personal respiratory protection.

Administrative controls refers to:

- identifying areas in the facility at risk of TB (e.g. respiratory ward, laboratory)
- drawing up an infection control plan to address the areas of susceptibility
- educating healthcare workers
- ensuring that high-risk patients are identified and isolated early on

Without effective administrative controls, the efficacy of environmental controls and personal respiratory equipment will be reduced (Granich et al., 1999).

If John is still infectious, a number of measures can be taken to reduce transmission of TB. Once again, these measures will vary according to national guidelines and the availability of resources. One approach in a well-resourced country, involving protective equipment and negative-pressure air condition, is outlined below (Jensen et al., 2005; NSW Health Quality and Safety Branch, 2007).

- Everyone entering the room must wear an appropriate respirator. As a minimum, this should be an N95 mask.
- The patient must wear an appropriate respirator whenever leaving the room.
- People transporting the patient from the room must wear an appropriate respirator.
- The patient should be in a negative-pressure room with an anteroom. The negative-pressure room means that the air will be drawn from the outside to the inside of the room, thereby preventing infectious particles from leaving the room. The anteroom provides a further barrier to the escape of infectious particles into the corridor.
- The room should have at least six but ideally 12 air changes per hour (all renovated or new facilities should aim for at least 12 air changes per hour).
- Air should be discharged outside but a high efficiency particulate air (HEPA) filter must be used if the air is going to be recirculated.

In areas with limited resources, high-tech measures may not be possible. However, natural ventilation can be an effective means of diluting and removing air with infectious particles. Natural ventilation can be achieved by having open windows at either end of the room. Mechanical fans can facilitate the movement of air through the windows. Also, outpatient waiting areas can be covered but be otherwise left open to the environment, thereby diluting the air. In fact one study showed that facilities with open doors and windows, especially those with large windows and high ceilings, can achieve more air changes per hour than a negative-pressure room and potentially have lower infection rates then negative-pressure rooms (Escombe et al., 2007). Unfortunately, such measures are only possible in a tropical or temperate climate (Granich et al., 1999).

Two days later, John's CD4 count comes through. It is $300 \times 10^6/L$, so Julius is happy to commence ARV therapy for HIV once he has completed therapy for TB.

> By the end of two weeks of therapy, John is feeling much better. His fevers and sweats have almost completely disappeared and he no longer has a headache. His most recent consecutive sputum samples are all smear-negative, so he is no longer infectious. Julius prepares John for discharge.
>
> John says, 'In my country, TB patients have to come in to the TB clinic everyday and take their tablets in front of the nurse. I am a diplomat—I refuse to do that.'

In DOT—directly observed therapy—a healthcare worker supervises every dose of anti-TB medication taken. The rationale is to prevent treatment failures, relapses and the emergence of drug resistance by ensuring compliance during the many months of therapy. However, a meta-analysis comparing DOT to unsupervised therapy concluded there was no significant improvement in cure and completion rates with DOT (Volmink and Garner, 2006).

Confusion can arise because there is also a DOTS (directly observed therapy, short course) strategy, of which DOT is only one component. According to the American Thoracic Society et al. (2003), the other components of DOTS are:

- government commitment to sustained TB control activities
- case detection by sputum smear microscopy from symptomatic patients self-reporting to health services
- a standardised treatment regimen of at least 6–8 months for at least all confirmed sputum smear-positive cases with DOT for at least the initial two months
- a regular, uninterrupted supply of all essential anti-TB drugs
- a standardised recording and reporting system for assessing treatment results for each patient and the TB control program overall

It is therefore important not to attribute failure of the DOT component of DOTS to the whole DOTS strategy itself.

Other ways to improve compliance with anti-TB therapy are the provision of incentives to patients, such as opiate substitution for injecting drug users, shelter for the homeless and peer assistance and repeated motivation of both staff and patients (Tuberculosis Coalition for Technical Assistance, 2006).

In Julius's country, DOT is mandatory but the TB nurse comes to the patient's home in the morning, providing a discrete service with little inconvenience to the patient. John accepts this and is discharged back to his consulate.

Ms Stella Poulos, the chief TB nurse for the hospital and surrounding regions, has been involved in contact tracing ever since John was found to have pulmonary TB. Alex, keen to know more about contact tracing, calls her.

Public health notification and response

The general principles of contact tracing for TB should not vary much around the world. The differences in practice probably relate to the fine details of policies and the availability of resources.

In broad terms, Stella needs to:

- categorise the infectiousness of the index case
- categorise the priority of the contacts (low, medium or high-risk)
- identify infected contacts

The two-step policy developed by one health department reflects a reasonable approach to contact tracing (NSW Health Communicable Diseases Branch, 2005b):

Step 1 Assess the infectiousness of the index case as high, medium or low (Table 22.1).

Step 2 Categorise contacts into risk groups, usually based on a minimum three-month period prior to diagnosis (Table 22.2).

Table 22.1 Assessing the infectiousness of the index case

High	Medium	Low
Cavitating lung disease Sputum smear-positive has already transmitted TB to a contact	Sputum culture-positive but smear-negative PCR-positive but smear-negative Smear-positive bronchial lavage	Smear-positive and clinically unlikely to be TB Sputum smear and culture-negative

CASE 22 TUBERCULOSIS

Table 22.2 Categorising contacts into risk groups

High	Medium	Low
Household contacts Friends, sexual contacts and relatives outside the household but with prolonged, close and frequent contact People who have prolonged contact in a closed environment	All the groups in the high-risk category (apart from household contacts) who have frequent but less prolonged contact[†]	Other school, work or social contacts

[†] It is difficult to ascribe an exact duration of contact that discriminates between those people who have 'frequent and prolonged' contact compared to those who have 'less frequent and prolonged' contact. One study found that being exposed to the index case for >120 hours increased a contact's risk of infection (Gerald et al., 2002).

The level of risk of the contact and the degree of infectiousness of the index case determine how quickly a contact should be assessed after first being identified. For example, high-risk contacts of highly infectious index cases should be screened within seven days and high-risk contacts of index cases of low infectiousness should be screened within 14 days. Furthermore, evaluation of the former group's status should be completed more quickly than those in the latter group, for example, five versus 10 days (National Tuberculosis Controllers Association and Centers for Disease Control and Prevention, 2005).

Broadly speaking, absence of infection in one risk category of contacts should remove the need to screen contacts in a lower risk group. For example, if infected contacts are found in the high-risk contacts but not in the medium-risk contacts, then the low-risk contacts do not have to be screened (NSW Health Communicable Diseases Branch, 2005b). This highlights the importance of categorising the contacts into the correct group.

'Are there groups of people who should be categorised as high-risk, irrespective of the level and frequency of contact with the index case?' Alex asks.

According to some guidelines, there may be high-risk groups no matter what the level and frequency of contact with the index case. They have an inherently increased risk of being infected with TB and/or developing TB disease. According to the National Tuberculosis Controllers Association and Centers for Disease Control and Prevention (2005), two of the most important groups are:

- children <5 years, because they are more likely to develop TB disease and the disease is more likely to be aggressive and widespread
- HIV patients and those on immunosuppressive medications or with immunosuppressive conditions

> Stella conducted a contact tracing investigation in an efficient manner. She identified three high-risk contacts (two household, one social), five medium-risk contacts and 20 low-risk contacts. Alex asks what will happen next.

Contacts need to be evaluated for active TB disease or LTBI. The cornerstone for diagnosing LTBI has been the tuberculin skin test (TST), although that may be superseded in the future by blood interferon assays (see below). In high-risk contacts such as children <5 years and HIV-positive individuals, a chest X-ray would also be recommended as part of the initial evaluation (National Tuberculosis Controllers Association and Centers for Disease Control and Prevention, 2005).

The window period from being infected with TB to developing a reactive TST is around 8–10 weeks (National Tuberculosis Controllers Association and Centers for Disease Control and Prevention, 2005). Therefore, if more than 10 weeks have elapsed since the last contact with the index case, a single TST should be adequate to exclude LTBI. However, this is often not the case because the contacts would have been exposed to the index case right up to the time of the hospital admission. Consequently, two TSTs may have to be done, the first test as a baseline and a second 10 weeks after the last exposure. The second TST does not have to be performed if the first TST is positive for LTBI.

While most countries would broadly agree with this approach, there will be some differences, for example, regarding the time interval between the first and second TSTs. Contacts with a positive TST need to have active TB disease excluded before being diagnosed with LTBI.

According to the NSW Health Communicable Diseases Branch (2005a), TST should only be avoided in those who have had:

- a previously positive TST
- previous TB

- serious adverse reactions to the TST
- recent infection or immunisation with a live vaccine

> 'How does TST work?' Alex asks.

The objective of a TST is to induce a delayed hypersensitivity skin reaction in people infected with TB. There are different techniques for the test (e.g. tine test, Heaf test) but the Mantoux test is the recommended test for screening or clinical assessment (Lee and Holzman, 2002).

The Mantoux test involves the intradermal injection of purified protein derivative (PPD) usually into the left forearm. PPD contains a mixture of proteins from TB and non-tuberculous mycobacteria. The amount of PPD used varies in different countries. After 48–72 hours, the amount of induration present at the injection site is determined. It is this degree of induration that is the basis for diagnosing LTBI. While this sounds fairly simple, it is a tricky test to carry out and needs to be performed by someone with experience in the area. It is also important to remember that the induration and not the erythema at the injection site is what must be measured.

It generally is a well-tolerated test although some vigorous reactions can result in skin necrosis, lymphangitis and regional adenitis. False-negative results for LTBI can occur due to old age, immunosuppression due to medications or illness (e.g. HIV, lymphoma, sarcoidosis, recent surgery, recent immunisation with a live vaccine or current viral infections (National Health and Medical Research Council, 2003). Previous BCG immunisation can result in false-positive reactions.

> Stella promptly reviews the three high-risk contacts. They consist of John's wife (Claudia), his three-year-old son and a work contact. His family have been tested for HIV and were negative and his son had a normal chest X-ray. At 48 hours, his son and the work contact had TSTs with 0 mm induration while Claudia had a 16 mm reaction.
> 'What does that mean for my son?' John asks.

Since children <5 years are at particular risk of developing aggressive TB disease, this is one situation where the contact should be empirically treated for LTBI. If the second TST 10 weeks after the last exposure is still unreactive, then treatment can be ceased. A similar approach would be taken to an immunosuppressed older contact (National Tuberculosis Controllers Association and Centers for Disease Control and Prevention, 2005).

> 'What treatment will he need?'

Unless isoniazid resistance is suspected or proven, isoniazid is traditionally used. Although the duration may vary slightly with different national guidelines, the treatment for LTBI consists of isoniazid for a period of 6–9 months (Jasmer et al., 2002). Another alternative is three months of rifampicin and isoniazid, which has a similar efficacy, mortality and rate of adverse reactions (Ena and Valls, 2005).

> Stella did indeed commence the boy on isoniazid and will repeat his TST 10 weeks later.
> 'So what do my test results mean?' Claudia asks.

The TST is not easy to interpret because the cut-off values for LTBI vary according to the situation. In general, there are three different cut-off values under which different categories are regarded as having LTBI: ≥ 5 mm, ≥ 10 mm and ≥ 15 mm (Jasmer et al., 2002) (Table 22.3).

Claudia's reading of 16 mm is clearly consistent with LTBI. She now needs a chest X-ray and clinical evaluation to exclude active TB disease.

> Claudia wants some clarification before accepting the diagnosis of LTBI. 'I had the BCG vaccine when I was a young child. Could that be giving a false reaction?'

Table 22.3 Examples of cut-off values for different categories of LTBI

≥ 5mm	close contacts of an index case with TB disease all HIV-positive people
≥ 10mm	injecting drug users
≥ 15mm	everyone else

SOURCE Jasmer et al., 2002

The BCG vaccine contains a live attenuated strain of *M. bovis* and can indeed result in false-positive TSTs. Even 1–3 years after vaccination, some people with no exposure to TB still have positive Mantoux reactions ≥15mm (Hoft and Tennant, 1999). However, Claudia's BCG remote vaccination as a child is unlikely to be responsible for her positive response now.

> Claudia notes, 'Well, it mustn't be a very good vaccine.'

Overall, BCG vaccination reduces the risk of TB by only 50% (Colditz et al., 1994), which is similar to its efficacy against leprosy (Zodpey et al., 2005). Its effect may last only 10 years and it can cause a number of side effects (National Health and Medical Research Council, 2003).

> 'Anyway, isn't there a new blood test for TB which isn't affected by the BCG?'

The QuantiFERON-TB Gold test (QFT-G) and the ELISPOT test are blood tests primarily used for detecting LTBI. The US Food and Drug Administration recently approved the use of QFT-G (Mazurek et al., 2005). Blood is collected and incubated overnight in the presence of MTB-specific proteins. People previously exposed to TB (i.e. those with LTBI) will produce gamma-interferon from T cells, which will be detected by the overnight assay (Diel et al., 2006).

A number of studies suggest this test is more specific than TST in patients previously vaccinated with BCG. The proteins used in the QFT-G assay—ESAT-6 and CFP-10—arise from genes in the region of difference 1 (RD1) of the MTB genome. The genes encoded in RD1 are supposedly not found in any of the BCG substrains and in very few non-tuberculous mycobacteria (*M. kansasii, M. szulgai* and *M. marinum*) (Mazurek et al., 2005; Pai et al., 2004). It appears to achieve this increase in specificity without sacrificing sensitivity (Pai et al., 2004).

But it is important to remember that there is no gold standard test for diagnosing LTBI. As a result, the evidence for this new assay's superiority over TST is based on solid arguments rather than definitive proof. This does not mean that the QFT-G assay is not superior to TST, but one cannot be 100% certain that it is. Having said that, some countries have already recommended its use in screening for LTBI (Mazurek et al., 2005).

> Claudia is also placed on isoniazid therapy.
> Alex calls up to check on Stella's progress. 'How are you going to deal with the work contact with an unreactive TST?' he wants to know.

Since he is a high-risk contact, he will require a second TST in 8–10 weeks. If this is positive but there is no evidence of active TB disease on a chest X-ray or clinical evaluation, he will be treated for LTBI. If the second test is negative, he will be cleared.

> 'Can TST and QFT-G be used to diagnose active TB infection in addition to LTBI?'

Both tests will be positive in people with active TB disease but this could be due either to active disease or LTBI. Also, there is a significant false-negative rate: 11% for QFT-G and 10–20% for TST (Jasmer et al., 2002; Mori et al., 2004). However, in a patient with a high pre-test probability of TB (e.g. a migrant originally from a high-prevalence area for TB who has necrotising granulomatous lymphadenitis), a positive TST or QFT-G can add weight to a decision to treat empirically for TB while a biopsy specimen is being cultured.

> Stella goes on to test the medium-risk contacts, none of whom have LTBI; therefore, she doesn't need to perform TST for the low-risk contacts.
> Around this time, she receives a call about a new case of pulmonary TB who flew for 10 hours while symptomatic. 'Is there a risk to the passengers?'

TB transmission on a flight is very uncommon but can occur. Transmission requires an index case who is infectious during the flight and a flight that is ≥8 hours in duration. In general, those at greatest risk are passengers sitting in the same row as the index case as well as those sitting two rows behind and in front of the index case. However, others might be at risk depending on the index case's movements and activities during the flight (World Health Organization, 2006a).

> Four weeks later, John's sputum becomes culture-positive for AFBs. The isolate is identified as MTB and is found to be fully sensitive to first-line agents. Staff are relieved that it isn't MDR-TB or XDR-TB. 'What is MDR-TB?' John asks.

MDR-TB is a TB isolate resistant to at least rifampicin and isoniazid. Isolates resistant to only one first-line drug are monoresistant and isolates resistant to more than one first-line drug (other than both rifampicin and isoniazid) are polyresistant (World Health Organization, 2006b). The strongest risk factor for MDR-TB is previous treatment, with previously treated individuals 10 times more likely to have MDR-TB or four times more likely to have resistance (Tuberculosis Coalition for Technical Assistance, 2006). This is likely to reflect inappropriate treatment regimens coupled with poor compliance.

> 'Is MDR-TB a global problem?' Alex asks his boss.

Cases of MDR-TB are found all over the world but the prevalence is low in many countries. The nations associated with high levels of MDR-TB include many of the former states of the Soviet Union, China, Ecuador and Israel (World Health Organization, 2004b).

> 'So what medications can be used to treat MDR-TB?'

There are a number of possibilities, which can be classified into four groups (Group 1 are the first-line oral agents) (World Health Organization, 2006b):

- Group 2—injectable agents (capreomycin, kanamycin, streptomycin, viomycin)
- Group 3—fluoroquinolones
- Group 4—oral bacteriostatic second-line drugs (ethionamide, protionamide, cycloserine, thioacetazone, terizidone)
- Group 5—drugs with unknown efficacy (linezolid, clarithromycin, clofazimine, amoxycillin/clavulanate)

> 'I've also heard of XDR-TB. What exactly is that?'

XDR-TB is extensively drug-resistant TB. Specifically, an XDR-TB isolate is MDR-TB with resistance to any fluoroquinolone plus resistance to at least one of the following antimicrobials: amikacin, kanamycin or capreomycin (Raviglione and Smith, 2007).

> After two months of therapy, John is feeling great but still has culture-positive (but smear-negative) sputum.
> 'Does that mean the treatment isn't working?' he asks.

The definition for failed treatment of pulmonary TB is positive sputum after five months of therapy (Tuberculosis Coalition for Technical Assistance, 2006).

References

Alisjahbana, B. van Crevel, R. (2007) Improved diagnosis of tuberculosis by better sputum quality. *Lancet* 369(9577), 1908–09.

American Thoracic Society, Centers for Disease Control, Infectious Diseases Society of America (2003) Treatment of tuberculosis. *Morbidity and Mortality Weekly Reports Recommendations and Reports* 52(RR-11), 1–77.

Chan, E.D., Iseman, M.D. (2002) Current medical treatment for tuberculosis. *British Medical Journal* 325(7375), 1282–86.

Colditz, G.A., Brewer, T.F., Berkey, C.S. et al (1994) Efficacy of BCG vaccine in the prevention of tuberculosis. Meta-analysis of the published literature. *Journal of the American Medical Association* 271(9), 698–702.

Conde, M.B., Soares, S.L., Mello, F.C. et al. (2000) Comparison of sputum induction with fiberoptic bronchoscopy in the diagnosis of tuberculosis: experience at an acquired immune deficiency syndrome reference center in Rio de Janeiro, Brazil. *American Journal of Respiratory and Critical Care Medicine* 162(6), 2238–40.

Corbett, E.L., Watt, C.J., Walker, N. et al. (2003) The growing burden of tuberculosis: global trends and interactions with the HIV epidemic. *Archives of Internal Medicine* 163(9), 1009–21.

Dean, G.L., Edwards, S.G., Ives, N.J. et al. (2002) Treatment of tuberculosis in HIV-infected persons in the era of highly active antiretroviral therapy. *AIDS* 16(1), 75–83.

Diel, R., Nienhaus, A., Lange, C., Meywald-Walter, K. et al. (2006) Tuberculosis contact investigation with a new, specific blood test in a low-incidence population containing a high proportion of BCG-vaccinated persons. *Respiratory Research* 7, 77.

Ena, J., Valls, V. (2005) Short-course therapy with rifampin plus isoniazid, compared with standard therapy with isoniazid, for latent tuberculosis infection: a meta-analysis. *Clinical Infectious Diseases* 40(5), 670–76.

Escombe, A.R., Oeser, C.C., Gilman, R.H. et al. (2007) Natural ventilation for the prevention of airborne contagion. *PLos Med* 4(2), e68.

Evans, J.T., Smith, E.G., Banerjee. A et al. (2007) Cluster of human tuberculosis caused by *Mycobacterium bovis*: evidence for person-to-person transmission in the UK. *Lancet* 369(9569), 1270–76.

Gerald, L.B., Tang, S., Bruce, F. et al. (2002) A decision tree for tuberculosis contact investigation. *American Journal of Respiratory and Critical Care Medicine* 166(8), 1122–27.

Goto, M., Noguchi, Y., Koyama, H. et al. (2003) Diagnostic value of adenosine deaminase in tuberculous pleural effusion: a meta-analysis. *Annals of Clinical Biochemistry* 40(Pt 4), 374–81.

Granich, R., Binkin, N., Jarvis, W. et al. (1999) *Guidelines for the prevention of tuberculosis in health care facilities in resource-limited settings.* World Health Organization; Geneva

Hoft, D.F., Tennant, J.M. (1999) Persistence and boosting of bacille Calmette-Guerin-induced delayed-type hypersensitivity. *Annals of Internal Medicine* 131(1), 32–36.

Horsburgh Jr, C.R. (2004) Priorities for the treatment of latent tuberculosis infection in the United States. *New England Journal of Medicine* 350(20), 2060–67.

Huard, R.C., De Oliveira Lazzarini, L.C., Butler, W.R. et al. (2003) PCR-based method to differentiate the subspecies of the *Mycobacterium tuberculosis* complex on the basis of genomic deletions. *Journal of Clinical Microbiology* 41(4), 1637–50.

Jasmer, R.M., Nahid, P., Hopewell, P.C. (2002) Clinical practice. Latent tuberculosis infection. *New England Journal of Medicine* 347(23), 1860–66.

Jensen, P.A., Lambert, L.A., Iademarco, M.F. et al. (2005) Guidelines for preventing the transmission of *Mycobacterium tuberculosis* in health-care settings, 2005. *Morbidity and Mortality Weekly Reports Recommendations and Reports* 54 (17), 1–141.

Jeren, T., Beus, I. (1982) Characteristics of cerebrospinal fluid in tuberculous meningitis. *Acta Cytologica* 26(5), 678–80.

Kashyap, R.S., Kainthla, R.P., Mudaliar, A V. et al. (2006) Cerebrospinal fluid adenosine deaminase activity: a complimentary tool in the early diagnosis of tuberculous meningitis. *Cerebrospinal Fluid Research*, 3, 5.

Kennedy, D. H., Fallon, R.J. (1979) Tuberculous meningitis. *Journal of the American Medical Association* 241(3), 264–8.

Khan, M.S., Dar, O., Sismanidis, C. et al. (2007) Improvement of tuberculosis case detection and reduction of discrepancies between men and women by simple sputum-submission instructions: a pragmatic randomised controlled trial. *Lancet* 369(9577), 1955–60.

Lee, E., Holzman, R.S. (2002) Evolution and current use of the tuberculin test. *Clinical Infectious Diseases* 34(3), 365–70.

Lipman, M., Breen, R. (2006) Immune reconstitution inflammatory syndrome in HIV. *Current Opinion in Infectious Diseases* 19(1), 20–25.

Mazurek, G.H., Jereb, J., Lobue, P. et al. (2005) Guidelines for using the QuantiFERON-TB Gold test for detecting *Mycobacterium tuberculosis* infection, United States. *Morbidity and Mortality Weekly Reports Recommendations and Reports* 54(RR-15), 49–55.

McGregor, M.M., Olliaro, P., Wolmarans, L. et al. (1996) Efficacy and safety of rifabutin in the treatment of patients with newly diagnosed pulmonary tuberculosis. *American Journal of Respiratory and Critical Care Medicine* 154(5), 1462–67.

Mori, T., Sakatani, M., Yamagishi, F. et al. (2004) Specific detection of tuberculosis infection: an interferon-gamma-based assay using new antigens. *American Journal of Respiratory and Critical Care Medicine* 170(1), 59–64.

National Collaborating Centre For Chronic Conditions (2006) *Tuberculosis: clinical diagnosis and management of tuberculosis, and measures for its prevention and control.* Royal College of Physicians; London. Available from www.library.nhs.uk/respiratory/ViewResource.aspx?resID=123634 (Accessed 2 July, 2007)

National Health and Medical Research Council (2003) *Australian Immunisation Handbook. 8th Edition.* National Health and Medical Research Council; Canberra. Available from www9.health.gov.au/immhandbook (Accessed 20 September, 2006)

National Tuberculosis Controllers Association and Centers for Disease Control and Prevention (2005) Guidelines for the investigation of contacts of persons with infectious tuberculosis. Recommendations from the National Tuberculosis Controllers Association and CDC. *Morbidity and Mortality Weekly Reports Recommendations and Reports* 54(RR-15), 1–47.

NSW Health Communicable Diseases Branch (2005a) *Tuberculin Skin Testing.* Available from www.health.nsw.gov.au/policies/pd/2005/PD2005_580.html (Accessed 1 July, 2007)

NSW Health Communicable Diseases Branch (2005b) *Tuberculosis Contact Tracing.* Available from www.health.nsw.gov.au/archive/policies/pd/2005/PD2005_212.html (Accessed 1 July, 2007)

NSW Health Quality and Safety Branch (2007) *Infection Control Policy.* Available from www.health.nsw.gov.au/policies/pd/2007/pdf/PD2007_036.pdf (Accessed 16 July, 2007)

Ormerod, L.P., Campbell, I.A., Davies, P.D. (2003) Current medical treatment for tuberculosis. Aspects of chemotherapy and management need clarifying. *British Medical Journal* 326(7388), 550

Pai, M., Riley, L.W., Colford Jr, J.M. (2004) Interferon-gamma assays in the immunodiagnosis of tuberculosis: a systematic review. *Lancet Infectious Diseases* 4(12), 761–76.

Pai, M., Flores, L.L., Pai, N. et al. (2003) Diagnostic accuracy of nucleic acid amplification tests for tuberculous meningitis: a systematic review and meta-analysis. *Lancet Infectious Diseases* 3(10), 633–43.

Public Health Agency of Canada (1996) Guidelines for preventing the transmission of tuberculosis in Canadian Health Care Facilities and other institutional settings. *Canadian Communicable Disease Report* 22(Suppl1), i–iv, 1–55.

Raviglione, M.C., Smith, I.M. (2007) XDR tuberculosis—implications for global public health. *New England Journal of Medicine* 356(7), 656–59.

Thwaites, G.E., Tran, T.H. (2005) Tuberculous meningitis: many questions, too few answers. *Lancet Neurology* 4(3), 160–70.

Thwaites, G.E., Chau, T T., Farrar, J.J. (2004a) Improving the bacteriological diagnosis of tuberculous meningitis. *Journal of Clinical Microbiology* 42(1), 378–79.

Thwaites, G.E., Nguyen, D.B., Nguyen, H.D. et al. (2004b) Dexamethasone for the treatment of tuberculous meningitis in adolescents and adults. *New England Journal of Medicine* 351(17), 1741–51.

Thwaites, G.E., Chau, T.T., Stepniewska, K. et al. (2002) Diagnosis of adult tuberculous meningitis by use of clinical and laboratory features. *Lancet* 360(9342), 1287–92.

Tuberculosis Coalition For Technical Assistance (2006) *International Standards for Tuberculosis Care*. Available from www.who.int/tb/publications/2006/istc/en/index.html (Accessed 2 July, 2007)

Van Deun, A., Salim, A. H., Cooreman, E. et al. (2002) Optimal tuberculosis case detection by direct sputum smear microscopy: how much better is more? *International Journal of Tuberculosis and Lung Disease* 6(3), 222–30.

Volmink, J., Garner, P. (2006) Directly observed therapy for treating tuberculosis. Cochrane Database of Systematic Reviews (2), CD003343.

Wilson, R.J., Pillay, D.G., Sturm, A.W. (1999) *Mycobacterium tuberculosis* is not an obligate aerobe. *Journal of Infection* 38(3), 197–98.

World Health Organization (2006a) *Tuberculosis And Air Travel. Guidelines For Prevention And Control*. World Health Organization; Geneva. Available from www.who.int/tb/publications/2006/who_htm_tb_2006_363.pdf (Accessed 10 January, 2007).

World Health Organization (2006b) *Guidelines For The Programmatic Management Of Drug-Resistant Tuberculosis*. World Health Organization; Geneva. Available from whqlibdoc.who.int/publications/2006/9241546956_eng.pdf (Accessed 10 January, 2007)

World Health Organization (2004a) *TB/HIV: A Clinical Manual*. World Health Organization; Geneva. Available from www.who.int/tb/publications/who_htm_tb_2004_329/en/index.html (Accessed 20 September, 2006)

World Health Organization (2004b) *Anti-tuberculosis Drug Resistance In The World. Third Global Report*. World Health Organization; Geneva. Available from www.who.int/tb/publications/who_htm_tb_2004_343/en/ (Accessed 20 June, 2007)

Zodpey, S.P., Ambadekar, N.N., Thakur, A. (2005) Effectiveness of Bacillus Calmette Guerin (BCG) vaccination in the prevention of leprosy: a population-based case-control study in Yavatmal District, India. *Public Health* 119(3), 209–16.

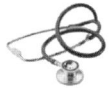

Index

abattoir workers, 303–4, 311
abscesses, 3–4, 6, 8–9
aches, *see* headache; myalgia
acid-fast bacilli (AFB), 367, 369, 371
acute confusional state, 318
acute flaccid paralysis (AFP), 290–3, 296, 321, 323
aerophobia, in rabies, 319
agglutination testing, 34–5, 113–15, *see also* serology
agitation, *see* acute confusional state
AIDS, *see* immunocompromised patients
allergies, *see* hypersensitivity
anaerobic bacteria, 1, 3–5, 9, 353
animal transmission, *see* zoonoses
antibiotic resistance
  enteric fever, 110, 115
  meningococcus, 238
  Staphylococcus aureus, 179
  tuberculosis, 386
antibiotics, *see* 'Treatment' section in each chapter
antibody enhancement hypothesis, 84
antibody testing, *see* serology
anticoagulants, 237–8
antigenic shift, 157–8, 285
antiretroviral therapy (ART), 55, 67, 373–4
antitoxins, 7–8, 100, 359
antiviral agents, 83, 149–50, 218, 227, 324–5, 328, 342–343
arboviruses, 76
atypical pneumonia, *see* SARS
Australian bat lyssavirus, 327–9
autoantibodies, 306
avian influenza, 153–4

bacteraemia, 232, 234, 237, 239
bacterial meningitis, *see* meningitis
bacterial pneumonia, *see* pneumonia
bacteriophages, 120, 205

Bairnsdale ulcer, *see* Buruli ulcer
bats, 320, 327–8, 347
biliary cryptosporidiosis, 68
bilirubin, 132
biopsies, of ulcers, 19
bioterrorism, 9–11, 314
bird flu, *see* avian influenza
bites, *see* zoonoses
bleeding, *see* haemorrhage
blood tests
  dengue fever, 77–8
  diphtheria, 97
  enteric fever, 106, 108–9
  Legionnaire's disease, 182
  mumps, 253–4, 257
  pertussis, 276
  pneumococcal disease, 164
  Q fever, 307
  SARS, 337–8
blurred vision, 2, 7
border entry screening, 343–4
Bordetella pertussis, 267, 285
botulinum antitoxin, 7–8, 12
botulism, 1–13, 291
'break-bone fever', *see* dengue fever
bulbar paralytic polio, 300
Buruli ulcer, 15–28
  recurrence and follow up, 23

camp, in outbreak investigation, 61–3
canned food, 5–6, 11, 291
capsular switching, 247–8
carriers, 69–70, 123–4, *see also* contacts
case control studies, 60, 121, 142
case definitions, 153
  mumps, 255
  pertussis, 272
  Pontiac fever, 192
  SARS, 335–6
cerebrospinal fluid, *see* CSF testing
cheesecake, in enteric fever, 121–3
chemoprophylaxis, *see* prophylaxis
chest X-rays, *see* radiological investigations
children, *see also* infants
  cholera, 37–9, 43
  cryptosporidiosis, 51, 54–6, 65–9
  dengue fever, 76, 84

diphtheria, 94, 103
enteric fever, 108, 126
giardiasis, 47, 51, 65–6
hepatitis A, 132, 142–3
infant botulism, 4–5, 12–13
measles, 227
meningococcal disease, 231–3, 242
neonatal listeriosis, 201–2
neonatal tetanus, 356, 361
pertussis, 269, 281
pneumococcal disease, 165, 170–2
SARS, 346–347
tuberculosis, 381–2
chlorination, 63–5, 191
cholera, 29–43
  chronic carriage of, 41
  pandemics, 42
cholera cots, 39
circulating vaccine-derived polioviruses (cVDPV), 298, 300
cirrhosis, 136
Clostridium botulinum, 1, 3–4, 9
Clostridium tetani, 352, 355, 361
clusters, *see* pandemics; 'Public health notification and response' section in each chapter
cochlear implants, 174–5
community-acquired pneumonia, 152, 180–181, 304–5, 313
confusion, 199–201, 318
conjunctivitis, 248
constipation, 108
contacts, *see also* carriers
  diphtheria, 98–9, 102–3
  educating, 239–40
  enteric fever, 118–19
  hepatitis A, 138–40
  measles, 219, 221–6
  meningococcal disease, 233, 237, 239–41, 246–7
  pertussis, 273, 279–84
  rabies, 326
  SARS, 340, 347–348
  tuberculosis, 379–85
contagion, *see* infectivity
contaminated food and water, *see* foodborne disease; waterborne disease
cooling towers, 188–9

Coronavirus, 334
corticosteroids, 117, 166–7, 192, 324–5, 342, 374
corynebacteriophage, 96
Corynebacterium diphtheriae, 92–3, 103
Corynebacterium ulcerans, 95
cough, *see* influenza; Q fever; SARS; whooping cough
Coxiella burnetii, 302, 304–5, 310, 312, 314–15
cross-reactive immunity, 174
cryptosporidiosis, 45, 50–70
  HIV/AIDS and, 66–9
  infectivity, 50, 65, 70
  outbreaks, 47–8, 50–3, 57–65
Cryptosporidium, 45, 49, 62, 64
  oocysts and sporozoites, 49–50, 65, 70
CSF testing
  botulism and, 6
  listeriosis, 198
  meningococcal disease, 236
  mumps, 253–4
  pneumococcal disease, 163–4
  poliomyelitis, 294–5
  rabies, 318–19, 322
  tuberculosis, 365–8
culture (microbiological)
  cholera, 33–4
  diphtheria, 95–6
  enteric fever, 112–14
  influenza, 147
  Legionnaire's disease, 184–5
  listeriosis, 207–8
  measles, 217–18
  meningococcal disease, 235–6
  pertussis, 273–4, 277
  poliomyelitis, 298
  Q fever, 305
  SARS, 339
  tuberculosis, 367, 369–70
cutaneous diphtheria, 102–3
cycles, *see* outbreaks

Daintree ulcer, *see* Buruli ulcer
Dakar score, 357–8
dehydration, 31–2, 38–9
delayed hypersensitivity skin reactions, 382
dementia, 179, 185–6

INDEX

dengue fever, 74–89
dengue haemorrhagic fever (DHF), 81–7
dengue shock syndrome (DSS), 82–4
descending motor paralysis, 3
diarrhoea
  cholera, 31–2, 37–9
  enteric fever, 108
  giardiasis and cryptosporidiosis, 47, 49–50, 56, 66–7
  Legionnaire's disease, 179–80
  listeriosis, 207–8
  measles, 219–20
  SARS, 340–1
diphtheria, 92–103
  cardiac complications, 100–1
diphtheria antitoxin, 100
disseminated intravascular coagulation (DIC), 237
dot-blot immunoassays, 80
DOT (directly observed therapy), 378–9
drowsiness, 177–8
drug resistance, *see* antibiotic resistance
drug susceptibilities, Vitek® determination of, 113–14
drugs, *see* antibiotics
dysautonomia, 359

eggs, in enteric fever, 121–3
elderly patients, 187–8, 202–3
electrolytes, 38–9
electrophysiological studies, 6–7, 294–5, 355
ELISA, *see* serology
encephalitis, 226–7, 319–21, 323
endocarditits, 101, 192–3, 309, 314–15
enteric fever, 105–27
  complications, 116–17
Enterobacteriaceae, 105
enterotoxins, *see* toxins
enteroviruses, 288, 291, 297
enzyme immunoassays, *see* serology
epidemics, *see* pandemics
epidemiology, *see* outbreaks
erythema, *see* rashes

faecal accidents, 63–5
fatigue, *see* drowsiness

fever, 3, 146, 177–8, 199, 201, 211, 213, 219, 290, 344, *see also* dengue fever; enteric fever; hepatitis A
flaviviruses, 74, 79–80, 86
flu, *see* influenza
food inspectors, 10, 205–6
foodborne disease
  botulism, 4–5, 7, 9–11
  cholera, 40
  diphtheria, 103
  enteric fever, 121–4
  giardiasis and cryptosporidiosis, 69
  hepatitis A, 136
  listeriosis, 203–5

gall bladder removal, 124–5
gardening, 193, 354–5
gastrointestinal conditions, 130–43, 181–2, 206–8, *see also* cholera; diarrhoea
genotypes, 84, 143
Giardia lamblia (*G. duodenalis*, *G. intestinalis*), 46, 62, 64
  cysts and trophozoites, 47, 65, 70
giardiasis, 46–70
  acute syndrome, 47
  lactose intolerance, and relapses, 66
  median infective dose, 65
  outbreak investigations, 47–8, 50–3, 57–65
Global Polio Eradication Initiative, 290
Gram negative bacteria, 30, 42, 106–7, 179–180, 237, 268
Gram positive bacteria, 1, 3–4, 9, 167, 198, 353
granulomas in liver, 306–7
Guillain–Barré syndrome (GBS), 293–5, 323

Haemophilus influenzae, 152
haemorrhage, 81–2, 233, 236
handwashing, *see* hygienic practices
headache, 253, 303, 364
health–care associated infections, *see* nosocomial transmission
heat therapy for ulcers, 21
hepatitis A, 130–43
  complications, 134–5

hepatitis A virus (HAV), 131
hepatitis, in Q fever, 306
herd immunity, 43, 140, 172
HIV/AIDS, *see* immunocompromised patients
holidays, *see* travellers
hospital transmission, *see* nosocomial transmission
hospital water supplies, 188–91
Howell-Jolly bodies, 164–5
hydration, 31–2, 38–9
hydrophobia (water avoidance), 318–19, 321, 323
hydrotherapy spas, 190–1
hygienic practices, 119, 123–4, 126, 328
  handwashing, 62, 68, 173, 308, 314
hypersensitivity, 8, 100, 226, 228, 311, 359, 382
hypothesis-generating questionnaires, 60–1, 121, 141–2

IgA deficiency, 139
IgM and IgG, *see* serology
immigrants, *see* travellers
immune reconstitution disease (IRD), 373
immunisation, *see* vaccination
immunity
  cholera, 32, 38
  diphtheria, 94–5, 103
  hepatitis A, 136, 140
  invasive pneumococcal disease, 170–2
  listeriosis, 202–3
  meningococcal disease, 247–8
  mumps vaccine failure, 262–3
  pertussis, 283
  poliomyelitis, 298
  tetanus, 354
immunoassays, *see* serology
immunocompromised patients, 185–6, 201, 224
  cryptosporidiosis and, 49–50, 55–6, 66–9
  pneumococcal disease, 173–4
  tuberculosis and, 368, 372–4, 381
  vaccination and, 157–8, 263–4
immunoglobulins, *see also* serology
  botulinum immunoglobulin, 8
  NHIG for hepatitis A, 138–40

rabies, 324–5, 327, 329–30
tetanus, 359
infants, *see* children
infection control measures, *see* hygienic practices; 'Isolation measures' section in each chapter; masks
infectivity
  cryptosporidiosis, 50, 70
  mumps, 257, 261
  tuberculosis, 376, 379–80
inflammation, *see* corticosteroids
influenza, 145–59, *see also* avian influenza
  complications, 149–52
influenza-like illness (ILI), 146–7, 290
inhalational botulism, 4–5, 8–9, 11, 13
insect vectors, *see* mosquito vectors
insecticides, 88–9
invasive pneumococcal disease (IPD), 162–75
  after cochlear implants, 174–5
  after influenza, 151–2
  complications, 167–8
  nosocomial pneumonia, 179, 181
investigations, *see* CSF testing; culture (microbiological); 'Investigations' section in each chapter; outbreaks; PCR testing; radiological investigations; serology
isolation measures, *see* 'Isolation measures' section in each chapter
itching (pruritis), in rabies, 320–1
IV fluids, in cholera, 38–9

jaundice, 141, *see also* hepatitis A

Koplik's spots, 214

lactose intolerance, in *Giardia*, 66
larvicidal treatment, 88–9
leg ulcers, *see* Buruli ulcer
Legionella, 177, 184, 193
Legionnaire's disease, 177–93, 313
  complications, 192–3
  extrapulmonary features, 181–2, 187–8
  risk factors for, 185–6, 188
leukopenia, 77–8

INDEX

Listeria monocytogenes, 120, 197, 199, 207
   as meningitis cause, 165–6
listeriosis, 197–208
   complications, 201
   pregnancy and, 202
LTBI (latent TB infection), 381–5
lumbar puncture, *see* CSF testing
Lyssavirus, 317, 327–8, 331

M2 protein ion channel inhibitors, 149, 156
MacConkey agar, 112–13
malaria, 110
malnutrition, 47, 50, 56, 84
Mantoux test, 382, 384
masks, 336–7, 345, 366, 369, 377
MDR-TB, 386
measles, 210–28
   complications, 218, 220–1, 224–7
meningitis, 163, 165–6, 198, 365–6
   after cochlear implants, 174–5
   meningococcal, 231–2, 234, 239
   mumps, 253–4, 258–9
   poliomyelitis second stage, 290
   tuberculous, 366
meningococcal disease, 230–48
   risk factors for, 244
   septicaemia, 232
meningococcus, 165–6, 175
microbiological diagnosis, *see* culture (microbiological); stool specimens
microscopy, 33, 52, 235–6, 370
molecular testing, *see* PCR testing
monoclonal antibodies, in SARS, 343
Morbillivirus, 210
mortality, *see* 'Prognosis' section in each chapter
mosquito vectors, 25, 75–6, 85–9, 102–3
multiplex kit for CSF testing, 254
multiresistant methicillin-resistant *Staphylococcus aureus* (MRSA), 179
mumps, 252–64
   complications, 259–60
   infectivity, 257, 261
mumps/measles/rubella (MMR) vaccine, 212–13, 221, 224–5, 227–8
myalgia (muscle pain), 232, 289, 303, 356
Mycobacterium tuberculosis, 364, 366, 371

Mycobacterium ulcerans, 15, 17
mycolactone, 22

needlestick injuries, *see* prophylaxis
negative predictive values (NPV), 148
Neisseria meningitidis, 230, 234
neonates, *see* children
neurological symptoms, *see* paralysis
neutralisation tests, 80
nodules, *see* Buruli ulcer
normal human immunoglobulin (NHIG), 138–40, 221, 224, 359
norovirus infections, 31–2
nosocomial transmission, 85, 179, 181, 188–90, 204–5
notifiable diseases, *see* 'Public health notification and response' section in each chapter

oral rehydration solutions (ORS), 38–9
oral testing kits for measles, 218
orchitis, 260–2
otitis media, 170, 172
outbreaks, *see* pandemics; 'Public health notification and response' section in each chapter
overseas, *see* travellers

pandemics, 42, 157, *see also* outbreaks
paradoxical reactions, 373
paraesthesias, in rabies, 320
paralysis, 3, 101, 321
paralytic polio, 290–4, 296–300
paralytic rabies, 293, 321, 323
parasites, *see Cryptosporidium*; *Giardia lamblia*
paratyphoid fever, 107, *see also* enteric fever
parotitis, 254–5, 258, 261
passive immunisation, 138–40, 221, 224, 343, 359
PCR testing, 19, 53, 96, 115, 185, 236, 273–4, 276, 297, 305, 367, 371
   RT (reverse transcriptase)-PCR, 80, 154, 217–18, 322
percussion myoedema, 323
peripheral neuropathy, 374–5
personal protective equipment (PPE), 335–7, 376–7

395

INDEX

pertussis (whooping cough), 267–85
phages, 120, 205
pharyngitis (sore throat), 92–103, 230
phobic spasms, 319, 321, 323
pneumonia, 151–2, *see also* invasive pneumococcal disease (IPD); Legionnaire's disease; Q fever; SARS
poliomyelitis, 288–300
polymerase chain reaction, *see* PCR testing
Pontiac fever, 191–2
positive predictive values (PPV), 148
post-antibiotic effects, 187
post-exposure prophylaxis (PEP), *see* prophylaxis
potting mixes, *Legionella* in, 193
poultry, in avian influenza, 154
pre-exposure prophylaxis for rabies (PEPR), 330
pregnant women, 54, 202, 225, 242, 262–3, 281–2, 312, 361
preserved foods, 5–6, 11, 291
prognosis, *see* 'Prognosis' section in text
prophylaxis, 85, 137–8, 219, 221, 224–6, 239–41, 246–7, 260–1, 279–80, 320, 325–9, 360–1, *see also* vaccination
   cholera, 41
   cryptosporidiosis, 69
   diphtheria, 99, 103
   influenza, 149
   nasopharynx carriage of meningococcus, 239
protein C, 237
protozoans, 46, 49, 180, 190–1
pseudomembranes, 93, 95–8
public health responses, *see* 'Public health notification and response' section in each chapter
pulmonary TB, 366, 368–70, 376, 387
purpura fulminans (coagulopathy), 163–5, 168, 237

Q fever, 302–15
QuantiFERON-TB Gold test (QFT-G), 384–5
quarantine, *see* 'Isolation measures' section in each chapter

Quellung reaction, 174

rabies, 317–31
radiological investigations, 80–1, 167, 183–4, 294, 305–6, 337–8, 381, 383
rapid tests for influenza, 147
rashes (erythema), 81, 106–8, *see also* measles; meningococcal disease
refugees, *see* travellers
replacement disease, 174
reportable diseases, *see* 'Public health notification and response' section in each chapter
resistant organisms, *see* antibiotic resistance
retrospective cohort studies, 60–1, 63–4
rhAPC (recombinant human activated protein C), 237–8
rigidity, 353, 356–7, 360
RNA viruses, 131, 212, 254, 288, 335
RT (reverse transcriptase)-PCR, *see* PCR testing
Rubulavirus (mumps virus), 252, 254

salivary gland swelling, 254–5, 258, 261
Salmonella enterica, 105, 112–15, 120
SARS, *see* Severe Acute Respiratory Syndrome
school camps, *see* camp, in outbreak investigation
screening for tuberculosis, 382, 384
sensitivity of tests (SnNOUT), 148
septic shock, 163, 167–8, 238
septicaemia, 232, 234, 237, 239
sera, 8
serology (antibody testing), 79–80
   antibody kits, 114–15
   cholera, 34–6, 42
   dengue fever, 78–80
   enteric fever, 113–15
   hepatitis A, 133–4, 143
   influenza, 147, 155–7
   Legionnaire's disease, 184–5
   measles, 216–17, 226
   meningococcal disease, 236
   mumps, 256
   pertussis, 273, 275–6

Q fever, 305–6, 310–11, 313
SARS, 339
Severe Acute Respiratory Syndrome (SARS), 334–48
   specimen collection, 339
shell vial cell culture system, 305
shivers, 106
shortness of breath, see SARS
skin biopsies, 322
smoking, meningococcal disease and, 244
SnNOUT (sensitivity of tests), 148
sore throat (pharyngitis), 92–103, 230
spatula test, 355
specificity of tests (SpPIN), 148
splenectomised patients, 165, 173–4
SpPIN (specificity of tests), 148
sputum analysis, 368–70
sputum induction, 369
Staphylococcus aureus, 152
statistics (sensitivity and specificity), 148
stepladder pattern of fever, 108
stiff jaw, see tetanus
stiff neck, see mumps
stool specimens, 33–4, 51–3, 63, 119, 207–8
streptococcal pharyngitis, 97, 100
Streptococcus pneumoniae, see invasive pneumococcal disease (IPD)
subacute sclerosing panencephalitis (SSPE), 226–7
supportive measures, 83, 135–6, 218–19, 262–3, 297
surgery, for ulcers, 20–2
surgical masks, see masks
swabs, 19, 95–6, 99, 236, 339–40
swimming pools, 63–5

TB clinics, 378–9
tellurity-containing culture media, 95
tetanus, 352–62
tetanus immunisation, 284
thrombocytopenia, 78
ticks, 293, 312
Tinsdale medium, 95
tiredness, see drowsiness
tourists, see travellers
tourniquet test for capillary fragility, 77–8

toxins, 5–7, 10–12, 22, 39, 43, 96, 99–101, 353, 355, 358–9
transmission, see hygienic practices; 'Isolation measures' in each chapter; masks; 'Transmission' in each chapter
travellers (overseas infection)
   acute flaccid paralysis (AFP), 293
   border entry screening for SARS, 343–4
   cholera, 32, 41–3
   dengue fever, 85–7
   diphtheria, 94, 102
   enteric fever, 107–8, 116, 125–6
   influenza, 159
   measles, 213
   meningococcal disease, 241–2
   poliomyelitis, 290
   SARS, 337, 347–348
   travellers' diarrhoea, 43
   tuberculosis, 365–6
treatment, see 'Treatment' section in each chapter
trismus (lockjaw), 355, 356, 358
tuberculin skin test (TST), 228, 381–5
tuberculosis (TB), 364–87
   compliance with therapy, 378–9
   HIV/AIDS and, 372–4
   infectivity, 376, 379–80
   LTBI (latent TB infection), 381–5
two-by-two tables, 121–2, 142
typhoid fever, 107, see also enteric fever

ulcers, 76–7, 102–3, see also Buruli ulcer
urinary antigen testing, 184

vaccination, see also prophylaxis
   ABL lyssavirus, 328–9
   Buruli ulcer, 25
   cholera, 42–3
   dengue fever, 86
   diphtheria, 94–5, 102–3
   given with other vaccinations, 140
   hepatitis A, 138–40
   hepatitis A virus, 132
   influenza, 157–9
   listeriosis, 203
   lyssavirus, 328–9

measles, 212–13, 216, 221, 227
meningococcal disease, 245–8
mumps, 260–4
mumps investigations and, 256
paratyphoid fever, 126
pertussis, 269, 283–4
pneumococcal disease, 170–5
poliomyelitis, 291, 293, 295, 298, 300
Q fever, 311, 314
rabies, 322, 324–31
SARS, 343
tetanus, 354, 360–2
tuberculosis, 383–4
typhoid, 125–7
vaccine-associated paralytic poliomyelitis (VAPP), 291, 300
vectors, see mosquito vectors
Vibrio cholerae, 29–30, 34–6, 40–2
viral meningitis, 253–4
viral pneumonia, see SARS
viral shedding, 156, 339
viral URTIs, 232
Vitek® (automated machine), 113–14
vomiting, 31, 270–2
water refusal in rabies, 318
waterborne disease, 23–5, 40–1, 49, 62, 64, 68–70, 88–9, 136–7, 188–91

weakness, in poliomyelitis, 289, 299
whooping cough, see pertussis
Widal test, 114–15
Winthrop-University Hospital Score, 183
wounds, 4, 8, 328, 358

XDR-TB, 386–7
XLD (xylose-lysine-deoxycholate) agar, 112–13

zoo, in outbreak investigation, 61–3
zoonoses (animal transmitted diseases)
  Corynebacterium ulcerans, 95
  Cryptosporidium, 62
  Giardia lamblia (G. duodenalis, G. intestinalis), 62
  meningococcal disease, 246
  paralysis, 293
  pertussis, 283
  Q fever, 308–9, 311–14
  rabies, 320, 326–7, 330
  SARS, 347